Vision Science and Optometry

Vision Science and Optometry

Guest Editors

Elvira Orduna-Hospital
Ana Sanchez-Cano

MDPI

Basel • Beijing • Wuhan • Barcelona • Belgrade • Novi Sad • Cluj • Manchester

Guest Editors
Elvira Orduna-Hospital
Department of Applied Physics
University of Zaragoza
Zaragoza
Spain

Ana Sanchez-Cano
Department of Applied Physics
University of Zaragoza
Zaragoza
Spain

Editorial Office
MDPI AG
Grosspeteranlage 5
4052 Basel, Switzerland

This is a reprint of the Special Issue, published open access by the journal *Life* (ISSN 2075-1729), freely accessible at: https://www.mdpi.com/journal/life/special_issues/1PVL35F9YK.

For citation purposes, cite each article independently as indicated on the article page online and as indicated below:

Lastname, A.A.; Lastname, B.B. Article Title. *Journal Name* **Year**, *Volume Number*, Page Range.

ISBN 978-3-7258-7322-7 (Hbk)
ISBN 978-3-7258-7323-4 (PDF)
https://doi.org/10.3390/books978-3-7258-7323-4

Contents

About the Editors

Elvira Orduna Hospital

Elvira Orduna Hospital is an Associate Professor at the University of Zaragoza, Spain. She holds a degree in Optics and Optometry, a Master's in Vision Science Research, and a PhD in Biomedical and Biotechnological Sciences. Her research interests focus on clinical optometry, ophthalmology, and binocular vision, with a growing involvement in the study of lighting and its effects on the visual system. She has authored numerous peer-reviewed publications, book chapters, and over two hundred conference presentations. She collaborates actively with the Retina and Visual System Research Group at IIS Aragón, where she contributes to projects spanning different population groups and visual conditions. She also supervises numerous student projects and participates in both national and international collaborations. Her current lines of work include ocular aberrations, retinal morphology, sports vision, and the impact of light on neuroprotection, reflecting a multidisciplinary approach that bridges basic science with clinical practice.

Ana Sanchez-Cano

Ana Sanchez-Cano is an Associate Professor in the Department of Applied Physics at the University of Zaragoza, Spain. She holds degrees in Physical Sciences and Optics and Optometry, as well as a PhD. Her research interests focus on circadian light, vision science, and the visual system, combining a physics-based approach with clinical insights from optometry. She integrates teaching and research and actively contributes as Co-Principal Investigator to the Retina and Visual System Research Group, leading and collaborating on national and international projects. She also supervises doctoral theses and undergraduate research, taking a multidisciplinary approach that bridges fundamental optics, visual perception, and circadian health. She is a member of the Spanish Lighting Committee (CEI) and the Spanish Society of Optics (SEDOPTICA), has served in leadership roles within national vision science committees, and has been recognized with multiple teaching and research merit awards.

Preface

The Reprint Vision Science and Optometry brings together a diverse set of contributions that reflect the breadth and depth of current research in visual science and clinical optometry. Its subject matter covers fundamental aspects of vision, ranging from optical quality and retinal function to binocular vision, accommodation, ocular biomechanics, visual ergonomics, and clinical applications in eye care. The aim of this Reprint is to provide an accessible and coherent reference that highlights scientific progress, encourages translation into practice, and fosters dialogue across related disciplines.

Our motivation in compiling this Reprint was to collect the most relevant and innovative findings recently published in this Special Issue, offering readers a consolidated source of knowledge that advances both theory and clinical practice. The Reprint is intended for researchers, clinicians, educators, and students who wish to broaden their understanding of vision science and to keep pace with rapid developments in optometry. We hope that the works included here will inspire further research and strengthen interdisciplinary collaboration within the field.

Elvira Orduna-Hospital and Ana Sanchez-Cano
Guest Editors

life

MDPI

Article

The Interaction between Vergence and Accommodation Cues in the Assessment of Fusional Vergence Range

Marc Argilés [1,2,*] and Genis Cardona [1,3,*]

1 Departament d'Òptica i Optometria (DOO), Universitat Politècnica de Catalunya (UPC), Campus de Terrassa, Edifici TR8, C.Violinista Vellsolà, 37, 08222 Terrassa, Spain
2 Centre for Sensors, Instruments and Systems Development (CD6), Universitat Politècnica de Catalunya (UPC), 08222 Terrassa, Spain
3 Applied Optics and Image Processing Group (GOAPI), School of Optics and Optometry of Terrassa, Universitat Politècnica de Catalunya (UPC), 08222 Terrassa, Spain
* Correspondence: marc.argiles@upc.edu (M.A.); genis.cardona@upc.edu (G.C.)

Abstract: Fusional vergence range tests are commonly used in optometric practice. The aim of this study was to investigate the possible contribution of CA/C, AC/A, and proximal cues (PCT) to the magnitude and presence of blur and recovery during the measurement of fusional vergence ranges and to determine whether the occurrence of blur is influenced by these vergence and accommodation cues. A total of 27 participants with normal binocular vision were included and AC/A, CA/C, and PCT ratios were evaluated. Blur, break, and recovery values in convergence and divergence were assessed with base-out and base-in prisms, respectively. No statistical correlations were found between AC/A, CA/C, and PCT ratios and the magnitude of blur, break, and recovery values in neither far, near, convergence, nor divergence testing conditions. However, better near point of convergence values were related to higher break values in convergence at far distances, but not at near distances. In addition, for convergence and far distance, a statistical difference was found between groups reporting and not reporting blur in AC/A stimulus and PCT ratios. The present results cannot confirm whether vergence and accommodation cues, such as AC/A, CA/C, and PCT ratios, may play an active role during the assessment of fusional vergence range.

Keywords: fusional vergence range; accommodation; vergence; proximal vergence

1. Introduction

Clinical evaluation of horizontal fusional vergence range is an important part of optometric testing. It can be evaluated for horizontal vergence, stimulating the range of convergence with a base-out (BO) prism, or for divergence, with a base-in (BI) prism, at both near (usually at 0.4 meters (m)) and far (usually at 6.0 m) distances [1–3]. The vertical fusional vergence range may also be evaluated, especially in the presence of vertical phoria. This study focuses on the horizontal fusional vergence range, which will be referred to simply as the fusional vergence range.

The balance between the magnitude of fusional vergence range and phoria determines the risk of increased visual symptoms at both near and far distances [4–10]. Clinical criteria to determine this balance have been explored and are commonly used in clinical practice for exophoria (Sheard criteria) and esophoria (Percival criteria) [11]. In addition, at each distance and vergence demand (BO and BI), the typical recording points for fusional vergence range with increasing vergence demand are blur (the patient reports blur of the presented visual stimulus) and break (the patient reports double vision). At this point, the clinician decreases the vergence demand, and the patient reports the recovery point (single and clear vision). Normative values for vergence range have been studied and published to guide clinicians in the management of their patients [6,7].

Interestingly, the physiological basis for the magnitude and presence of blur and recovery during the evaluation of fusional vergence is not fully understood. The magnitude of the break point has a central mechanism component. Some authors have referred to a vergence controller gain (VCG) and to the extraocular muscle function [12–15]. The vergence and accommodation interaction, which is represented by some components such as the AC/A ratio, CA/C ratio, and proximal vergence may influence the final output for vergence and accommodation response. Theoretical models have been studied to explain this interaction, which is represented by a negative feedback (loop) for both the vergence and accommodative systems, and includes phasic (fast) and tonic (slow) components (Figure 1). The AC/A and CA/C ratio represents the cross-link between those systems, with proximal vergence and accommodation cues providing a smaller contribution to the final add-up visual response.

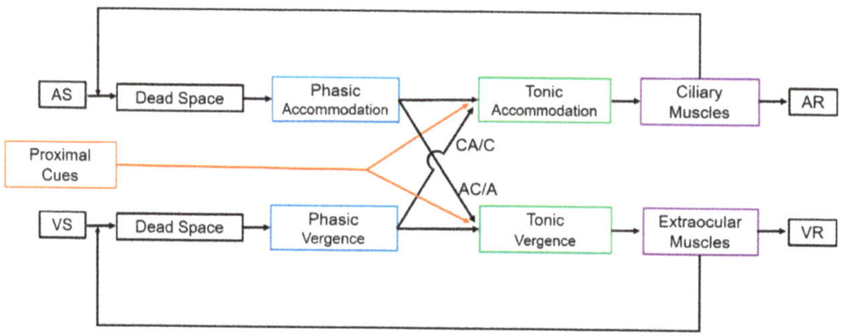

Figure 1. Schematic of the dual-static accommodation and vergence system. This model is based on the classical work of Hung, Ciuffreda, and Rosenfield [15]. For a viewing distance of 0.4 m, the accommodative stimulus (AS) is 2.50 D, and for a standard pupillary distance of 6.0 cm, the vergence stimulus (VS) is $6 \times 2.5 = 15$ prism diopters (Δ). Some authors prefer to use a meter angle (MA), which represents the reciprocal distance for the stimulus (MA = 1/distance (m)). The ocular convergence in prism diopters is the interpupillary distance (IPD) multiplied by MA. Thus, for example, for an IPD of 6 cm and a stimulus at 0.4 m, the ocular convergence is $6 \times 2.5 = 15$ Δ. Dead Space for accommodation corresponds to the depth of focus and for vergence to the Panum's area. The phasic and tonic accommodation for each system is represented, as well as the negative loops. The VCG gain is shown as the flow arrow between VS and VR. Proximal cues contribute to the dual system. AS = Accommodative Stimulus, VS = Vergence Stimulus, AR = Accommodative Response, VR = Vergence Response.

The AC/A ratio is commonly measured in clinical practice, and can be evaluated using heterophoria or the gradient technique [1,2]. This value shall be employed to determine the best treatment option for each patient and for the diagnosis of binocular anomalies such as convergence insufficiency, which has a low AC/A ratio, or excess of divergence, where this ratio is abnormally high [16,17]. Conversely, the CA/C ratio is not commonly evaluated in daily clinical routines, although some studies have shown its importance for the diagnosis of binocular and accommodative anomalies [18–23]. This ratio is often overlooked. Indeed, to evaluate the sole contribution of vergence to the accommodation response, the accommodative system must be static (or not responsive) during the test, which is commonly known as "open-loop" in the negative feedback (Figure 1). For the AC/A ratio, it is easier to open-loop the vergence system using a prism to dissociate and obtain double vision (Von Graefe technique), or to assess it monocularly (with the Cover Test or Maddox Rod methods).

Some studies have used a Difference of Gaussians (DoG) stimulus to open-loop the accommodative system, with good agreement between stimulus and response CA/C ratios [24]. One study found that the AC/A gradient, rather than the calculated AC/A, correlated better with the CA/C ratio [25], although it must be noted that in clinical practice the stimulus rather than the response is commonly determined for both CA/C and AC/A ratios. Sweeney et al. (2014) found a good agreement between stimulus and response for both the AC/A and CA/C ratios, although poorer for CA/C, and noted that the results of the CA/C assessment displayed high variability, thus justifying the fact that this ratio is not often determined [26]. Indeed, the clinician needs experience to detect minimal changes in accommodation (using the MEM or NOTT techniques to evaluate the accommodative error). In addition, CA/C values are very small, ranging from 0.040 D/Δto 0.580 D/Δ, with a mean of 0.080 D/Δ [3,20].

Hence, when evaluating fusional vergence, an increase in vergence demand is added, and the amount of prism in the vergence cross-links to the accommodation response due to the effective CA/C ratio. For instance, with a BI prism, the slow mechanism adapts to the new vergence demand when surpassing the accommodative lag (usually +0.50 D), and the overall contribution of the CA/C could determine the magnitude of the blur and recovery points. In the case of convergence, with increasing vergence demand, the effective contribution of the CA/C ratio determines the ability of the patient to increase the accommodative system response to maintain single vision. Two assumptions, untested until now, may be put forward at this point: the larger the CA/C ratio, the more likely a blur will be reported; and the lower this ratio, the more likely that break is reported without a previous blur [27].

In addition, patients can use different cues (blur or disparity-driven) to adjust their visual system. A series of studies conducted by Horwood and Riddell revealed that in cases of esotropia and exotropia, near responses to cues differed from those in a non-strabismic population [25,28–32], and one study concluded that proximal vergence contributes to the control of intermittent exotropia [33]. Likewise, the actual mechanism influenced by the CA/C and AC/A ratios and proximal cues, which determines the magnitude or presence of break and recovery during the assessment of fusional vergence ranges, in either BI or BO conditions, remains poorly understood.

The interplay between the AC/A, CA/C, and proximal vergence cues and the fusional vergence range is complex and essential for maintaining binocular vision. Understanding these relationships is crucial for clinicians when diagnosing and treating binocular vision disorders. Therefore, the aim of this study was to investigate the possible contribution of CA/C, AC/A, and proximal cues to the magnitude and presence of blur and recovery when using BO and BI prisms to determine the fusional vergence range. In addition, it explores whether the occurrence of blur is influenced by high or low cross-link ratios.

2. Materials and Methods

2.1. Participants Selection

Participants between 18 and 25 years, all university students, were recruited for the study. No random sampling was used in this research. Subjects willing to participate in the study were recruited by order of attendance following a complete optometric examination to determine whether they satisfied the inclusion and exclusion criteria. The inclusion criteria were visual acuity at far and near distances equal or superior to 20/20, and stereoacuity, as measured with the Random Dot test, with both random points and lateral disparity, better than 40 s of arc. Participants with any ocular pathology were excluded, as were those with systemic pathologies or taking medications that could affect vision. All participants needed to fulfill the Sheard criteria in case of exophoria and the Percival criteria in case of esophoria, and display normal values of near point of convergence (NPC) and amplitude of accommodation (AA), with their habitual correction. All participants agreed to participate in the study and signed an informed consent after the nature of the investigation was explained to them. This study was approved by the Institutional Review Board of the UPC (06/2023).

2.2. Fusional Vergence Range, Heterophoria, Near Point of Convergence, and Amplitude of Accommodation

All tests were performed in the same order, but taking into account the possible influence of vergence adaptation when determining fusional vergence range. Dissociate phorias at far (6 m) and near (0.4 m) distances were evaluated with the Von Graefe method. Each measure was repeated 3 times, and the median value was calculated. Fusional vergence ranges were measured at distance and near with a phoropter. Patients were particularly instructed to report the first occurrence of blur, break, and recovery conditions. The fusional vergence range was determined starting with divergence at far and near distances, followed by convergence at far and near distances. Near point of convergence was measured with the Royal Air Force (RAF) rule, and breakup values (double vision) were recorded. Monocular amplitude of accommodation was measured in both eyes with the push-up Donder's technique, using the same RAF rule. We used the minimum amplitude of accommodation of Hofstetter to calculate the threshold for normal amplitude of accommodation [1–3].

2.3. CA/C Stimulus Ratio

The CA/C ratio was measured using the method described by Tsuetaki and Schor [24], traditionally used in clinical practice. Briefly, a Difference of Gaussians stimulus, included in the reverse of a Wesson chart (Bernell Corporation, Mishawaka, IN, USA), was used for this purpose, which has been shown to display good clinical repeatability. This image subtended 21 degrees of visual angle at 0.4 m. Accommodative error was measured using the modified NOTT technique by calculating the accommodative lag (in D) with and without a 6 Δ BO prism. The CA/C ratio was then calculated as the difference between accommodative errors in both conditions, divided by 6 (expressed in D/Δ units).

2.4. AC/A Stimulus Ratio

Interpupillary distance (IPD) was measured with an auto refractometer. The AC/A stimulus ratio was calculated as described in the literature [1,2]. The AC/A stimulus gradient was measured using the Thorington modified test and the Maddox rod. Phoria was measured with and without +2.00 D binocular addition lenses. Each phoria was measured three times and the median value was obtained. The AC/A stimulus gradient ratio was then calculated as the difference in phorias in absolute value, divided by 2 (expressed in Δ/D units).

2.5. Proximal Cues (PCT Ratio)

Inputs for proximity in the vergence and accommodative system may include static cues, such as relative size, overlap, perspective, shading, and texture gradients, and dynamic cues, such as motion parallax and loom. Other non-visual cues related to stimulus position may include proprioceptive information such as touch and memory about object distance [15,34–36]. Proximal vergence can be expressed as the proximal convergence to testing distance ratio (PCT), that is, the percentage contribution of proximal vergence to the overall vergence response [37,38], and can be calculated from the difference between the AC/A stimulus and gradient ratios [37]. This method was used to calculate the PCT ratio in the present study.

2.6. Data Analysis

Data distribution was first analyzed using the Shapiro–Wilk test. Parametric data were expressed as mean and standard deviation (SD) and nonparametric data as median and range or interquartile range (IQR). To study the statistical significance of differences between the two groups, the paired or unpaired *t*-test was employed for parametric data, and the Wilcoxon's rank test or the Mann–Whitney U test for paired or unpaired non-parametric data, respectively, or when the sample size was under 10, irrespective of normality. Parametric ANOVA or the non-parametric Kruskal–Wallis test were used when three or more groups were compared. For correlation analysis, the Pearson or Spearman correlation tests were used, according to data normality. The IBM SPSS Statistics for Windows, Version 27.0 (Armonk, NY, USA: IBM Corp) was used for data analysis and the G*Power software, Version 3.1, was employed to calculate the post hoc sample size [39]. A p-value < 0.05 denoted statistical significance.

3. Results

3.1. Participants and Descriptive Values

A total of 35 subjects were screened, of whom 27 satisfied the inclusion and exclusion criteria and were finally included in the study, with a mean age ± SD of 21.3 ± 1.4 years, ranging from 18 to 24 years, and 57% were female. The mean refractive spherical error was −0.50 ± 1.29 D for the right eye, ranging from −4.00 D to +3.50 D, and −0.56 ± 1.32 D for the left eye, ranging from −4.00 D to +3.25 D. Astigmatism values were 0.36 ± 0.67 D, ranging from 0.00 D to 3.25 D, and 0.40 ± 0.71 D, ranging from 0.00 D to 3.50 D, for the right and left eyes, respectively. Median and IQR values were 4.00 cm (4.00, 6.00) for NPC; 13.00 D (12.00, 20.00) for AA; 4.40 Δ/D (3.30, 5.40) for the AC/A stimulus; 1.00 Δ/D (1.00, 2.00) for the AC/A gradient; 3.30 Δ/D (2.00, 4.00) for the PCT ratio; and 0.030 D/Δ (0.025, 0.041) for the CA/C ratio. Descriptive values for fusional vergence ranges are shown in Table 1.

Table 1. Descriptive statistics for the results of blur (b), break (B), and recovery (r) values using base-out (BO) and base-in (BI) prisms for the convergence and divergence range, respectively. Median and interquartile range (25% and 75%) values are shown. All units are prism diopters (Δ).

	Far (6.0 m)						Near (0.4 m)					
	BI			BO			BI			BO		
	b	B	r	b	B	r	b	B	r	b	B	r
Median	6.00	8.00	4.00	12.00	20.00	12.00	18.00	20.00	14.00	21.00	28.00	18.00
IQR (25%)	4.00	6.00	3.50	8.00	14.00	6.00	12.00	16.00	10.00	12.00	24.00	12.00
IQR (75%)	7.00	12.00	6.00	18.00	30.00	18.00	18.00	22.00	18.00	28.50	32.00	22.00

3.2. Incidence of Blur Reporting during Fusional Vergence Test

At far, 20 participants reported blur (74.1%) during BO testing, and 10 (37.0%) during BI. At near distances, 10 participants (37.0%) reported blur during BO, and 15 participants (55.5%) during BI. At far and near distances, 6 (22.2%) and 8 (29.6%) participants, respectively, reported blur at both BI and BO (Table 2).

Table 2. Incidence, expressed in number of participants and percentage (%), of blur at far, near, and divergence (BI) and convergence (BO) conditions.

Far (6.0 m)				Near (0.4 m)			
BI		BO		BI		BO	
Blur	No blur	Blur	No blur	Blur	No blur	Blur	No blur
10 37.0%	17 63.0%	20 74.1%	7 25.9%	15 55.5%	12 44.5%	10 37.0%	17 63.0%

3.3. Correlation between CA/C and AC/A

The CA/C ratio did not show statistical significant correlations with the AC/A stimulus ratio (rho(27) = 0.34, p = 0.084), nor with the AC/A gradient ratio (rho(27) = −0.15, p = 0.461). The AC/A stimulus and AC/A gradient ratio were not significantly correlated (rho(27) = 0.13, p = 0.514).

3.4. Correlations between CA/C, AC/A, and PCT with Break and Recovery Values

At far and divergence, no statistically significant correlations were found between CA/C ratio values and the points of blur (rho(10) = 0.31, p = 0.409), break (rho(27) = 0.00, p = 0.99), and recovery (rho(27) = −0.06, p = 0.765). Similar results were found in convergence conditions for blur (rho(20) = 0.30, p = 0.187), break (rho(27) = 0.28, p = 0.211), and recovery (rho(27) = 0.22, p = 0.273) values. Neither the AC/A nor the PCT ratios presented any statistical correlation with the divergence and convergence blur, break, and recovery values (all $p > 0.100$).

At near distances, the CA/C ratio was not significantly correlated with the divergence blur (rho(15) = 0.11, p = 0.681), break (rho(27) = −0.07, p = 0.725) and recovery (rho(27) = 0.16, p = 0.405) values, nor with the convergence blur (rho(10) = 0.07, p = 0.833), break (rho(27) = 0.07, p = 0.714), and recovery (rho(27) = 0.07, p = 0.833) values.

A statistically significant moderate negative correlation was found between the NPC and break point values at far (rho(27) = −0.43, p = 0.025) in convergence conditions. No further correlations were found between NPC and AA values and break and recovery point values at far or near in convergence or divergence conditions. Figure 2 displays all the correlations between CA/C, AC/A, and PCT values, at far and near distances, and break, recovery, and blur values for both convergence (BO) and divergence (BI) conditions.

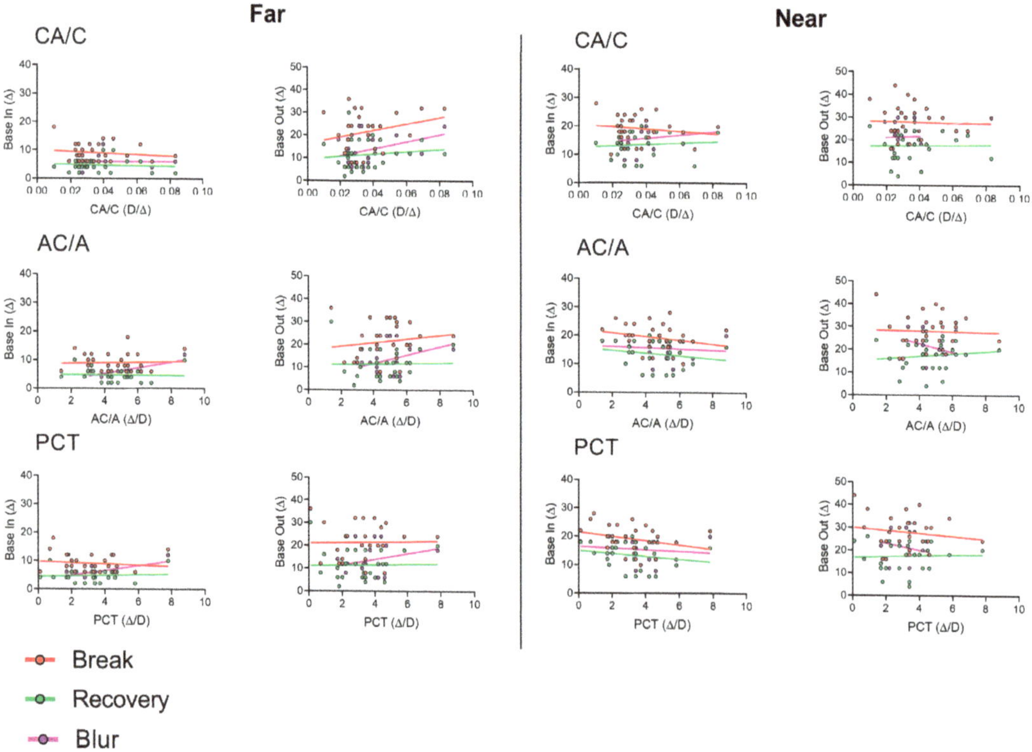

Figure 2. Correlations between CA/C (top), AC/A (middle), and PCT (below) and values of break (red), recovery (green), and blur (purple) at far (6 m) and near (0.4 m) distances in convergence (Base Out) and divergence (Base In) conditions.

3.5. AC/A, CA/C, and PCT Values and the Occurrence of Blur

As noted above, at far distance and divergence conditions, 10 participants reported blur. No statistically significant differences were found between subjects reporting and not reporting blur in the AC/A stimulus ratio, $p = 0.824$, AC/A gradient ratio, $p = 0.863$, PCT ratio, $p = 0.863$, and CA/C ratio, $p = 0.359$.

For convergence and far distance, 20 participants reported blur. Statistical differences were found between subjects reporting and not reporting blur in the AC/A stimulus ratio, $p = 0.033$, and PCT ratio, $p = 0.005$, but not in the AC/A gradient ratio, $p = 0.299$, nor in the CA/C ratio, $p = 0.135$. Overall, higher AC/A stimulus and PCT ratios were found in participants who did not report blur, with a difference in medians of 2.00 Δ/D in both parameters.

For near distance and divergence conditions, 15 participants reported blur. No statistically significant differences were found between groups and AC/A stimulus ratio, $p = 0.494$, AC/A gradient ratio, $p = 0.628$, PCT ratio, $p = 0.328$, and CA/C ratio, $p = 0.510$. Finally, at near and convergence conditions, 10 participants reported blur, with no statistical differences between groups in AC/A stimulus ratio, $p = 0.744$, AC/A gradient ratio, $p = 0.824$, PCT ratio, $p = 0.615$, and CA/C ratio, $p = 0.451$.

4. Discussion

The aim of this study was to investigate whether independent AC/A, CA/C, and PCT ratios contribute to the magnitude of break and recovery values when assessing the fusional vergence range, and whether the occurrence of blur is influenced by these ratios as a result of the cross-links between the vergence and accommodation systems. In a theoretical, static model, these factors act as cues that contribute to the vergence and accommodative response; however, to the best of our knowledge, the possible contribution of these ratios to the fusional vergence range has not been studied.

The theoretical hypotheses for the contribution of AC/A and CA/C ratios are as follows: with the introduction of BI prisms, patients need to adjust (relax) their accommodative system while increasing divergence, whereas with BO prisms, the accommodative system needs to adjust (activate) while increasing convergence. The effective contribution of both ratios can determine the magnitude of breaking and recovery when assessing the fusional vergence range. In addition, the higher the CA/C ratio, the more likely blur will be reported [27]. The possible contribution of the PCT ratio has not been studied.

The median of AC/A stimulus was 4.40 Δ/, IQR (3.30,5.40), which is the normal value according to the literature [40,41]. The values of the AC/A gradient described in this study were also in agreement with previous research [25]. Albeit this parameter is commonly assessed in clinical practice, its range of normality exhibits high variability depending on the method used to evaluate near and far phoria [42,43].

The present study found a median CA/C ratio of 0.030 D/Δ and IQR (0.025,0.041) with the method proposed by Tsuetaki and Schor [24], who found a mean of 0.050 D/Δ. Scheiman and Wick indicated a normal CA/C ratio of approximately 0.080 D/Δ [3], which is close to that reported in other studies [26], although other authors observed a range of normality from 0.040 to 0.220 D/Δ [20]. While some studies have shown that the CA/C ratio could be a clinically useful measure for the diagnosis of binocular and accommodative anomalies [19,21,22], there is a lack of normative values using the same methodology available in common clinical testing. In addition, the CA/C ratio has been found to be influenced by age [23]; therefore, this factor should be considered when comparing normative values of different populations.

The present findings revealed that the closer the NPC, the greater the break magnitude with BO prisms at far distances but not at near distances. These findings suggest that near vision involves a much more complex interaction of the vergence and accommodation systems than far vision. For convergence and far distance, a statistical difference was found in the AC/A stimulus and PCT ratios between groups reporting and not reporting blur, which highlights the role of AC/A in convergence: the higher the AC/A ratio, the lower the possibility of reporting blur. This can be explained by the fact that a high AC/A ratio and better proximal cues can compensate for the vergence and accommodation interactions while increasing the convergence demand, increasing the ability to detect blur at far distances.

This study did not find any correlation between the CA/C and AC/A stimulus ratios, in contrast with previous research authors [25], although measurement procedures for the determination of the CA/C ratio were different. Finally, the PCT values have been seldom investigated [37,38], with only one study analyzing the differences between measurement methods [38]. However, a recent study found that proximal cues contribute significantly to the control of intermittent exotropia and divergence excess [33], as these patients tend to have a high AC/A ratio [3].

No statistical correlations were found between AC/A, CA/C, and PCT ratios and the magnitude of blur, break, and recovery values in neither far, near, BI, nor BO testing conditions. These results are in agreement with the investigations conducted by Horwood et al. [28,31,32], which showed a different use of blur, vergence, and proximity cues among individuals, and an influence of factors such as visual experience and genetic factors. While it is normal to report blur at far distances [6], reporting blur at near distances is highly dependent on each observer. Whereas approximately the same percentage of participants reported blur at near distances in divergent conditions, in convergence, most participants (63.0%) did not report blur. At far distances and convergence, most participants reported blur (74.1%). Therefore, it would seem that each individual exhibits different levels of sensitivity to blur responses that cannot be explained from specific cues alone; however, the higher the AC/A and PCT ratios, the better the ability to detect blur at far vision and convergence. It is known that high or low AC/A and CA/C ratios may lead to binocular dysfunctions, such as convergence insufficiency [1–3], which is characterized by high exophoria, low AC/A ratios, high CA/C ratios, and a low convergence fusional vergence range at near distances. In this particular case, the theory indicates that, with a high CA/C ratio, accommodation exceeds vergence, which in turn explains the high exophoria at near distances. Thus, the present findings may be of relevance for individuals with low AC/A ratios and convergence insufficiency, a dysfunction that may be improved with vision therapy [44]. Future studies could assist in explaining how individuals use different cues to adjust their visual system while assessing fusional vergence range. Moreover, although the clinical evaluation of the PCT ratio may contribute to understanding clinical outcomes in far and convergence, the actual impact of this ratio in other visual demands, such as near vision and divergence, remains elusive.

This study is not devoid of limitations. Thus, it may be acknowledged that the current sample size (n = 27) could not be sufficient to reach solid conclusions. Indeed, a post hoc analysis using G*Power [39] to calculate the sample size necessary to detect a difference of 0.010 D/Δ in the CA/C ratio evidenced that a minimum sample size of 120 was needed to achieve 95% power. Therefore, the present findings must be interpreted with caution, given the possibility of Type II statistical error, that is, of failing to detect significant intergroup differences due to insufficient sample size, and the high variability in the methods of measuring the CA/C ratio, and consequent range of normative values, reported in the literature. Other published research studying the interactions of CA/C and AC/A ratios used a sample of n = 25 [26], n = 16 [19], n = 27 [25], n = 26 [20], and even 10 participants to evaluate the change in these parameters obtained with vision therapy [18]. These factors prevent verifying the initial assumptions of this study.

Notwithstanding these limitations, this study opens a new research avenue to explore the theoretical assumptions related to the vergence and accommodative interactions underpinning fusional vergence range testing in normal binocular vision, and pave the way for future work comparing these relationships in normal and binocular disorders, such as convergence insufficiency or accommodative insufficiency.

In conclusion, the evaluation of AC/A, CA/C, and PCT ratios demonstrates high variability among individuals, with implications in clinical practice. The present results cannot confirm whether vergence and accommodation cues, such as AC/A, CA/C, and PCT ratios, are involved in the assessment of the fusional vergence range, particularly in the magnitude of blur, break, and recovery values, nor the actual presence of a blur point. However, these findings highlight that at far distance and convergence conditions, lower NPC and higher AC/A stimulus ratios contribute to a larger magnitude of the break point. These results may be of interest to clinicians when exploring the fusional vergence range, and give support to the recommendation of exploring AC/A, CA/C, and proximal vergence in clinical practice, particularly in patients with convergence insufficiency.

Author Contributions: M.A. initiated and managed the study. M.A. and G.C. led the manuscript preparation together. M.A. performed the statistical analysis. M.A. and G.C. coordinated the experimental measurements. All authors have read and agreed to the published version of the manuscript.

Funding: This research received no external funding.

Institutional Review Board Statement: The study was conducted in accordance with the Declaration of Helsinki, and approved by the Institutional Review Board of the UPC (06/2023).

Informed Consent Statement: Informed consent was obtained from all subjects involved in the study.

Data Availability Statement: The data that support the findings of this study are available from the corresponding author, M.A., upon reasonable request.

Acknowledgments: We thank Paula Gil and Eulàlia Montoliu and Eric Bezis for the laboratory support during the experimental measurements.

Conflicts of Interest: The authors declare no conflicts of interest.

References

1. Grosvenor, T.; Grosvenor, T.P. *Primary Care Optometry*; Elsevier Health Sciences: Amsterdam, The Netherlands, 2007.
2. Rosenfield, M.; Logan, N. *Optometry: Science, Techniques and Clinical Management*; Elsevier Health Sciences: Amsterdam, The Netherlands, 2009.
3. Scheiman, M.; Wick, B. *Clinical Management of Binocular Vision: Heterophoric, Accommodative, and Eye Movement Disorders*; Lippincott Williams & Wilkins: Philadelphia, PA, USA, 2008.
4. Antona, B.; Barrio, A.; Barra, F.; Gonzalez, E.; Sanchez, I. Repeatability and agreement in the measurement of horizontal fusional vergences. *Ophthalmic Physiol. Opt.* **2008**, *28*, 475–491. [CrossRef]
5. Fray, K.J. Fusional amplitudes: Developing testing standards. *Strabismus* **2017**, *25*, 145–155. [CrossRef] [PubMed]
6. Lança, C.C.; Rowe, F.J. Measurement of fusional vergence: A systematic review. *Strabismus* **2019**, *27*, 88–113. [CrossRef] [PubMed]
7. Palomo Álvarez, C.; Puell, M.C.; Sánchez-Ramos, C.; Villena, C. Normal values of distance heterophoria and fusional vergence ranges and effects of age. *Graefes Arch. Clin. Exp. Ophthalmol.* **2006**, *244*, 821–824. [CrossRef] [PubMed]
8. Rovira-Gay, C.; Mestre, C.; Argiles, M.; Vinuela-Navarro, V.; Pujol, J. Feasibility of measuring fusional vergence amplitudes objectively. *PLoS ONE* **2023**, *18*, e0284552. [CrossRef]
9. Rowe, F.J. Fusional vergence measures and their significance in clinical assessment. *Strabismus* **2010**, *18*, 48–57. [CrossRef]
10. Sreenivasan, V.; Babinsky, E.E.; Wu, Y.; Candy, T.R. Objective measurement of fusional vergence ranges and heterophoria in infants and preschool children. *Investig. Opthalmology Vis. Sci.* **2016**, *57*, 2678–2688. [CrossRef]
11. Moon, B.-Y.; Kim, S.-Y.; Yu, D.-S. Receiver operating characteristic curve analysis of clinical signs for screening of convergence insufficiency in young adults. *PLoS ONE* **2020**, *15*, e0228313. [CrossRef]
12. Hung, S.S.; Fisher, A.G.; Cermak, S.A. The performance of learning-disabled and normal young men on the test of visual-perceptual skills. *Am. J. Occup. Ther.* **1987**, *41*, 790–797. [CrossRef]
13. Hung, G.K. Linear model of accommodation and vergence can account for discrepancies between AC/A measures using the fixation disparity and phoria methods. *Ophthalmic Physiol. Opt.* **1991**, *11*, 275–278. [CrossRef]
14. Hung, G.K. Adaptation model of accommodation and vergence. *Ophthalmic Physiol. Opt.* **1992**, *12*, 319–326. [CrossRef] [PubMed]
15. Hung, G.K.; Ciuffreda, K.J.; Rosenfield, M. Proximal contribution to a linear static model of accommodation and vergence. *Ophthalmic Physiol. Opt.* **1996**, *16*, 31–41. [CrossRef] [PubMed]
16. Gwiazda, J.; Thorn, F.; Held, R. Accommodation, accommodative convergence, and response AC/A ratios before and at the onset of myopia in children. *Optom. Vis. Sci.* **2005**, *82*, 273–278. [CrossRef]
17. Arnoldi, K.A.; Reynolds, J.D. Diagnosis of pseudo-divergence excess exotropia secondary to high accommodative convergence to accommodation ratio. *Am. Orthopt. J.* **2006**, *56*, 133–137. [CrossRef]
18. Brautaset, R.L.; Jennings, A.J.M. Effects of orthoptic treatment on the CA/C and AC/A ratios in convergence insufficiency. *Investig. Opthalmology Vis. Sci.* **2006**, *47*, 2876–2880. [CrossRef]
19. Fukushima, T.; Torii, M.; Ukai, K.; Wolffsohn, J.S.; Gilmartin, B. The relationship between CA/C ratio and individual differences in dynamic accommodative responses while viewing stereoscopic images. *J. Vis.* **2009**, *9*, 21. [CrossRef] [PubMed]

20. Hirani, K.J.; Firth, A.Y. Convergence accommodation to convergence (CA/C) ratio: Stability with different levels of convergence demand. *Br. Ir. Orthopt. J.* **2009**, *6*, 60–64. [CrossRef]
21. Neveu, P.; Roumes, C.; Philippe, M.; Fuchs, P.; Priot, A.-E. Stereoscopic viewing can induce changes in the CA/C ratio. *Investig. Opthalmology Vis. Sci.* **2016**, *57*, 4321–4326. [CrossRef]
22. Rosenfield, M.; Gilmartin, B. Assessment of the CA/C ratio in a myopic population. *Am. J. Optom. Physiol. Opt.* **1988**, *65*, 168–173. [CrossRef] [PubMed]
23. Rosenfield, M.; Ciuffreda, K.J.; Chen, H.-W. Effect of age on the interaction between the AC/A and CA/C ratios. *Ophthalmic Physiol. Opt.* **1995**, *15*, 451–455. [CrossRef]
24. Tsuetaki, T.K.; Schor, C.M. Clinical method for measuring adaptation of tonic accommodation and vergence accommodation. *Am. J. Optom. Physiol. Opt.* **1987**, *64*, 437–449. [CrossRef] [PubMed]
25. Horwood, A.M.; Riddell, P.M. The clinical near gradient stimulus AC/A ratio correlates better with the response CA/C ratio than with the response AC/A ratio. *Strabismus* **2013**, *21*, 140–144. [CrossRef] [PubMed]
26. Sweeney, L.E.; Seidel, D.; Day, M.; Gray, L.S. Quantifying interactions between accommodation and vergence in a binocularly normal population. *Vis. Res.* **2014**, *105*, 121–129. [CrossRef]
27. Benjamin, W.J. *Borish's Clinical Refraction*; Elsevier Health Sciences: Amsterdam, The Netherlands, 2006.
28. Horwood, A.M.; Riddell, P.M. The use of cues to convergence and accommodation in naïve, uninstructed participants. *Vis. Res.* **2008**, *48*, 1613–1624. [CrossRef]
29. Horwood, A.M.; Riddell, P.M. Decreased accommodation during decompensation of distance exotropia. *Br. J. Ophthalmol.* **2012**, *96*, 508–513. [CrossRef] [PubMed]
30. Horwood, A.M.; Riddell, P.M. Evidence that convergence rather than accommodation controls intermittent distance exotropia. *Acta Ophthalmol.* **2012**, *90*, e109–e117. [CrossRef] [PubMed]
31. Horwood, A.M.; Riddell, P.M. Accommodation and vergence response gains to different near cues characterize specific esotropias. *Strabismus* **2013**, *21*, 155–164. [CrossRef]
32. Horwood, A.M.; Riddell, P.M. Disparity-driven vs blur-driven models of accommodation and convergence in binocular vision and intermittent strabismus. *J. AAPOS* **2014**, *18*, 576–583. [CrossRef]
33. Mestre, C.; Neupane, S.; Manh, V.; Tarczy-Hornoch, K.; Candy, T.R. Vergence and accommodation responses in the control of intermittent exotropia. *Ophthalmic Physiol. Opt.* **2023**, *43*, 598–614. [CrossRef]
34. Joubert, C.; Bedell, H.E. Proximal vergence and perceived distance. *Optom. Vis. Sci.* **1990**, *67*, 29–35. [CrossRef]
35. Wick, B. Clinical factors in proximal vergence. *Am. J. Optom. Physiol. Opt.* **1985**, *62*, 1–18. [CrossRef] [PubMed]
36. Wick, B.; Bedell, H.E. Magnitude and velocity of proximal vergence. *Investig. Opthalmology Vis. Sci.* **1989**, *30*, 755–760.
37. Fogt, N.; Toole, A.J.; Rogers, D.L. A review of proximal inputs to the near response. *Clin. Exp. Optom.* **2016**, *99*, 30–38. [CrossRef]
38. Fogt, N. Comparisons of proximal vergence measures. *Vis. Dev. Rehabil.* **2020**, *6*, 252. [PubMed]
39. Faul, F.; Erdfelder, E.; Lang, A.-G.; Buchner, A. G* Power 3: A flexible statistical power analysis program for the social, behavioral, and biomedical sciences. *Behav. Res. Methods* **2007**, *39*, 175–191. [CrossRef]
40. Murray, C.; Newsham, D. The normal accommodative convergence/accommodation (AC/A) ratio. *J. Binocul. Vis. Ocul. Motil.* **2018**, *68*, 140–147. [CrossRef]
41. Gwiazda, J.; Grice, K.; Thorn, F. Response AC/A ratios are elevated in myopic children. *Ophthalmic Physiol. Opt.* **1999**, *19*, 173–179. [CrossRef]
42. Bhoola, H.; Bruce, A.S.; Atchison, D.A. Validity of clinical measures of the AC/A ratio. *Clin. Exp. Optom.* **1995**, *78*, 3–10. [CrossRef]
43. Rainey, B.B.; Goss, D.A.; Kidwell, M.; Feng, B. Reliability of the response AC/A ratio determined using nearpoint autorefraction and simultaneous heterophoria measurement. *Clin. Exp. Optom.* **1998**, *81*, 185–192. [CrossRef] [PubMed]
44. Singh, N.K.; Mani, R.; Hussaindeen, J.R. Changes in stimulus and response AC/A ratio with vision therapy in Convergence Insufficiency. *J. Optom.* **2017**, *10*, 169–175. [CrossRef]

life

MDPI

Article

The Role of Visual Performance in Fine Motor Skills

Pilar Granados-Delgado, Miriam Casares-López, Francesco Martino, Rosario González Anera and José Juan Castro-Torres *

Laboratory of Vision Sciences and Applications, Department of Optics, Faculty of Sciences, University of Granada, Avenida Fuentenueva s/n, 18071 Granada, Spain; pilargrd@ugr.es (P.G.-D.); clmiriam@ugr.es (M.C.-L.); francesco@ugr.es (F.M.); rganera@ugr.es (R.G.A.)
* Correspondence: jjcastro@ugr.es

Abstract: The aim of this study was to analyse the relationship between fine motor skills (FMSs) and visual performance. Thirty young participants with normal binocular vision performed five fine motor tasks: Purdue, Grooved, and O'Connor pegboards, a needle threading task, and a water pouring task, which were characterised by the time taken to complete the task, the number of pegs inserted, the error made in pouring the water, and the volume spilled. To evaluate visual performance, near visual acuity, near contrast sensitivity (CS), and disability glare were assessed. Fine motor skills and visual performance were assessed under monocular and binocular viewing conditions. An overall visual performance score (OVPS) and an overall fine motor skills score (OFMSS) were calculated. All visual functions measured binocularly were better than in monocular conditions, and all FMSs tasks were performed worse monocularly than binocularly ($p < 0.001$), except for the error made in the water pouring task ($p = 0.024$). There was a positive correlation between OVPS and OFMSS (rho = 0.329; $p = 0.010$). The regression model showed that the OFMSS can be predicted by age and CS at 21.3%. Individuals with normal binocular vision and better near visual function exhibit superior fine motor abilities. CS stands out as the visual function that has the greatest bearing on the performance of FMSs.

Keywords: visual performance; visual acuity; contrast sensitivity; disability glare; fine motor skills

1. Introduction

The visual system provides information about the objects in our environment through the interpretation of the images received by the eyes and subsequently processed by the brain. In daily activities, humans interact with objects using their hands. Thus, interactions between our visual system and hand movements have been studied in many disciplines, including optometry. In terms of vision, there are different metrics for quantifying visual performance. These include visual acuity (VA), contrast sensitivity (CS), and disability glare [1–3]. Contrast sensitivity (CS) is the ability to perceive sharp and clear outlines of very small objects. The term used to describe the visual impairment that occurs in the presence of bright light sources is "disability glare" [1]. Sometimes the loss of CS can be more disturbing than the loss of visual acuity because the real world is not constantly in high level of contrast. Additionally, it is well known that the human binocular visual system has the ability to fuse two images into a single image and to perceive depth through the disparity that exists between those two images. The loss of binocular vision negatively impacts the daily life of sufferers [4].

Visuomotor coordination is a hallmark of human evolution and a key aspect of manual dexterity [5], which is involved in several everyday tasks, such as sewing, cooking, or doing a puzzle. The manual dexterity factor is defined as the ability to make skilful, controlled arm–hand manipulations of larger objects [6] and the finger dexterity factor is defined as the ability to make rapid, skilful, controlled manipulative movements of small objects, primarily involving the fingers [7]. Thus, the literature suggests that there are multiple types of dexterity. According to factor analysis findings, pegboard dexterity and finger tapping assess different dimensions of manual dexterity. For this reason, there are several methods for analysing and evaluating manual dexterity and, within this, fine motor skills (FMSs). This dexterity can be quantified as the time required to complete a defined task, like pouring a fluid into a recipient or threading a needle, but it could also be the time needed to complete a pegboard test, such as the O'Connor test or Grooved pegboard test [8–11]. Most studies on this topic focus on examining the precise position of the hands during tasks involving FMSs, as well as assessing certain visual functions [12–15]. On the other hand, several studies have demonstrated that visual impairment affects the performance of tasks involving manual dexterity [12,16,17] as well as everyday tasks such as driving [18–20], thus showing the importance of binocular vision. Previous studies have used and compared different standardised manual and finger dexterity tests in populations with and without mental or physical conditions [10,21–23]. However, they did not assess the influence of vision on manual dexterity. Other studies found an association between visual performance and manual tasks simulating everyday tasks involving grasping [4,24,25], showing that the presence of some degree of binocular vision is beneficial for the performance of certain sensorimotor tasks [15]. Other authors monitored a bead threading task using a motion capture system, finding that a greater maximum reach velocity was linked to improved vergence function. Reduced stereoacuity thresholds correlated with a decrease in grip duration, and improved accommodative function was linked to a shorter duration of positioning [14].

In addition to the aforementioned binocular vision, some studies have demonstrated that CS and disability glare (DG) are associated with better performance in tasks that require an accurate visual function, such as driving [26,27]. Changes in visual quality (considering different visual functions) and their effect on binocular vision and driving performance have also been investigated. It has been observed that the greater the interocular differences, the lower the binocular summation of the visual functions (VA and CS) and the poorer the stereoacuity [28]. Therefore, we hypothesize that manual dexterity will be impaired when developing daily activities in monocular vision without the full benefit of binocular vision functions. In view of the above, we also hypothesize that visual quality, specifically contrast sensitivity, may have a relationship with the performance of manual dexterity tasks, particularly those involving FMSs, and which are visually demanding.

Thus, the aim of this study was to determine to what degree vision (including VA, CS, and binocular vision), particularly near vision, is involved in the performance of manual tasks involving FMSs, using five different tests and tasks performed by participants with normal binocular vision.

2. Materials and Methods

2.1. Subjects

A total of 30 subjects were enrolled in the study (10 males and 20 females) with a mean age of 24.7 ± 4.2 years. The inclusion criteria were age between 18 and 40 years (non-presbyopic), corrected binocular VA of at least 1.0 (decimal notation) for near and distance vision, normal binocular vision (fusion and stereopsis), fusional vergences within normal values, and no asthenopia. Additionally, the refractive history was evaluated, and participants with high astigmatism, amblyopia, or a history of treatment for visual abnormalities were excluded. The mean (±SD) spherical refractive error was −2.61 ± 3.03 D and the mean astigmatism was −0.74 ± 0.54 D, ranging from 0.00 D to −2.50 D. All the participants signed a written informed consent form in accordance with the Declaration of Helsinki [29]. The procedures described were approved by the Human Research Ethics Committee of the University of Granada (1256/CEIH/2020).

A thorough visual examination was carried out prior to the first measurement session to ensure that the participants had their best corrected visual acuity (BCVA) and balanced binocular vision. Stereopsis was evaluated using the Randot Stereotest (Stereo Optical, Inc., Chicago, IL, USA) at near vision (40 cm) to verify that there was good binocular integrity.

The average stereoacuity for the participants was 28.5 ± 12.4 arcsec, which is within the normal range (<40 arcsec) for correct binocular vision [30–33].

In addition, they had to complete two questionnaires to confirm that they had normal vision and no asthenopia: the visual discomfort scale (CONLON) and the Binocular Vision Discomfort Questionnaire (BVDQ). The CONLON questionnaire uses percentages: a total score of 24 points or less means that the participants can be classified in the low visual discomfort group [34]. The BVDQ does not have a standardised score; however, a lower score is associated with less discomfort [35]. For the CONLON and BVDQ questionnaires, we obtained average scores of 12.5 ± 8.1 points and 13.6 ± 8.6 points, respectively, confirming that our sample did not experience visual discomfort.

2.2. Visual Performance

Visual performance was assessed by means of different visual functions, including visual acuity, contrast sensitivity, and disability glare.

2.2.1. Visual Acuity

Near and distance VA was assessed in monocular and binocular viewing conditions using the OptoTab VA screening test (SmarThings4Vision, Zaragoza, Spain), a test used in previous studies [36]. The test was performed for near (0.5 m) and distance (5.5 m) vision. The software employs optotypes to identify wrong answers. It provides an exact calculation of the decimal visual acuity (VA).

2.2.2. Contrast Sensitivity

Contrast sensitivity (CS) was measured at 0.5 m using the OptoTab contrast sensitivity test (SmarThings4Vision), which comprises sinusoidal grids showing different orientations. Five spatial frequencies were assessed: 1.5, 3, 6, 12, and 18 cycles per degree (cpd) of visual angle. A total of nine contrast levels were evaluated for each spatial frequency as follows: the observers had to recognize and indicate whether the grid was inclined to the right, the left, or vertical; if they responded correctly, the contrast level decreased until they were no longer able to correctly indicate the inclination of the grating, reaching the contrast threshold for that condition and reporting the corresponding CS value. In order to establish correlations between this visual function and FMSs, the CS for each subject and condition was reported as the average of the CS for all of the spatial frequencies tested, as other works have done [28].

2.2.3. Disability Glare

Disability glare (DG) is the loss of retinal image contrast due to intraocular light scattering or straylight, which is caused by imperfections and loss of transparency of the optical media [37]. This value was obtained by evaluating CS at six target sizes (6.3, 4, 2.5, 1.6, 1, and 0.7 degrees, corresponding to spatial frequencies of 1.0, 1.7, 2.6, 4.2, 6.6, and 10.4 cpd, respectively) with and without the presence of glare using the CGT-1000 device (Takagi, Japan) [38]. The instrument evaluates 12-step contrast thresholds using a visual stimulus consisting of a central luminous ring. The glare source is composed of 8 LEDs distributed around the contrast stimulus (Figure 1). This device measures the monocular contrast threshold, which was determined by the lowest contrast level perceived by each participant. For each stimulus size, the DG was reported as the difference between the contrast threshold and the contrast threshold with the presence of glare, so that the higher the DG value, the greater the glare experienced by the subject and the poorer the visual performance in the presence of light sources [39]. For each subject and condition, the DG was reported as the DG averaged for all spatial frequencies (target sizes). Each subject was tested under monocular and binocular conditions with a modification of the instrument that enabled both eyes to be assessed simultaneously.

To obtain a single metric for visual function, the Overall Visual Performance Score (OVPS) was calculated. This score was obtained as the averaged z-scores obtained from each of the individual variables: VA, mean CS and DG. For each subject, the z-score of a variable is defined as the number of standard deviations below (negative) or above (positive) the group mean. The scores of DG were converted so that positive z-scores represented a better performance than the mean.

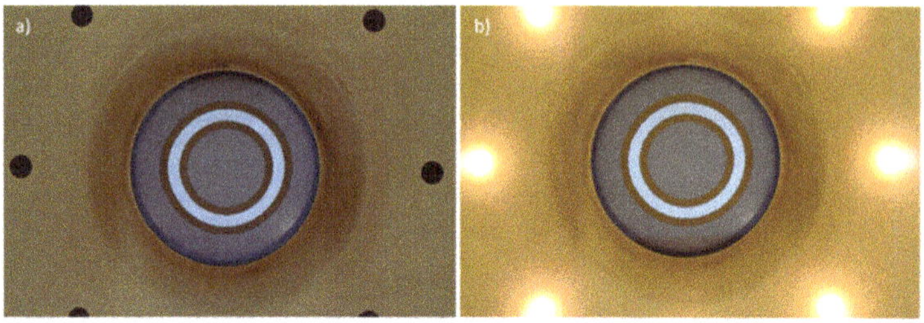

Figure 1. Central light ring used as a visual stimulus without (**a**) and with (**b**) the presence of glare in the Takagi CGT-1000 glare tester. Six of the eight LEDs composing the glare source can be observed.

2.3. Fine Motor Skills

A total of 5 different tests were performed to assess FMSs under three viewing conditions: monocularly (right and left eye) and binocularly (Figure 2). The task order and viewing conditions were randomised. The participants were seated in a chair 50 cm in front of the table. Training was performed for each test prior to the final measurement to minimise learning and fatigue effects. The tests were performed under photopic conditions. The illuminance on the test board was measured using a PCE-170A light meter (PCE Instruments, PCE Deutschland GmbH, Meschede, Germany), obtaining a mean illuminance of 753 ± 120 lux (measured in 9 points with the lux meter placed directly above the test board). The following FMSs tests were performed:

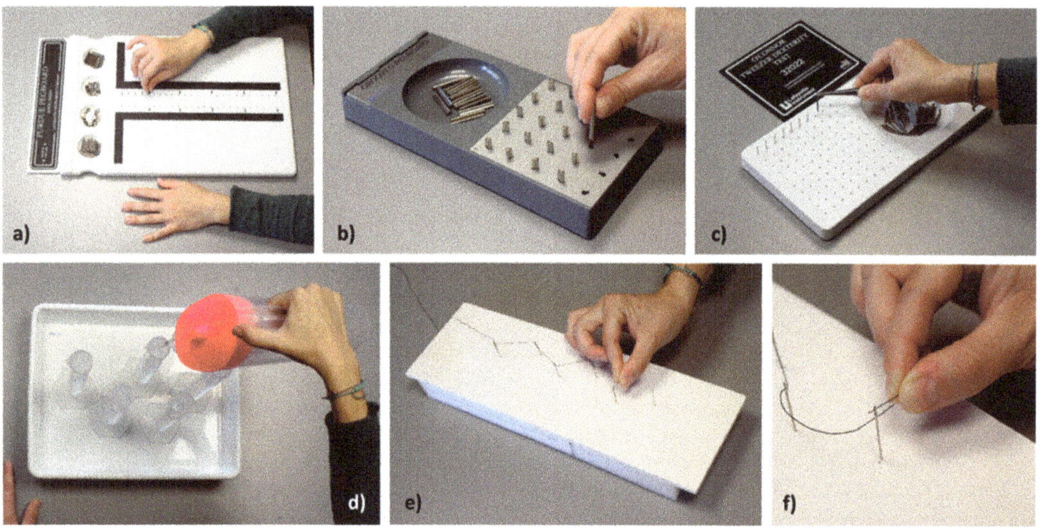

Figure 2. (**a**) Purdue Pegboard; (**b**) Grooved Pegboard; (**c**) O´Connor Pegboard; (**d**) water jug and test tubes to be used in the water pouring task; (**e**,**f**) sewing thread, needles and threading device for the threading task.

2.3.1. Purdue Pegboard (Lafayette Instruments, Lafayette, IN, USA)

This is a standardised test used to assess unimanual and bimanual motor skills [40–42]. The board presents two parallel vertical rows of 25 holes each (Figure 2a). Pegs are located in the extreme right-hand and left-hand wells at the top of the board, while collars and washers are put in the two middle wells. The main task in the test consists of placing as many pegs or pieces (pegs, collars, and washers) as possible into a row of holes on the board, from top to bottom, within a given time. Four different tasks (subtests) were performed with this test. Three of the subtests consisted of inserting as many pegs as possible (1) into the holes of the dominant-hand row using the dominant hand (first subtest), (2) into the non-dominant-hand row using the non-dominant hand (second subtest), and (3) into both rows using both hands simultaneously (third subtest). In these subtests, the number of pegs inserted in 30 s was recorded. In the fourth subtest, the participants used both hands alternately to construct assemblies in the dominant-hand row of the board. Each assembly included a total of four pieces: a peg, then a washer over it, then a collar, and then another washer. The subject had to complete as many assemblies as possible within 60 s. In this subtest, the number of pieces placed correctly was recorded.

2.3.2. Grooved Pegboard (Lafayette Instruments, Lafayette, IN, USA)

This is used to measure hand–eye coordination and motor speed. This is a strong predictor of motor performance in healthy adults [43]. The test board comprises a perforated board with 25 holes with the same asymmetrical profile but in different orientations, and a well containing the pegs (Figure 2b). The pegs have a protruding section that matches the shape of the holes so the pegs must be inserted so that the orientation of its section coincides with that of the hole. The participants had to use their dominant hand to insert the pegs row by row from left to right (right-handed), or in the opposite direction (right to left) if they were left-handed. The time taken to place all the pegs (in seconds) was measured using a stopwatch.

2.3.3. O'Connor Tweezer Dexterity Test (Lafayette Instruments, Lafayette, IN, USA)

This consists of a board with 100 holes and a well containing pegs (Figure 2c). This test measures the speed with which a subject is able to pick up pegs and insert them into the holes using a pair of tweezers [11]. In our experiment, the subject had to insert the pegs in the holes of the first row (one peg per hole, 10 holes in total) in the shortest possible time while holding the tweezers with the dominant hand. The time taken to place the pegs in the first row (in seconds) was recorded.

2.3.4. Water Pouring Task

This manual dexterity task consisted of pouring 450 mL of water into five test tubes (diameter 2.7 cm and capacity 100 mL) arranged in a zigzag pattern on a tray (Figure 2d). A similar test has been used in previous research [15]. Each test tube was marked at 90 mL. The participants had to hold a jug (containing 600 mL of water) with their dominant hand and fill the five test tubes, from right to left for right-handed participants (left to right for left-handed participants), up to the mark. We quantified the time taken to complete the task (in seconds), the error made in filling each tube (in mL), and the water spilled onto the tray (in mL).

2.3.5. Threading Task

In this task, the participants were asked to thread six needles with a black thread over a white background in the shortest possible time, using their dominant hand (Figure 2e,f). The participants were given specific instructions in order to avoid any tactile reference when performing the tasks. The time taken to thread the first four needles (hole size 1.3×8.0 mm) was recorded, as was the time taken to thread all of them. The last two needles presented a higher level of difficulty since the needle eye was smaller (1.0×4.0 mm).

To obtain an overall measure of FMSs, the Overall Fine Motor Skills Score (OFMSS) was calculated in the same way as described for the OVPS. This score was obtained as the averaged z-scores for each of the individual FMSs parameter variables for each participant. The scores were converted so that the more positive the score, the better the FMSs performance.

2.4. Statistical Analysis

Sample size was determined by power calculation using G*Power v.3.1.9.2 software. The analysis indicated that 21 participants were needed to achieve equivalent effect sizes (Cohen d [0.8–1.2]) with 95% power on all of the key measures in this study (vision and FMSs variables).

Statistical analyses were performed using the software SPSS 28.0 (SPSS Inc., Chicago, IL, USA). To analyse the relationship between FMSs performance and the visual parameters (near VA, near CS and DG), an eye was randomly selected and the means and standard deviations were calculated for each visual parameter and the FMSs metric. Prior to the data analysis, the Kolmogorov–Smirnov test was run on all variables (vision and tasks). Wilcoxson's Z-test was applied to determine if there were statistically significant differences between the monocular and binocular conditions. The relationship between visual function and FMSs was first explored with a bivariate correlation analysis. A Spearman correlation analysis was conducted when normality could not be assumed, and a Pearson correlation analysis was performed when the data were normally distributed. Finally, to determine how visual function and other factors predict the performance of FMSs tasks, a regression model (with a forward stepwise selection) was run with the OFMSS as a dependent variable, visual variables (DG, CS and VA) and age as covariates, and the total CONLON score as a fixed factor. The significance level was set at $p < 0.05$ for all tests.

3. Results

3.1. Visual Performance and FMSs

No biological-sex-related differences were found for visual function and the performance of FMSs ($p < 0.05$). The results from the visual assessment (by means of near visual acuity, contrast sensitivity, and disability glare) are summarised in Table 1. In the case of contrast sensitivity and disability glare, both the total average values and the average values for each of the spatial frequencies or angular sizes are shown. We obtained better results for VA and DG in the binocular condition, but there were no statistically significant differences between the two viewing conditions. However, significant results were obtained from the detailed analysis of DG when comparing the two conditions, specifically for the angle sizes of 6.3, 4, 2.5, and 1.6 degrees. Statistically significant differences were observed in CS measured under binocular conditions versus monocular measurements, with better contrast sensitivities obtained in binocular conditions ($p < 0.05$). The average CS for each spatial frequency measured is also shown in Table 1. A better CS was obtained in binocular conditions for all spatial frequencies except for 6 cpd ($p > 0.05$).

Table 1. Mean values for the visual parameters studied under the two viewing conditions.

		Viewing Condition		Statistic	
		Monocular	Binocular	Wilcoxon's Z-Test	p-Values
Near VA		1.21 ± 0.05	1.23 ± 0.04	−1.934	0.053
Mean DG		0.031 ± 0.029	0.019 ± 0.012	−1.635	0.102
DG for each stimulus size	6.3 deg	0.014 ± 0.012	0.004 ± 0.004	−4.345	<0.001 *
	4 deg	0.015 ± 0.014	0.005 ± 0.006	−3.804	<0.001 *
	2.5 deg	0.014 ± 0.027	0.007 ± 0.008	−3.351	0.001 *
	1.6 deg	0.024 ± 0.013	0.017 ± 0.012	−2.437	0.015 *
	1 deg	0.038 ± 0.038	0.0279 ± 0.018	−0.772	0.440
	0.7 deg	0.080 ± 0.123	0.053 ± 0.054	−0.285	0.776
Mean CS		115.96 ± 8.05	121.98 ± 4.64	−3.469	0.001 *
CS for each spatial frequency	1.5 cpd	80.70 ± 15.66	90.60 ± 10.35	−2.412	0.016 *
	3 cpd	149.57 ± 19.58	159.40 ± 11.77	−2.434	0.015 *
	6 cpd	163.43 ± 5.54	165.63 ± 2.01	−1.897	0.058
	12 cpd	124.10 ± 14.47	129.80 ± 4.475	−2.068	0.039 *
	18 cpd	60.83 ± 19.54	64.47 ± 6.91	−1.958	0.050 *

* Significant differences. VA, visual acuity; CS, contrast sensitivity; DG, disability glare.

Table 2 shows the results for the FMSs. The scores corresponding to the binocular viewing conditions obtained from the three validated tests (Purdue, O'Connor, and Grooved) are consistent with both the standardised scores provided by each manufacturer and by previous studies [22,40,44]. The time modification when performing the adapted O'Connor Tweezer Dexterity task was considered.

Table 2. Mean values of parameters characterizing the performance of fine motor skills in two different viewing conditions (monocular and binocular).

Test		Viewing Condition		Statistic	
		Monocular	Binocular	Wilcoxon's Z-Test	*p*-Values
Purdue pegboard	Dominant hand (no. pegs)	13.77 ± 1.92	15.40 ± 1.65	−4.307	<0.001 *
	Non-dominant hand (no. pegs)	12.43 ± 1.65	13.90 ± 1.90	−4.081	<0.001 *
	Both hands (no. pegs)	10.03 ± 1.43	11.63 ± 1.38	−4.523	<0.001 *
	Assemblies (no. pegs)	36.30 ± 6.57	40.37 ± 6.55	−3.949	<0.001 *
O'Connor tweezer dexterity	Performance time (s)	42.16 ± 6.58	36.40 ± 7.31	−3.960	<0.001 *
Grooved pegboard	Performance time (s)	63.48 ± 8.36	58.84 ± 7.88	−3.990	<0.001 *
Needle threading	4-needle performance time (s)	37.28 ± 14.40	18.84 ± 4.71	−4.782	<0.001 *
	All-needle performance time (s)	60.07 ± 22.76	30.81 ± 8.00	−4.782	<0.001 *
Water pouring	Performance time (s)	42.31 ± 10.64	37.33 ± 8.85	−3.671	<0.001 *
	Error made (mL)	9.23 ± 7.42	7.80 ± 4.92	−1.133	0.257
	Water spilled (mL)	13.47 ± 13.63	0.93 ± 1.93	−4.408	<0.001 *

* Significant differences.

The tasks for which the time required to complete them was assessed were performed significantly faster under binocular viewing conditions compared to monocular viewing ($p < 0.05$). When the task was performed under binocular viewing, less water was spilled ($p < 0.05$) and there was, on average, greater accuracy when filling the test tubes, although the differences were not significant ($p > 0.05$). Finally, performing the Purdue pegboard task binocularly resulted in more pegs inserted in 30 s for all conditions (dominant and non-dominant hand, and both hands) and more assemblies made within 60 s ($p < 0.05$). In addition, in the Purdue pegboard test, there were significant differences between the results using the dominant and non-dominant hand. The results were better when performing the peg insertion with the dominant hand ($Z = -5.864$; $p < 0.001$).

The correlation between the three standardised tests (Purdue, Grooved, and O'Connor) and the two tests that simulated everyday tasks (needle threading and water pouring) was also analysed. We obtained a significant correlation (rho = 0.412; $p = 0.024$), showing that the better the three standardised dexterity tests were performed, the better the simulated everyday tasks were performed.

3.2. Correlations Between Vision and FMSs

Only the following variables were normally distributed: Grooved test performance time, pieces inserted in the Purdue test assembly task, O'Connor test performance time, and water pouring time. We used Spearman's correlation index for our analysis as most of the variables were not normally distributed.

Figure 3 shows the parameters of the two daily visual tasks as a function of the averaged contrast sensitivity. We found significant descending correlations between the mean CS and the two FMSs tasks: the threading task for the two different levels of difficulty (rho = −0.547, $p < 0.001$; and rho = −0.486, $p < 0.001$, respectively) (Figure 3a), and the water spilled during the pouring task (rho = −0.385, $p = 0.002$) (Figure 3b). Each point represents the mean CS for each participant in each viewing visual condition (monocular and binocular) (abscissas), and their corresponding values of time spent to thread the needles (s) or amount of spilled water (mL) (ordinates in Figure 3a,b, respectively). The results indicated that the better the CS, the less time needed to complete the threading task and the lower the volume of water spilled.

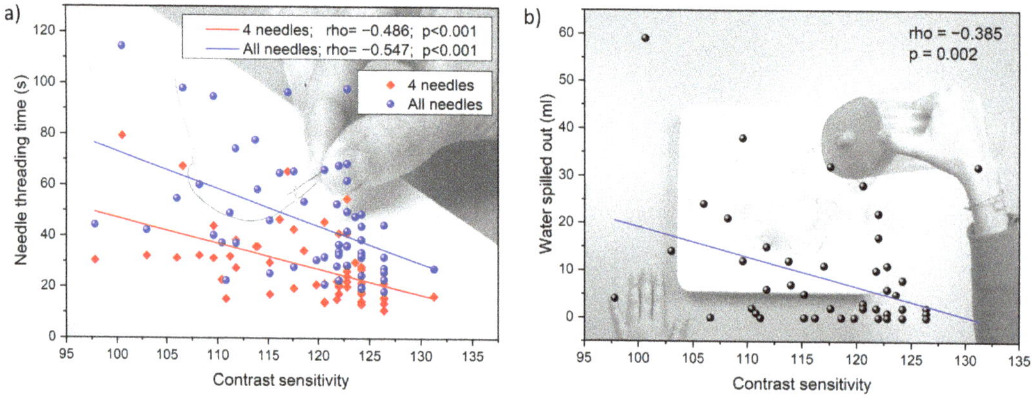

Figure 3. (**a**) Scatter plot showing the relationship between needle threading time (in seconds) and mean near CS for the two levels of difficulty (threading of 4 and 6 needles); (**b**) Scatter plot showing the relationship between water spilled (in mL) during the pouring task and mean near CS.

Significant correlations between the FMSs tasks and the spatial frequencies of the CS are shown in Table 3. The results indicate that CS correlates positively with the number of pegs inserted in the Purdue pegboard task, suggesting that better CS at the highest spatial frequency (18 cpd) is associated with a higher number of pegs inserted.

Table 3. Significant correlations between FMSs and contrast sensitivity at near distance, for each spatial frequency measured.

		CS Spatial Frequencies (cpd)				
		1.5	**3**	**6**	**12**	**18**
Purdue pegboard	Non-dominant hand (no. pegs)					rho: 0.278 *p*-value: 0.032
	Both hands (no. pegs)					rho: 0.255 *p*-value: 0.050
O'Connor tweezer dexterity	Performance time (s)		rho: −0.307 *p*-value: 0.017			
Needle threading	4-needle performance time (s)	rho: −0.354 *p*-value: 0.005	rho: −0.382 *p*-value: 0.003		rho: −0.351 *p*-value: 0.006	rho: −0.277 *p*-value: 0.032
	All-needle performance time (s)	rho: −0.337 *p*-value: 0.009	rho: −0.326 *p*-value: 0.011		rho: −0.336 *p*-value: 0.009	rho: −0.256 *p*-value: 0.048
Water pouring	Performance time (s)		rho: −0.344 *p*-value: 0.007			
	Water spilled (mL)	rho: −0.319 *p*-value: 0.013	rho: −0.345 *p*-value: 0.007	rho: −0.265 *p*-value: 0.040		

Significant negative correlations were found for the remaining tasks, indicating that as the CS improved, less time was needed to complete the FMSs tasks. Additionally, for the two tasks that simulate everyday tasks (water pouring and threading), there were significant correlations, especially at the low frequencies (1.5 and 3 cpd).

Table 4 reports the significant correlations obtained between DG and FMSs for each quantified stimulus size. These results revealed an association between the DG values obtained for each stimulus angle size in the contrast threshold test, with and without glare, and the performance of the manual tasks. Elevated DG values suggest a greater deterioration of CS under glare conditions. Overall, the findings demonstrated that greater impairment from glare leads to poorer performance of FMSs tasks. Specifically, more time was required to complete the Purdue pegboard tasks and fewer pieces were introduced when CS deteriorated. Significant correlations were found for almost all tasks for the 6.3 and 4-degree stimulus sizes; however, an association was observed for the 2.5-degree stimulus size only for the needle threading and water-pouring tasks. Correlations were found between DG for the 1.6-degree stimulus size and the Purdue pegboard tasks. DG was greater at this size and was associated with more water being spilled during the water-pouring task. For the smallest size, no correlations were found.

Table 4. Significant correlations between FMSs and disability glare at near distance, for each stimulus angle size measured.

		Disability Glare Stimulus Angle Sizes (Degree)				
		6.3	4	2.5	1.6	1
Purdue pegboard	Dominant hand (no. pegs)	rho: −0.311; *p*-value: 0.016	rho: −0.262; *p*-value: 0.043			
	Non-dominant hand (no. pegs)		rho: −0.265; *p*-value: 0.041		rho: −0.301; *p*-value: 0.020	
	Both hands (no. pegs)	rho: −0.361; *p*-value: 0.005	rho: −0.423; *p*-value: 0.001		rho: −0.292; *p*-value: 0.024	
O'Connor tweezer dexterity	Performance time (s)	rho: 0.331; *p*-value: 0.010	rho: 0.272; *p*-value: 0.035			
Needle threading	4-needle performance time (s)	rho: 0.447; *p*-value: 0.000	rho: 0.552; *p*-value: 0.000	rho: 0.378; *p*-value: 0.003		
	All-needle performance time (s)	rho: 0.433; *p*-value: 0.001	rho: 0.517; *p*-value: 0.000	rho: 0.360; *p*-value: 0.005		
Water pouring	Performance time (s)		rho: 0.271; *p*-value: 0.036	rho: 0.298; *p*-value: 0.021		
	Water spilled (mL)	rho: 0.427; *p*-value: 0.001	rho: 0.389; *p*-value: 0.002	rho: 0.343; *p*-value: 0.007	rho: 0.371; *p*-value: 0.004	

To analyse the relationship between visual performance and FMSs, first, the OVPS and OFMSS indices were calculated. Figure 4 shows the correlation between these two indices (rho = 0.329; *p*-value = 0.010). The higher the OVPS, the better the visual performance. Likewise, the higher the OFMSS, the better the performance of FMSs. This positive correlation suggests that individuals with better near visual function (in terms of VA, CS, and DG) exhibit superior fine motor abilities.

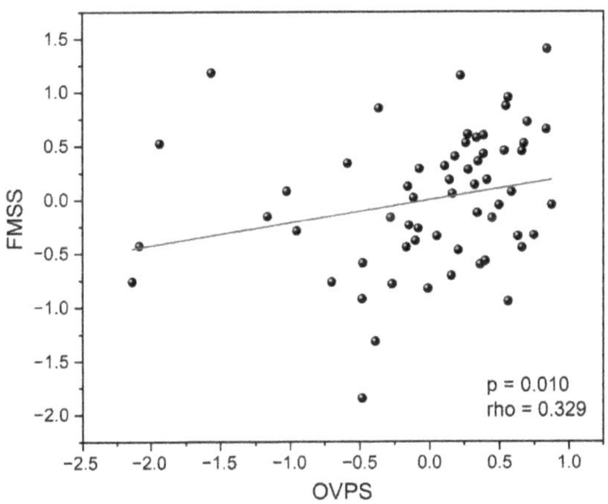

Figure 4. The overall fine motor skills score (OFMSS) as a function of the overall visual performance score (OVPS).

To find the best linear model to predict the FMSs score as a function of visual parameters and other variables, a multiple linear regression analysis was run with the OFMSS as the dependent variable and the different visual functions and age as covariates. The visual parameter included was the near CS. This forward stepwise method selected the age of the participants. The results of this analysis are shown in Table 5.

Table 5. Results of the multiple linear regression analysis. The coefficients, the standard deviation (SD), the t-statistic, the *p*-values, and the confidence interval (CI) are shown.

	Coefficient	SD	t-Statistic	*p*-Value	95% CI
OFMSS	−5.497	1.322	−4.158	0.000	[−8.143, −2.850]
Mean near CS	0.038	0.010	3.672	0.001	[0.017, 0.058]
Age (years)	0.042	0.017	2.385	0.020	[0.007, 0.077]

According to the R-squared value obtained, this model explains 21.3% of the *OFMSS*. The *OFMSS* would be given by the following regression line Equation (1)

$$OFMSS = 0.038 \times CS + 0.042 \times age(years) - 5.497 \quad (1)$$

The standard deviations were 0.010, 0.017, and 1.322, for the first, second, and third terms of the equation, respectively.

The *OFMSS*, i.e., the performance of FMSs, can therefore be predicted by this linear regression model at 21.3%. The predictive factors include age and the average *CS* measured for near vision, with *CS* being the most important contributor to the regression model.

4. Discussion

In this study, we investigated the relationship between visual function in healthy non-presbyopic adults, assessed by means of visual acuity (VA), contrast sensitivity (CS) and disability glare (DG), as well as fine motor skills (FMSs). We analysed adults instead of children because the cortical maturation of visual, somatosensory, and motor processing provides the neural substrate for refining FMSs in adolescence [5]. Firstly, our results from the clinical tests of visual function showed better outcomes for binocular viewing, in line with previous studies [24,26,45–47].

To evaluate FMSs, we analysed the performance of five different tasks: three standardised dexterity tests (Purdue, Grooved and O'Connor tests) and two everyday fine-motor tasks. The first three tests have been described in the literature as tests that allow us to measure motor function. In particular, factor analysis studies have shown that the Purdue pegboard test is supported by a finger dexterity factor [7]. Meanwhile, the needle threading and the water pouring tests enabled us to characterise two everyday fine-motor tasks performed using the dominant hand, similar to that reported in a previous work [4]. In our research, we obtained a correlation between the two types of tests (standardised dexterity tests and daily tasks). These results may indicate that these two types of tests can be used to reliably assess FMSs. However, further research into this issue is needed to reach a solid conclusion.

The improvement when performing FMSs binocularly is in line with previous studies [9,16,17,48]. These results suggest that the contribution of depth vision and binocular summation is reflected in improved performance in all tasks related to controlling the terminal reach and grasp. According to Melmoth and Grant [12], these benefits derive from binocular disparity processing linked to changes in relative hand–pegboard distance, and this depth information is independently used to regulate the progress of the approaching hand and to guide the task, thereby ensuring that the grip is securely applied.

We also found differences when comparing the results of the Purdue pegboard test with the dominant and non-dominant hand. The results were better when inserting the pegs with the dominant hand, as reflected in previous studies [49,50].

As mentioned above, the main aim of our research was to investigate the relationship between VA, CS, DG, and FMSs. We focused on these three visual functions because, in clinical practice, VA is the parameter most commonly used to characterise vision, and CS defines important characteristics that are not captured by VA alone. Previous studies have shown that CS plays an important role in the performance of daily tasks that involve visuomotor skills, including driving [26], endoscopic surgery [51], and sports [52,53]. In addition, previous studies on amblyopic participants have shown that even after the total recovery of VA following refractive amblyopia treatment, interocular differences in CS were not equalised and stereopsis did not return to normal values [54]. Previous studies have shown that optical correction would improve refractive amblyopia but may nevertheless present an impairment in fine motor skills [55] or have poor visual development due, for example, to high astigmatism [56]. This aspect shows the importance of taking into consideration the refractive history of the subjects and whether they have presented any type of vision anomaly such as amblyopia. In the present study, subjects with high astigmatism, amblyopia, or a history of treatment for visual abnormalities were excluded. Furthermore, subjects included in the study showed normal values in the results of the standardized manual dexterity tests. In our study we also analysed DG, incorporating information on how CS is affected by glare. It is known that visual performance is more sensitive to glare in central vision than in peripheral vision [57]. We found decreased DG in both monocular and binocular vision because all our participants were healthy, but with significant differences for the bigger stimulus sizes.

In general, more significant correlations were obtained for the needle threading and water pouring, which represent real daily tasks that are visually demanding, particularly the needle threading task. We found that the better the CS, the less time was needed to complete the needle threading task, and the less water was spilled during the pouring task. Meanwhile, for DG, the correlations indicated that greater glare-induced disability leads to poorer performance in the FMSs tasks. These findings support our initial hypothesis, confirming the influence of CS in daily fine-motor tasks involving near vision and are in line with the previous studies discussed above [58]. In each of the five tasks, we observed varying levels of contrast that define, for example, the holes in the pegboards and the components to be retrieved and inserted, as well as the edges of the test tubes or the eyes of the needles used. This might suggest that improved CS is related to a stronger visual signal, resulting in a faster initial movement impulse.

Correlations between FMSs and CS and DG for each spatial frequency and angle size were analysed. Although correlations were found for both high and low frequencies in the case of the standardised tests, more correlations were found for low spatial frequencies in the needle threading and water pouring tasks. These findings could be explained by the fact that, although the sizes subtended by the different stimuli were smaller, the five FMSs tasks performed in our study presented a high degree of difficulty and involved spatial vision for planning and performance. CS performance appears to be a determinant in visuospatial processing [59]. Grandjean et al. suggested that the performance of CS tests is mediated, in part, by visuospatial skills, and they showed that the designs used in the test to assess CS may require different types of skills. According to our results, this seems reasonable since our FMSs tasks also involved visuospatial skills. On the other hand, the low spatial frequencies are much larger and easier for the eyes to detect, and the eyes would be most sensitive to detecting objects under low contrast objects when the spatial frequencies are around 3 to 5 cpd. In our study, the difference between monocular and binocular contrast sensitivity (under normal conditions, CS, and assessing glare, DG) is significantly higher for low and medium spatial frequencies, so these spatial frequencies could have a greater impact on the performance of some FMSs. This would explain why the DG correlates better with FMSs for lower spatial frequencies (higher angle sizes, 6.3

and 4.0 degrees) so that the higher the DG value, the worse the FMSs performance. These correlations are also observed for CS and daily tasks, further showing that the highest spatial frequency evaluated in this work (18 cpd) also plays an important role. In addition, the results provided by Grandjean et al. suggest that attention and executive system functioning may also contribute to performance in CS tests [59]. Similarly, these functions are present in our FMSs tasks. Another interesting factor to be considered is the sensory feedback from low-threshold receptors in the skin. This feedback plays a crucial role in hand control in FMSs [43].

On the other hand, we calculated the OFMSS, enabling us to group different FMSs tasks into a single metric. By incorporating all the variables that characterise these tests, we were able to jointly evaluate the different dimensions of manual dexterity involved in the FMSs, providing a more complex characterisation. The correlations are only used to identify the relationship between two variables; however, a regression analysis is required to determine the value of one variable in terms of another [60,61]. Our results indicated that the near CS and age predict the FMSs in 21.3% of cases. We found that age is a predictor of FMSs performance. Therefore, according to our results, there seems to be an age-related improvement in the performance of FMSs in adults aged 18 to 40. However, according to the literature, from the ages of 60 to 65, there is a deterioration in these abilities [62,63]. Thus, the regression model obtained in this study would only apply to young adults up to 40 years of age, and further studies would be needed to report a regression model covering a wider age range. These results may be related and supported by other findings. Recent research has shown that medium spatial frequency ranges are most optimal for testing visual function, such as 3 cpd in age macular degeneration (AMD) [64] and 4 cpd in amblyopia [56]. In line with the predictions for FMSs, measuring CS at intermediate spatial frequencies may be a good way to proceed. At the visual level, along the lines suggested previously, additional visual measures, among which we highlight CS, are necessary to understand the impact of vision and therefore of vision loss in daily life [58].

It should also be noted that we only analysed healthy participants and is important to analyse other groups of subjects, such as those with any type of non-strabismic binocular anomaly, amblyopia, or degrading visual function, using filters or lenses. It would also be interesting to study the influence of visual performance on FMSs in older subjects, who suffer from deteriorated fine motor skills but also decreased contrast sensitivity, especially at high frequencies [58].

Recent studies have monitored FMSs performance and yielded promising preliminary results using new systems [65]. The combination of these findings and the measured visual functions can offer further insight into the role of the visual system in the various motor skills. Additionally, analysing relevant visual variables alongside FMSs performance could enhance our understanding of that role.

5. Conclusions

Binocular vision is superior to monocular vision for the visual functions studied (visual acuity, contrast sensitivity, and disability glare) and results in better performance in the execution of various fine motor tasks. There is also a correlation between visual performance and fine motor skills, so that the better the visual performance, the better the fine motor skills. The results of this study provide important insights into the role of near contrast sensitivity in the performance of complex manipulation tasks in non-presbyopic adults. In individuals with normal binocular vision, contrast sensitivity stands out as the visual function with the greatest relevance in terms of fine motor performance. In particular, low-medium spatial frequencies correlate more closely with daily tasks in healthy adults, suggesting the implication of spatial vision in the planning and execution of these tasks. These results highlight the importance of visual functions, such as contrast sensitivity, indicating that this should be included in routine ophthalmology or optometry vision screenings. The assessment of these visual functions may also be useful in other clinical areas such as psychology or neurology, where manual dexterity or fine motor skills are often analysed.

Author Contributions: Conceptualization, J.J.C.-T., M.C.-L. and P.G.-D.; Data curation, P.G.-D.; formal analysis, P.G.-D. and F.M.; Funding acquisition, J.J.C.-T. and R.G.A.; Methodology, J.J.C.-T., M.C.-L., and P.G.-D.; Supervision, J.J.C.-T. and M.C.-L.; Writing—original draft, P.G.-D.; Writing—reviewing and editing, J.J.C.-T., M.C.-L., F.M., and R.G.A. All authors have read and agreed to the published version of the manuscript.

Funding: Grant PID2020-115184RB-I00 was funded by MCIN/AEI/10.13039/501100011033 and A-FQM-532-UGR20 was funded by FEDER/Junta de Andalucía-Consejería de Transformación Económica, Industria, Conocimiento y Universidades.

Institutional Review Board Statement: The study was conducted in accordance with the Declaration of Helsinki and approved by the Human Research Ethics Committee of the University of Granada (1256/CEIH/2020) for studies involving humans.

Informed Consent Statement: Informed consent was obtained from all subjects involved in the study.

Data Availability Statement: The data that support the findings of this study are available from the corresponding author upon reasonable request.

Conflicts of Interest: The authors declare no conflicts of interest. The funders had no role in the design of the study; in the collection, analyses, or interpretation of data; in the writing of the manuscript; or in the decision to publish the results.

References

1. Patterson, E.J.; Bargary, G.; Barbur, J.L. Understanding disability glare: Light scatter and retinal illuminance as predictors of sensitivity to contrast. *J. Opt. Soc. Am. A-Opt. Image Sci. Vis.* **2015**, *32*, 576–585. [CrossRef] [PubMed]
2. Gilbert, M. Definition of visual acuity. *Br. J. Ophthalmol.* **1953**, *37*, 661–669. [CrossRef] [PubMed]
3. Peli, E. Contrast in complex images. *J. Opt. Soc. Am. A-Opt. Image Sci. Vision.* **1990**, *7*, 2032–2040. [CrossRef] [PubMed]
4. Piano, M.E.F.; O'Connor, A.R. The Effect of Degrading Binocular Single Vision on Fine Visuomotor Skill Task Performance. *Investig. Ophthalmol. Vis. Sci.* **2013**, *54*, 8204–8213. [CrossRef]
5. Niechwiej-Szwedo, E.; Colpa, L.; Wong, A. The role of binocular vision in the control and development of visually guided upper limb movements. *Philos. Trans. R. Soc. B-Biol. Sci.* **2023**, *378*, 11. [CrossRef]
6. Fleishman, E.A.; Hempel, W.E. A Factor Analysis of Dexterity Tests. *Pers. Psychol.* **1954**, *7*, 15–32. [CrossRef]
7. Fleishman, E.A.; Ellison, G.D. A factor-analysis of fine manipulative tests. *J. Appl. Psychol.* **1962**, *46*, 96–105. [CrossRef]
8. Almuklass, A.M.; Feeney, D.F.; Mani, D.; Hamilton, L.D.; Enoka, R.M. Peg-manipulation capabilities of middle-aged adults have a greater influence on pegboard times than those of young and old adults. *Exp. Brain Res.* **2018**, *236*, 2165–2172. [CrossRef] [PubMed]
9. Alramis, F.; Roy, E.; Christian, L.; Niechwiej-Szwedo, E. Contribution of binocular vision to the performance of complex manipulation tasks in 5–13 years old visually-normal children. *Hum. Mov. Sci.* **2016**, *46*, 52–62. [CrossRef]
10. Tolle, K.A.; Rahman-Filipiak, A.M.; Hale, A.C.; Andren, K.A.K.; Spencer, R.J. Grooved Pegboard Test as a measure of executive functioning. *Appl. Neuropsychol. Adult* **2020**, *27*, 414–420. [CrossRef]
11. Lundergan, W.P.; Soderstrom, E.J.; Chambers, D.W. Tweezer dexterity aptitude of dental students. *J. Dent. Educ.* **2007**, *71*, 1090–1097. [CrossRef] [PubMed]
12. Melmoth, D.R.; Grant, S. Advantages of binocular vision for the control of reaching and grasping. *Exp. Brain Res.* **2006**, *171*, 371–388. [CrossRef]
13. Suttle, C.M.; Melmoth, D.R.; Finlay, A.L.; Sloper, J.J.; Grant, S. Eye-Hand Coordination Skills in Children with and without Amblyopia. *Investig. Ophthalmol. Vis. Sci.* **2011**, *52*, 1851–1864. [CrossRef] [PubMed]
14. Niechwiej-Szwedo, E.; Thai, G.; Christian, L. Contribution of stereopsis, vergence, and accommodative function to the performance of a precision grasping and placement task in typically developing children age 8–14 years. *Hum. Mov. Sci.* **2020**, *72*, 10. [CrossRef] [PubMed]
15. O'Connor, A.R.; Birch, E.E.; Anderson, S.; Draper, H. Relationship between Binocular Vision, Visual Acuity, and Fine Motor Skills. *Optom. Vis. Sci.* **2010**, *87*, 942–947. [CrossRef]
16. Servos, P.; Goodale, M.A.; Jakobson, L.S. The role of binocular vision in prehension—A kinematic analysis. *Vis. Res.* **1992**, *32*, 1513–1521. [CrossRef]
17. Gnanaseelan, R.; Gonzalez, D.A.; Niechwiej-Szwedo, E. Binocular advantage for prehension movements performed in visually enriched environments requiring visual search. *Front. Hum. Neurosci.* **2014**, *8*, 11. [CrossRef] [PubMed]
18. Wood, J.M. Age and visual impairment decrease driving performance as measured on a closed-road circuit. *Hum. Factors* **2002**, *44*, 482–494. [CrossRef]

19. Ortiz-Peregrina, S.; Ortiz, C.; Martino, F.; Casares-Lopez, M.; Castro-Torres, J.J.; Anera, R.G. Speed management across road environments of varying complexities and self-regulation behaviors in drivers with cataract. *Sci. Rep.* **2022**, *12*, 12. [CrossRef]
20. Martino, F.; Castro-Torres, J.J.; Casares-Lopez, M.; Ortiz-Peregrina, S.; Ortiz, C.; Anera, R.G. Deterioration of binocular vision after alcohol intake influences driving performance. *Sci. Rep.* **2021**, *11*, 8904. [CrossRef]
21. Liu, S.; Zou, L.L.; Wen, W.; Wang, S.; Liu, G.S.; Li, Y.L.; Guoke, Y.; Chang, X.; Liu, H.; Liao, R.; et al. Binocular treatment in adult amblyopia is based on parvocellular or magnocellular pathway. *Eur. J. Ophthalmol.* **2020**, *30*, 658–667.
22. Strenge, H.; Niederberger, U.; Seelhorst, U. Correlation between tests of attention and performance on grooved and purdue pegboards in normal subjects. *Percept. Mot. Ski.* **2002**, *95*, 507–514. [CrossRef]
23. Berger, M.A.M.; Krul, A.J.; Daanen, H.A.M. Task specificity of finger dexterity tests. *Appl. Ergon.* **2009**, *40*, 145–147. [CrossRef] [PubMed]
24. Gonzalez, D.A.; Niechwiej-Szwedo, E. The effects of monocular viewing on hand-eye coordination during sequential grasping and placing movements. *Vis. Res.* **2016**, *128*, 30–38. [CrossRef]
25. Keefe, B.D.; Watt, S.J. Viewing geometry determines the contribution of binocular vision to the online control of grasping. *Exp. Brain Res.* **2017**, *235*, 3631–3643. [CrossRef]
26. Casares-Lopez, M.; Castro-Torres, J.J.; Martino, F.; Ortiz-Peregrina, S.; Ortiz, C.; Anera, R.G. Contrast sensitivity and retinal straylight after alcohol consumption: Effects on driving performance. *Sci. Rep.* **2020**, *10*, 12. [CrossRef]
27. Ortiz-Peregrina, S.; Casares-Lopez, M.; Ortiz, C.; Castro-Torres, J.J.; Martino, F.; Jimenez, J.R. Comparison of the effects of alcohol and cannabis on visual function and driving performance. Does the visual impairment affect driving? *Drug Alcohol Depend.* **2022**, *237*, 9. [CrossRef]
28. Martino, F.; Castro-Torres, J.J.; Casares-Lopez, M.; Ortiz-Peregrina, S.; Ortiz, C.; Jimenez, J.R. Effect of interocular differences on binocular visual performance after inducing forward scattering. *Ophthalmic Physiol. Opt.* **2022**, *14*, 730–743. [CrossRef]
29. World Medical Association. Declaration of Helsinki. Ethical principles for medical research involving human subjects. *J. Indian Med. Assoc.* **2009**, *107*, 403–405.
30. Adams, W.E.; Leske, D.A.; Hatt, S.R.; Holmes, J.M. Defining Real Change in Measures of Stereoacuity. *Ophthalmology* **2009**, *116*, 281–285. [CrossRef]
31. Garnham, L.; Sloper, J.J. Effect of age on adult stereoacuity as measured by different types of stereotest. *Br. J. Ophthalmol.* **2006**, *90*, 91–95. [CrossRef] [PubMed]
32. Simons, K. Stereoacuity norms in young-children. *Arch. Ophthalmol.* **1981**, *99*, 439–445. [CrossRef]
33. Fielder, A.R.; Moseley, M.J. Does stereopsis matter in humans? *Eye* **1996**, *10*, 233–238. [CrossRef]
34. Conlon, E.G.; Lovegrove, W.J.; Chekaluk, E.; Pattison, P.E. Measuring visual discomfort. *Vis. Cognition.* **1999**, *6*, 637–663. [CrossRef]
35. Feinberg, D.L.; Rosner, M.S.; Rosner, A.J. Validation of the Binocular Vision Dysfunction Questionnaire (BVDQ). *Otol. Neurotol.* **2021**, *42*, E66–E74. [CrossRef] [PubMed]
36. Consejo, A.; Trillo-Moreno, I.; Remon, L. Corneal tissue changes following short-term soft contact lens wear of different materials. *Ophthalmic Physiol. Opt.* **2023**, *43*, 35–45. [CrossRef]
37. Aslam, T.M.; Haider, D.; Murray, I.J. Principles of disability glare measurement: An ophthalmological perspective. *Acta Ophthalmol. Scand.* **2007**, *85*, 354–360. [CrossRef]
38. Castro-Torres, J.J.; Martino, F.; Casares-Lopez, M.; Ortiz-Peregrina, S.; Ortiz, C. Visual performance after the deterioration of retinal image quality: Induced forward scattering using Bangerter foils and fog filters. *Biomed. Opt. Express* **2021**, *12*, 2902–2918. [CrossRef]
39. Pesudovs, K. Takagi Glare Tester CGT-1000 for contrast sensitivity and glare testing in normal individuals and cataract patients. *J. Refract. Surg.* **2007**, *23*, 492–498. [CrossRef]
40. Tiffin, J.; Asher, E.J. The Purdue Pegboard: Norms and Studies of Reliability and Validity. *J. Appl. Psychol.* **1948**, *32*, 234–247. [CrossRef]
41. Chen, S.; Mao, M.; Zhu, G.; Chen, Y.; Qiu, Y.; Ye, B.; Xu, D. Cortical activity in patients with high-functioning ischemic stroke during the Purdue Pegboard Test: Insights into bimanual coordinated fine motor skills with functional near-infrared spectroscopy. *Neural Regen. Res.* **2024**, *19*, 1098–1104. [CrossRef] [PubMed]
42. Buddenberg, L.A.; Davis, C. Test-retest reliability of the purdue pegboard test. *Am. J. Occup. Ther.* **2000**, *54*, 555–558. [CrossRef]
43. Bowden, J.L.; McNulty, P.A. The magnitude and rate of reduction in strength, dexterity and sensation in the human hand vary with ageing. *Exp. Gerontol.* **2013**, *48*, 756–765. [CrossRef] [PubMed]
44. Hamm, N.H.; Curtis, D. Normative data for the purdue pegboard on a sample of adult candidates for vocational-rehabilitation. *Percept. Mot. Ski.* **1980**, *50*, 309–310. [CrossRef]
45. Campbell, F.W.; Green, D.G. Monocular versus binocular visual acuity. *Nature* **1965**, *208*, 191. [CrossRef] [PubMed]
46. Rose, D. Monocular versus binocular contrast thresholds for movement and pattern. *Perception* **1978**, *7*, 195–200. [CrossRef]
47. Niechwiej-Szwedo, E.; Cao, M.; Barnett-Cowan, M. Binocular Viewing Facilitates Size Constancy for Grasping and Manual Estimation. *Vision* **2022**, *6*, 23. [CrossRef]
48. Zhu, X.J.; Li, Y.H.; Liu, L.Q. Functional significance of stereopsis in professional table-tennis players. *J. Sports Med. Phys. Fit.* **2019**, *59*, 1798–1804. [CrossRef]

49. Annett, M.; Hudson, P.T.W.; Turner, A. Reliability of differences between hands in motor skill. *Neuropsychologia* **1974**, *12*, 527–531. [CrossRef]
50. Triggs, W.J.; Calvanio, R.; Levine, M.; Heaton, R.K.; Heilman, K.M. Predicting hand preference with performance on motor tasks. *Cortex* **2000**, *36*, 679–689. [CrossRef]
51. Olive, T. Optometric Testing in the Laparoscopic Surgeon. *J. Am. Assoc. Gynecol. Laparosc.* **1996**, *3* (Suppl. S4), S36–S37. [CrossRef] [PubMed]
52. Burris, K.; Liu, S.C.; Appelbaum, L. Visual-motor expertise in athletes: Insights from semiparametric modelling of 2317 athletes tested on the Nike SPARQ Sensory Station. *J. Sports Sci.* **2020**, *38*, 320–329. [CrossRef] [PubMed]
53. Gao, Y.P.; Chen, L.P.; Yang, S.N.; Wang, H.Y.; Yao, J.X.; Dai, Q.; Chang, S. Contributions of Visuo-oculomotor Abilities to Interceptive Skills in Sports. *Optom. Vis. Sci.* **2015**, *92*, 679–689. [CrossRef] [PubMed]
54. Jia, Y.; Ye, Q.Q.; Zhang, S.L.; Feng, L.; Liu, J.; Xu, Z.X.; Zhuang, Y.; He, Y.; Zhou, Y.; Chen, X.; et al. Contrast Sensitivity and Stereoacuity in Successfully Treated Refractive Amblyopia. *Investig. Ophthalmol. Vis. Sci.* **2022**, *63*, 6. [CrossRef]
55. Yap, T.P.; Boon, M.Y. Electrodiagnosis and Treatment Monitoring of Children with Refractive Amblyopia. *Adv. Ophthalmol. Optom.* **2020**, *5*, 1–24. [CrossRef]
56. Yap, T.P.; Luu, C.D.; Suttle, C.; Chia, A.; Boon, M.Y. Effect of Stimulus Orientation on Visual Function in Children with Refractive Amblyopia. *Investig. Ophthalmol. Vis. Sci.* **2020**, *61*, 5. [CrossRef]
57. Wu, D.; Liu, N.; Xu, P.B.; Sun, K.W.; Xiao, W.; Li, C.X. Reduced Contrast Sensitivity Function in Central and Peripheral Vision by Disability Glare. *Perception* **2020**, *49*, 1348–1361. [CrossRef] [PubMed]
58. Rubin, G.S.; Bandeen-Roche, K.; Huang, G.H.; Muñoz, B.; Schein, O.D.; Fried, L.P.; West, S.K. The association of multiple visual impairments with self-reported visual disability: SEE project. *Investig. Ophthalmol. Vis. Sci.* **2001**, *42*, 64–72.
59. Grandjean, P.; White, R.F.; Sullivan, K.; Debes, F.; Murata, K.; Otto, D.A.; Weihe, P. Impact of contrast sensitivity performance on visually presented neurobehavioral tests in mercury-exposed children. *Neurotoxicol. Teratol.* **2001**, *23*, 141–146. [CrossRef]
60. Armstrong, R.A.; Eperjesi, F.; Gilmartin, B. The use of correlation and regression methods in optometry. *Clin. Exp. Optom.* **2005**, *88*, 81–88. [CrossRef]
61. McAlinden, C.; Khadka, J.; Pesudovs, K. Statistical methods for conducting agreement (comparison of clinical tests) and precision (repeatability or reproducibility) studies in optometry and ophthalmology. *Ophthalmic Physiol. Opt.* **2011**, *31*, 330–338. [CrossRef] [PubMed]
62. Baweja, H.S.; Kwon, M.; Onushko, T.; Wright, D.L.; Corcos, D.M.; Christou, E.A. Processing of visual information compromises the ability of older adults to control novel fine motor tasks. *Exp. Brain Res.* **2015**, *233*, 3475–3488. [CrossRef] [PubMed]
63. Voelcker-Rehage, C. Motor-skill learning in older adults—A review of studies on age-related differences. *Eur. Rev. Aging Phys. Act.* **2008**, *5*, 5–16. [CrossRef]
64. Anders, P.; Traber, G.L.; Hall, U.; Garobbio, S.A.; Chan, E.J.; Gabrani, C.; Camenzind, H.; Pfau, M.; Herzog, M.; Scholl, H.P. Evaluating contrast sensitivity in early and intermediate age-related macular degeneration with the quick contrast sensitivity function. *Investig. Ophthalmol. Vis. Sci.* **2023**, *64*, 7. [CrossRef] [PubMed]
65. Kim, B.; Neville, C. Accuracy and feasibility of a novel fine hand motor skill assessment using computer vision object tracking. *Sci. Rep.* **2023**, *13*, 14. [CrossRef]

life

MDPI

Article

Utility of Fundus Autofluorescence and Optical Coherence Tomography in Measuring Retinal Vascular Thickness, Macular Density, and Ophthalmic Manifestations in Women with Gestational Diabetes Mellitus

Rami Al-Dwairi [1,*], Omar Altal [2], Marwa Fares [1], Sharaf H. Adi [1], Shahed A. Said [2], Asmaa Shurair [1], Rania Al-Bataineh [3], Ihsan Aljarrah [4], Seren Al Beiruti [1], Ahmed H. Al Sharie [5] and Abdelwahab Aleshawi [1,*]

1 Department of Special Surgery, Division of Ophthalmology, Faculty of Medicine, Jordan University of Science & Technology, Irbid 22110, Jordan; marwa11kf@gmail.com (M.F.); dr.sharafadi@gmail.com (S.H.A.); asmaashurair@gmail.com (A.S.); seren.beiruti@yahoo.com (S.A.B.)
2 Department of Obstetrics and Gynecology, Faculty of Medicine, Jordan University of Science & Technology, Irbid 22110, Jordan; altal_omar@yahoo.com (O.A.); shahdazmii2018@gmail.com (S.A.S.)
3 Department of Family Medicine, Faculty of Medicine, Jordan University of Science & Technology, Irbid 22110, Jordan; raniabataineh123@gmail.com
4 Thin Films and Nanotechnology Lab, Department of Physics, Jordan University of Science & Technology, Irbid 22110, Jordan; ihsanaljarrah@gmail.com
5 Department of Pathology and Microbiology, Faculty of Medicine, Jordan University of Science & Technology, Irbid 22110, Jordan; ahmedalsharie3@gmail.com
* Correspondence: ramialdwairi@yahoo.com (R.A.-D.); abdelwahhabjamal@yahoo.com (A.A.)

Abstract: Background: Gestational diabetes mellitus (GDM) is a transient elevation of blood glucose during pregnancy. It is typically not associated with diabetic retinopathy. However, certain investigators revealed retinal microvascular injury. In this study, we aimed to assess the ophthalmic findings, optical coherence tomography (OCT) parameters, and retinal vascular thickness and macular density through fundus autofluorescence (FAF). **Methods**: Prospectively, women diagnosed with GDM were enrolled in this study. All the participants underwent comprehensive ophthalmic examination. Furthermore, macular OCT with analysis of the central subfield thickness (CST) and total thickness was carried out. Moreover, FAF was performed, and the macular density and retinal vascular thickness were extracted using ImageJ software. **Results**: Thirty-four women were enrolled. The mean maternal age was 32.7 years. No participant had diabetic retinopathy, nine eyes had early cataract, and two eyes had keratoconus. Higher levels for the 1 h oral glucose tolerance test (OGTT) were associated with a drop in the CST and total thickness. Moreover, women who underwent CS had higher levels of total thickness. Higher levels for the fasting OGTT were associated with a thinner inferior temporal retinal artery. Pregnant women with miscarriages had lower macular density on FAF, as represented by lower values of integrated density and mean gray values. Higher levels for the fasting OGTT were associated with higher values of integrated density. **Conclusions**: Although GDM is typically not associated with diabetic retinopathy, microscopic changes involving the microvascular environment and the macula may occur. Regular ophthalmic screening for women with GDM may be advised. Larger studies with more investigations may reveal further findings.

Keywords: gestational diabetes; diabetic retinopathy; OCT; OGTT

1. Introduction

Gestational diabetes mellitus (GDM) is one of the most common medical complications of pregnancy. It is characterized by the onset of hyperglycemia or impaired glucose tolerance during gestation, typically diagnosed between 24 and 28 weeks of pregnancy. Unlike other forms of diabetes, GDM usually resolves postpartum [1,2]. Numerous risk factors for GDM have been identified, including a history of GDM in a previous pregnancy, macrosomia, congenital anomalies, neonatal death, low educational status, smoking, a body mass index (BMI) $\geq$ 25, a family history of type 2 diabetes mellitus, and pregnancy-induced hypertension [1,3].

Although GDM typically resolves postpartum, it is associated with significant short- and long-term complications for both the mother and the fetus. The maternal complications include an increased likelihood of emergency cesarean delivery and preeclampsia, while the fetal complications may include macrosomia, neonatal hypoglycemia, birth asphyxia, shoulder dystocia, respiratory distress syndrome, and hyperbilirubinemia [4]. Additionally, GDM has been linked to an increased long-term risk of obesity, cardiovascular disease, and glucose intolerance, which may progress to type 2 diabetes in both the mother and her offspring [5]. Within 10 years postpartum, approximately 50% of women with a history of GDM develop type 2 diabetes [6].

Pregnancy induces a range of multi-organ changes, including alterations in the eyes. Some of these changes may exacerbate pre-existing conditions, while others may arise as a result of normal physiological processes or pregnancy-related complications [7]. Physiological changes during pregnancy, including metabolic, immunologic, vascular, and hormonal fluctuations, have been shown to exacerbate diabetic retinopathy, which, if left untreated, can lead to permanent vision loss [8]. GDM, as a common pregnancy complication, is associated with an increased incidence of pathological ophthalmic conditions. Specifically, the incidence of glaucoma, retinal detachment, and DR is significantly higher in GDM patients [6]. However, conflicting data exist in the literature regarding the necessity of including GDM patients in diabetic retinopathy screening [6,8], highlighting the need for further research to address policy changes concerning this matter.

This prospective observational study aims to investigate the ocular parameter changes in GDM patients. Specifically, we will discuss the effects of various gestational variables and optical parameters on optical coherence tomography (OCT), the retinal vascular thickness, and the macular density on fundus autofluorescence (FAF).

2. Methods

2.1. Participants and Data

This study was conducted at King Abdullah University Hospital, a tertiary clinical and research center affiliated with Jordan University of Science and Technology, during the period of June 2023 to February 2024. Prospectively and after obtaining the approval of the institutional review board, all pregnant women diagnosed GDM were invited to participate in this study, which aimed to investigate the ophthalmic findings in these women and to assess the OCT and FAF parameters in this group of patients. Electronic databases and interviews were utilized to collect data from the participants. Demographic data and the medical history were obtained. In addition, a detailed maternal and obstetric history was obtained from the participants. Furthermore, a comprehensive ophthalmic assessment and history were performed.

All pregnant women with GDM aged from 20 to 45 years were enrolled in this study. Females with singleton pregnancy between 20 and 33 weeks of gestation were included. The exclusion criteria included a chronic diabetes history prior to gestation, high blood pressure, a positive oral glucose tolerance test (OGTT) before 26–28 weeks of pregnancy, and albuminuria in pregnant women. Moreover, participants with renal or cardiorespiratory ailments and who were previously taking any hypoglycemic agents were excluded. Furthermore, a contraindication for metformin, a fetal anomaly on ultrasound examination, gestational hypertension, preeclampsia, fetal growth restriction (birth weight <10th centile for its gestational age on ultrasound comparing with a 1st dating or early 2nd trimester scan), and ruptured membranes were included in the exclusion list. Lastly, any women with ocular diseases that adversely affect the vision were excluded.

This study was carried out in compliance with the ethical guidelines in place at our institute, taking the Declaration of Helsinki as an ethical guideline for research involving human subjects. Written informed consent was obtained from all the participants.

2.2. Obstetrics Settings

The course and care of pregnancy was the responsibility of a single consultant in maternal–fetal obstetrical medicine. GDM was definition by the oral glucose tolerance test according to the World Health Organization criteria: using a 75 g OGTT after overnight fasting (8 to 10 h) at 26–28 weeks gestation. Diagnosis of GDM was made with at least two elevated readings for the OGTT, fasting glucose (>5.3 mmol/L), at one hour (10 mmol/L) and at two hours (8.6 mmol/L). These pregnant women were assessed for high risk factors, including a family history of diabetes, previous history of macrosomia, previous history of GDM, and previous history of poor obstetric outcome (miscarriage, intrauterine fetal death). Women who screened negative at the first antenatal visit had repeat screening at 28, 32 and 36 weeks of pregnancy.

The treatment commenced with similar guidelines. Metformin therapy was started at a dose of 500 mg once or twice daily with food and increased, typically over a period of 1 to 2 weeks, in intermittent doses dependent upon the glycemic control of the patient. If the targets were not achieved with metformin and dietary modification alone, subcutaneous insulin was commenced. Patients were asked to measure their blood sugar levels daily and note them in a diary, and after every week, their doses of metformin and insulin were adjusted according to the control of their blood sugar levels.

The mode of delivery depended on the antenatal course, the presence of antenatal complications, the experience of the obstetricians, and the choice of the pregnant women. The birth weight of the baby was calculated immediately after birth and was presented in grams.

2.3. Ophthalmological Examination Settings

All the patients underwent comprehensive ophthalmic examinations by a vitreoretinal consultant or well-trained residents during the follow-up visits with the obstetrics team, including the best-corrected visual acuity (BCVA) determined using a Snellen visual acuity chart by decimal unit. Then, the BCVA was converted to the LogMAR visual acuity. A Goldmann applanation tonometer was utilized to measure the intraocular pressure. Slit-lamp and indirect biomicroscopes were used to assess the lens status, anterior segment, and fundus conditions. The pupil was dilated with tropicamide eyedrops.

2.4. OCT Measurements

The acquisition of the OCT images was performed twice by two experienced optometrists to ensure the accuracy of the images. Then, the images were reviewed by a consultant vitreoretinal surgeon. Any image with low quality was repeated. Following the process of pupillary dilatation by tropicamide 1% eyedrops, each participant was seated in front of the OCT scanner and their head was stabilized on the chin rest. The macular area was analyzed using spectral domain (SD)-OCT (Retinascan RS-3000; NIDEK, Gamagori, Japan). Four radial scans, each measuring 6 mm in length, were positioned at the fovea in the macula at angles of 0°, 45°, 90°, and 135°. The scans comprised 1024 A-scans utilizing high-definition (50 HD) frame enhancement software. This equipment is equipped with a light source that emits electromagnetic radiation with a wavelength of 880 nm. The instrument had demonstrated excellent consistency and accuracy in measuring both healthy and diseased eyes. The Early Treatment Diabetic Retinopathy Study (ETDRS) was used to acquire nine consecutive macular sectors located in the foveal center [9]. Retinal thickness was determined by measuring the distance between two interfaces at each location along the x-axis of the scan. A low-intensity light source was utilized for internal fixation, and the procedure was performed in a dimly lit environment. Images exhibiting a signal strength below 7/10, inadequate centering, motion artifacts, and dark areas were removed, ensuring a minimum of 2 images of acceptable quality. The retinal thickness was defined as the distance between the vitreoretinal interface and the anterior surface of the retinal pigment epithelium along each A-scan. The central subfield thickness (CST) was the average thickness within a central 1 mm area from the inner limiting membrane to the retinal pigment epithelium layer. Other measurements performed in this study were the fovea minimum (representing the thinnest area at the fovea), total thickness (which is the summation of the thickness of the nine ETDRS areas), and total volume (which is the summation of the volume of the nine ETDRS areas). Figure 1 presents an example from one of the participant's OCT.

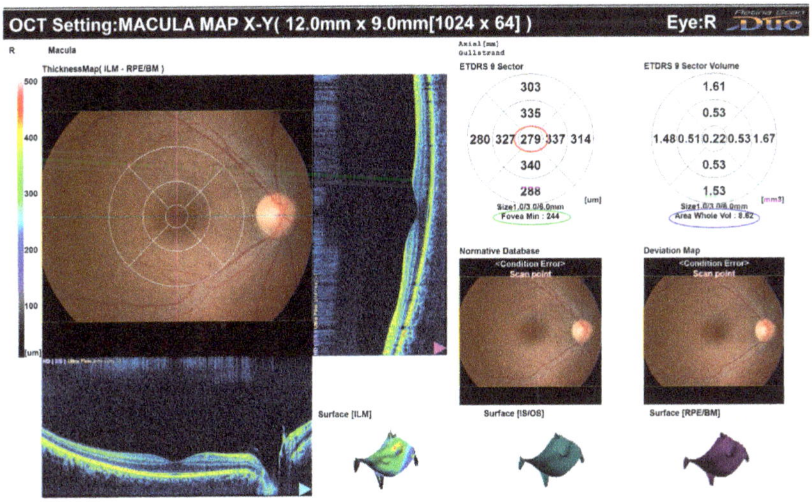

Figure 1. OCT of the macula of one of the participants, demonstrating the CST (in red circle), the foveal minimum (in green circle), and the volume of the whole area (in blue circle).

2.5. Fundus Autofluorescence (FAF) Acquisition

The acquisition and analysis of the FAF images were performed twice by the same two optometrists to ensure the accuracy and consistency, and to minimize the interobserver variability. Then, the images were reviewed by a consultant vitreoretinal surgeon. FAF imaging of the macula was obtained using a confocal scanning laser ophthalmoscope (Spectralis HRA, Heidelberg Engineering, Heidelberg, Germany). A 30 × 30° area centered at the fovea was scanned using excitation with a 488 nm argon laser and 500 nm filter. An image resolution of 1536 × 1536 pixels was used. The gain level was adjusted to delineate the major vessels and the disc on a single scan image, followed by averaging for sufficient quality. Macula-centered and optic-disc-centered images were acquired. The automatic real-time (ART) averaging mode was chosen, and 100 frames were captured to maximize the signal-to-noise ratio.

2.6. Retinal Vessel Diameter and Macular Density Measurements

The analysis of the FAF images was conducted by an experienced investigator through ImageJ software 1.53K (National Institutes of Health, Bethesda, MD, USA). First, the superior-temporal retinal artery and vein diameter, and the inferior-temporal retinal artery and vein diameter, were measured. The thickness was measured for both eyes at the point 2 mm away from the margin of the optic disc using the straight ruler tool of the software. Figure 2 shows the points where the measurements of the retinal vessel diameter were calculated.

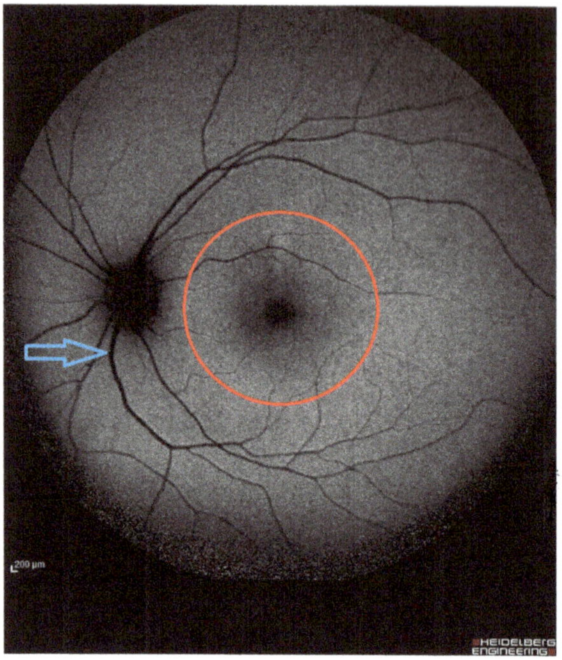

Figure 2. FAF of one of the participants showing the 5 mm macular area that was investigated for the density analysis. Also, it shows the place (in blue arrow) where the thickness of the major retinal vessels was measured (at 2 mm from the outer margin of the optic disc).

To quantitatively evaluate the FAF, the luminosity of the autofluorescence in a circle with a diameter of 5 mm at the center of the fovea was measured at each time point. Specifically, the average gray value of the autofluorescence in this area adjacent to the retinal vascular arcade was compared to that of the arcade vessels (veins). We quantified the mean signal intensity of 1000 pixels in the optic disc where the retinal pigmented epithelium and photoreceptors are absent as the zero point in individual images. This analysis allowed us to calculate the ratio of the autofluorescence intensity, providing a reliable indicator of the changes occurring in the treated areas. The following parameters were obtained: mean gray value, which is defined as the average gray value within the selection. This value is the summation of the gray values of all the pixels in the selection divided by the number of pixels. The minimum and maximum gray values are the minimum and maximum gray values within the selection, respectively. The integrated density is the summation of the values of the pixels in the image or selection and it is equivalent to the product of the area and mean gray value. The raw integrated density is the summation of the pixel values in the selected area. The following formulas summarize the measured parameters:

$$\text{The raw integrated density} = \text{sum of pixel values in the selected area}$$

$$\text{The mean gray value} = \text{raw integrated density}/(\text{area in pixels})$$

$$\text{The integrated density} = \text{raw integrated density} \times (\text{area in scaled units})/(\text{area in pixels})$$

2.7. Statistical Analyses

The collected data were entered into a spreadsheet and analyzed using the IBM SPSS statistical package for Windows v.29 (Armonk, NY, USA). Nominal variables were expressed as the frequency (percentage) and continuous variables as the mean ± standard error of the mean (SEM). Data normality was tested using the Kolmogorov–Smirnov test.

The statistical significance between the study groups was determined by the ANOVA test for continuous variables. A simple linear regression test was utilized to assess the relation between two continuous variables. A statistically significant result was considered if $p \leq 0.05$. The power of analysis equation was used to estimate the sample size with the assumption of the power of analysis at 90%, alpha level of 0.05, anticipated mean CST of 190 microns, and populational CST of 200 microns. The yielded required sample size was 51 eyes.

3. Results

3.1. General Demographic and Clinical Characteristics

A total of 34 pregnant women and 68 eyes were included in the analysis cohort. The mean maternal age was 32.7 ± 0.7 years, and the mean gestational age at delivery was 38.2 ± 0.2 weeks. The mean gestational age at the diagnosis of GDM was 30.3 ± 0.3 weeks, while the mean gestational age at the ophthalmic examination was 30.9 ± 0.7 weeks. The gestational parameters showed an average gravidity of 4.0 ± 0.2 and miscarriages of 0.88 ± 0.10. For GDM treatment, 5 participants (14.7%) were treated with diet only, 12 (35.3%) were treated with an oral hypoglycemic agent (OHGA)-based regimen, and 17 (50%) were treated with an insulin-based regimen. The mean values for the fasting, one-hour, and two-hour OGTT were 5.49 ± 0.10 mmol/L, 9.81 ± 0.30 mmol/L, and 8.38 ± 0.20 mmol/L, respectively. Regarding the mode of delivery, 28 participants (82.4%) delivered via cesarean section (CS), while 6 (17.6%) delivered through normal vaginal delivery (NVD). The cohort's birth weight was 2763.70 ± 0.10 g.

Ophthalmic examination of the cohort revealed cataracts in nine eyes (13.2%); these cataractous changes were very mild and did not interfere with the OCT or FAF acquisition. Corneal and anterior segment pathology was observed in two eyes (2.9%) (keratoconus), and no cases of posterior segment pathology (no diabetic retinopathy). The optical parameters included the uncorrected visual acuity (0.81 ± 0.03 LogMAR), best-corrected visual acuity (0.97 ± 0.01 LogMAR), intra-ocular pressure (IOP) (14.9 ± 0.2 mmHg), and spherical equivalent (−1.55 ± 0.20 diopter). The OCT parameters included the CST, foveal minimum, total thickness, and total volume, with means of 259.70 ± 5.50 microns, 200.70 ± 6.10 microns, 2692.60 ± 32.80 microns, and 8.30 ± 0.10 mm^3, respectively. Autofluorescence images were used to measure the retinal vascular thickness, with the following mean values: 0.1217 ± 0.003 mm for the superior-temporal retinal artery, 0.1507 ± 0.004 mm for the superior-temporal retinal vein, 0.1286 ± 0.003 mm for the inferior-temporal retinal artery, and 0.1535 ± 0.004 mm for the inferior-temporal retinal vein. Additionally, autofluorescence images were used to assess the macular density parameters, including the total area of investigation (28.06 ± 0.01 mm^2), mean gray value (135.54 ± 3.10 pixels), maximum gray value (231.89 ± 3.90 pixels), minimum gray value (37.82 ± 4.70 pixels), integrated density (3789.47 ± 86.40 pixels/mm), and raw integrated density (7702068.87 ± 1784.88 pixels/mm). Table 1 summarizes the general demographic and clinical characteristics of the study cohort.

Table 1. General demographical and clinical characteristics.

Variables	Number * Percentage (%)
	Mean ± SEM
Mother's age (years)	32.7 ± 0.7
Gestation age at delivery (weeks)	38.22 ± 0.2
Gestational age at diagnosis of GDM (weeks)	30.3 ± 0.3
Gestational age at ophthalmic examination (weeks)	30.9 ± 0.7
Gestational parameters	
Gravity	4.0 ± 0.2
Miscarriages	0.88 ± 0.1

Table 1. *Cont.*

Variables	Number *	Percentage (%)
	Mean ± SEM	
Mean values of OGTT (mmol/L):		
Fasting OGTT	5.49 ± 0.1	
One-hour OGTT	9.81 ± 0.3	
Two-hour OGTT	8.38 ± 0.2	
Method of GDM treatment (out of 34 participants)		
Diet only	5	14.7
OHGA-based regimen	12	35.3
Insulin-based regimen	17	50.0
Mode of delivery (out of 34 participants)		
CS	28	82.4
NVD	6	17.6
Fetal weight (grams)	2763.7 ± 0.1	
Ophthalmic examination findings (out of 68)		
Cataract	9	13.2
Corneal and anterior segment pathology	2	2.9
Posterior segment pathology	0	0.0
Optical parameters		
Uncorrected visual acuity (LogMAR)	0.81 ± 0.03	
Best-corrected visual acuity (LogMAR)	0.97 ± 0.01	
IOP (mmHg)	14.9 ± 0.2	
Spherical equivalent (Diopter)	−1.55 ± 0.2	
OCT parameters		
CST (micron)	259.7 ± 5.5	
Foveal minimum (micron)	200.7 ± 6.1	
Total thickness (micron)	2692.6 ± 32.8	
Total volume (mm^3)	8.3 ± 0.1	
Retinal vascular thickness through autofluorescence images (mm)		
Superior-temporal retinal artery	0.1217 ± 0.003	
Superior-temporal retinal vein	0.1507 ± 0.004	
Inferior-temporal retinal artery	0.1286 ± 0.003	
Inferior-temporal retinal vein	0.1535 ± 0.004	
Macular density parameters through autofluorescence images		
Total area of investigation (mm^2)	28.06 ± 0.01	
Mean gray value (pixel)	135.54 ± 3.1	
Maximum gray value (pixel)	231.89 ± 3.9	
Minimum gray value (pixel)	37.82 ± 4.7	
Integrated density (pixel/mm)	3789.47 ± 86.4	
Raw integrated density (pixel/mm)	7,702,068.87 ± 1784.88	

Abbreviations: GDM: gestational diabetes mellitus; OGTT: oral glucose tolerance test; OHGA: oral hypoglycemic agent; CS: cesarean section; NVD: normal vaginal delivery; OCT: optical coherence tomography; CST: central subfield thickness; SEM: standard error of mean. * N = 34.

3.2. Factors Affecting OCT Parameters

In examining the factors affecting the OCT parameters (i.e., CST and total thickness), none of the following showed a significant association: maternal age, gestational age at delivery, gestational age at ophthalmic examination, gestational parameters, method of GDM treatment, or fetal weight. Regarding the mean values for the OGTT, only the one-hour OGTT resulted in a significant decrease in the regression coefficient (B) in both the CST (−7.28 ± 3.10 microns, p = 0.024) and total thickness (−54.57 ± 17.20 microns, p = 0.030), whereas the fasting and two-hour OGTT had no significant effect. As for the mode of delivery, no significant effects were found on the CST; however, the mean total thickness in patients who underwent CS were significantly higher than those who had an

NVD (2763.47 ± 236.40 microns vs. 2395.10 ± 346.10 microns, p = 0.001). A statistically significant negative relationship was observed between the best-corrected visual acuity and CST (regression coefficient (B) = −277.27 ± 11.80 microns, p = 0.018), while no significant effect was observed on the total thickness. The IOP was not significantly associated with either the CST or total thickness. Lastly, a statistically significant negative association was found between the spherical equivalent and the total thickness (regression coefficient (B) = −97.05 ± 14.60 microns, p = 0.032), with no effect on the CST. Table 2 summarizes the factors affecting the OCT parameters.

Table 2. Factors affecting the OCT parameters.

	Mean ± SEM * or B Regression Coefficient ± SEM **			
Variables	**CST (Micron)**	***p*-Value**	**Total Thickness (Micron)**	***p*-Value**
Mother's age (years) **	−0.33 ± 0.9	0.73	−2.72 ± 5.4	0.62
Gestation age at delivery (weeks) **	−0.28 ± 2.1	0.89	−10.19 ± 7.0	0.43
Gestational age at ophthalmic examination (weeks) **	−2.32 ± 1.2	0.07	−4.47 ± 8.0	0.56
Gestational parameters **				
Gravity	−3.27 ± 2.3	0.17	−9.74 ± 14.1	0.49
Miscarriages	0.39 ± 5.4	0.94	0.40 ± 3.1	0.99
Method of GDM treatment *				
Diet only	249.75 ± 5.5		2681.36 ± 89.3	
OHGA-based regimen	280.35 ± 11.5	0.43	2757.00 ± 187.8	0.58
Insulin-based regimen	252.70 ± 19.1		2665.56 ± 196.7	
Mean values of OGTT (mmol/L) **				
Fasting OGTT	−12.02 ± 7.8	0.13	−75.96 ± 14.5	0.10
One-hour OGTT	−7.28 ± 3.1	0.024	−54.57 ± 17.2	0.03
Two-hour OGTT	−0.37 ± 3.9	0.93	10.927 ± 22.9	0.63
Mode of delivery *				
CS	263.57 ± 5.7	0.06	2763.47 ± 236.4	0.001
NVD	243.40 ± 4.6		2395.10 ± 346.1	
Fetal weight (grams) **	−7.10 ± 6.1	0.58	−97.45 ± 41.2	0.18
Optical parameters **				
Best-corrected visual acuity (LogMAR)	−277.27 ± 11.8	0.018	−228.65 ± 61.5	0.74
IOP (mmHg)	1.60 ± 3.2	0.62	−12.08 ± 11.4	0.30
Spherical equivalent (Diopter)	−12.99 ± 7.9	0.11	−97.048 ± 14.6	0.032

Abbreviations: GDM: gestational diabetes mellitus; OGTT: oral glucose tolerance test; OHGA: oral hypoglycemic agent; CS: cesarean section; NVD: normal vaginal delivery; CST: central subfield thickness; SEM: standard error of mean. * ANOVA test, ** linear regression analysis.

3.3. Factors Affecting Thickness of Retinal Vasculature

Our analysis of the association between several variables and the retinal vasculature thickness (i.e., superior-temporal retinal artery, superior-temporal retinal vein, inferior-temporal retinal artery, and inferior-temporal retinal vein) revealed several significant relationships. A statistically significant negative association was observed between the fasting OGTT and the inferior-temporal retinal artery thickness (regression coefficient (B) = −0.010 ± 0.004 mm, p = 0.010). The mode of delivery yielded a significantly thicker superior-temporal retinal vein in those who delivered via CS compared to those who had an NVD (0.155 ± 0.02 mm vs. 0.128 ± 0.03 mm, p = 0.018). Among the optical parameters, the best-corrected visual acuity was associated with a significant decrease in both the inferior-temporal retinal artery and vein thickness, with regression coefficients (B) of −0.160 ± 0.07 mm (p = 0.030) and −0.233 ± 0.09 mm (p = 0.020), respectively. In contrast, neither maternal age, gestational age at delivery, gestational age at ophthalmic examination, gestational parameters, methods of treating GDM, nor fetal weight yielded significance. Table 3 summarizes the factors affecting the thickness of the retinal vasculature.

Table 3. Factors affecting the thickness of the retinal vasculature.

Variables	Mean ± SEM * or B Regression Coefficient ± SEM **							
	Superior-Temporal Retinal Artery Thickness (mm)	***p*-Value**	**Superior-Temporal Retinal Vein Thickness (mm)**	***p*-Value**	**Inferior-Temporal Retinal Artery Thickness (mm)**	***p*-Value**	**Inferior-Temporal Retinal Vein Thickness (mm)**	***p*-Value**
Mother's age (years) **	0.001 ± 0.001	0.31	0.001 ± 0.001	0.30	0.0001 ± 0.001	0.72	0.0001 ± 0.001	0.64
Gestation age at delivery (weeks) **	0.002 ± 0.001	0.74	0.003 ± 0.002	0.11	0.0005 ± 0.001	0.74	0.002 ± 0.002	0.29
Gestational age at ophthalmic examination (weeks) **	0.0001 ± 0.002	0.83	0.003 ± 0.002	0.08	0.001 ± 0.001	0.26	0.001 ± 0.003	0.71
Gestational parameters **								
Gravity	0.001 ± 0.001	0.57	0.0001 ± 0.002	0.90	0.003 ± 0.001	0.72	0.001 ± 0.002	0.51
Miscarriages	−0.003 ± 0.003	0.42	−0.007 ± 0.004	0.09	−0.003 ± 0.004	0.42	−0.004 ± 0.005	0.43
Method of GDM treatment *								
Diet only	0.126 ± 0.02		0.143 ± 0.03		0.133 ± 0.01		0.160 ± 0.04	
OHGA-based regimen	0.115 ± 0.02	0.41	0.150 ± 0.02	0.65	0.130 ± 0.003	0.75	0.153 ± 0.001	0.77
Insulin-based regimen	0.123 ± 0.03		0.154 ± 0.03		0.126 ± 0.004		0.151 ± 0.005	
Mean values of OGTT (mmol/L) **								
Fasting OGTT	−0.004 ± 0.004	0.37	−0.005 ± 0.006	0.34	−0.01 ± 0.004	0.01	−0.009 ± 0.006	0.11
One-hour OGTT	0.001 ± 0.002	0.60	0.0001 ± 0.003	0.91	−0.002 ± 0.002	0.39	−0.002 ± 0.003	0.52
Two-hour OGTT	0.003 ± 0.002	0.12	0.0001 ± 0.003	0.89	0.0001 ± 0.002	0.85	0.001 ± 0.003	0.72
Mode of delivery *								
CS	0.126 ± 0.02	0.06	0.155 ± 0.02	0.018	0.129 ± 0.003	0.83	0.156 ± 0.005	0.15
NVD	0.107 ± 0.01		0.128 ± 0.03		0.127 ± 0.008		0.139 ± 0.007	
Fetal weight (grams) **	−0.004 ± 0.006	0.55	−0.006 ± 0.008	0.50	−0.004 ± 0.005	0.61	−0.008 ± 0.007	0.27
Optical parameters **								
Best-corrected visual acuity (LogMAR)	−0.11 ± 0.07	0.17	−0.007 ± 0.09	0.94	−0.16 ± 0.07	0.03	−0.233 ± 0.09	0.02
IOP (mmHg)	−0.003 ± 0.002	0.24	−0.005 ± 0.003	0.07	0.001 ± 0.002	0.75	0.003 ± 0.003	0.35
Spherical equivalent (Diopter)	−0.005 ± 0.003	0.17	−0.007 ± 0.003	0.06	0.001 ± 0.002	0.69	0.005 ± 0.003	0.98

Abbreviations: GDM: gestational diabetes mellitus; OGTT: oral glucose tolerance test; OHGA: oral hypoglycemic agent; CS: cesarean section; NVD: normal vaginal delivery; SEM: standard error of mean. * ANOVA test, ** linear regression analysis.

3.4. Factors Affecting Density Parameters of Autofluorescence Images

The examination of the relationship between several variables and the macular density parameters through autofluorescence images (i.e., mean gray value and integrated density) demonstrated several significant effects. Specifically, miscarriages, out of the gestational parameters, affected both density parameters, with regression coefficients (B) of −6.50 ± 3.10 pixels for the mean gray value (p = 0.042) and −173.75 ± 58.70 pixels/mm for the integrated density (p = 0.049). Moreover, the fasting OGTT was the only OGTT parameter to have a significant effect, with a significant increase in the integrated density (228.00 ± 89.40 pixels/mm, p = 0.040). Regarding the optical parameters, the spherical equivalent significantly affected both macular density parameters, with regression coefficients (B) of −10.95 ± 2.90 pixels for the mean gray value (p = 0.002) and −298.90 ± 81.30 pixels/mm for the integrated density (p = 0.001). The other variables (i.e., maternal age, gestational age at delivery, gestational age at ophthalmic examination, methods of GDM treatment, mode of delivery, and fetal weight) lacked significance in relation to the macular density parameters. Table 4 summarizes the factors affecting the density parameters of the autofluorescence images.

Table 4. Factors affecting the density parameters of the autofluorescence images.

Variables	Mean ± SEM * or B Regression Coefficient ± SEM **			
	Mean Gray Value (pixel)	p-Value	Integrated Density (pixel/mm)	p-Value
Mother's age (years) **	0.045 ± 0.05	0.40	13.04 ± 11.5	0.38
Gestation age at delivery (weeks) **	2.19 ± 1.2	0.07	57.22 ± 33.1	0.09
Gestational age at ophthalmic examination (weeks) **	−1.73 ± 1.5	0.29	−48.73 ± 43.4	0.28
Gestational parameters **				
Gravity	0.22 ± 1.3	0.87	13.26 ± 31.9	0.71
Miscarriages	−6.50 ± 3.1	0.042	−173.75 ± 58.7	0.049
Method of GDM treatment *				
Diet only	140.06 ± 6.0		3932.15 ± 169.1	
OHGA-based regimen	142.14 ± 4.9	0.28	3928.61 ± 125.1	0.37
Insulin-based regimen	131.12 ± 23.8		3681.34 ± 130.6	
Mean values of OGTT (mmol/L) **				
Fasting OGTT	7.29 ± 3.4	0.07	228.001 ± 89.4	0.04
One-hour OGTT	1.50 ± 2.1	0.49	50.25 ± 57.8	0.39
Two-hour OGTT	1.09 ± 2.1	0.61	28.58 ± 59.0	0.63
Mode of delivery *				
CS	136.63 ± 3.8	0.52	3815.45 ± 105.9	0.57
NVD	131.64 ± 4.1		3695.90 ± 116.1	
Fetal weight (grams) **	9.76 ± 6.1	0.16	264.16 ± 148.5	0.17
Optical parameters **				
Best corrected visual acuity (LogMAR)	35.89 ± 21.1	0.64	907.5 ± 1078.3	0.63
IOP (mmHg)	−0.71 ± 2.0	0.73	−30.3 ± 56.5	0.60
Spherical equivalent (Diopter)	−10.95 ± 2.9	0.002	−298.9 ± 81.3	0.001

Abbreviations: GDM: gestational diabetes mellitus; OGTT: oral glucose tolerance test; OHGA: oral hypoglycemic agent; CS: cesarean section; NVD: normal vaginal delivery; SEM: standard error of mean. * ANOVA test.** Linear regression analysis.

4. Discussion

To the best of our knowledge, this is the first study conducted to evaluate the clinical ophthalmic manifestations, macular OCT analyses, retinal vascular thickness, and FAF macular density analyses in pregnant women with GDM. It was revealed that no participant had clinical retinal changes. Furthermore, it was found that higher levels for the 1 h OGTT were associated with a drop in the CST and total thickness. Moreover, women who underwent CS had higher levels of total thickness. The superior-temporal retinal vein thickness was higher in women who underwent CS. In addition, higher levels of fasting OGTT were associated with a thinner inferior-temporal retinal artery. Interestingly, pregnant women with a previous history of miscarriage had lower macular density on FAF, as represented by lower values of integrated density and mean gray values. Furthermore, higher levels for the fasting OGTT were associated with higher values of integrated density.

Moreover, higher dioptric powers of the spherical equivalent were associated with lower values of both the integrated density and mean gray value.

Diabetic retinopathy plays a major role in public health. It is considered the major cause of blindness in diabetic patients. Microvascular complications, including retinopathy, are divided into the proliferative stage, which contains neovascularization, and non-proliferative stage, which is characterized by the presence of micro aneurysms, retinal hemorrhages, and intraretinal microvascular abnormalities together with soft and hard exudates [10,11]. Therefore, early screening and detection help in preventing blindness, with special consideration of pregnant women, as several studies were conducted on them. Regarding chronic (pre-existing diabetes recognized during pregnancy) diabetes mellitus in pregnancy, Temple et al. conducted a study reflecting the relation between the duration of diabetic retinopathy type 1 in addition to the baseline background retinopathy changes at the beginning of pregnancy and diabetic progression. The findings suggest that both increase the progression; however, moderate–severe retinopathy changes play a stronger role than the duration [12]. They found a significant progression by the end of the second trimester [12]. Moloney and Drunry compared the progression of retinopathy in pregnant and non-pregnant women and the results revealed increases in background retinopathy along with the appearance of new onset retinal lesions [13]. However, despite an exclusive finding, fundus autofluorescence imaging was not performed [13]. Pregnancy itself, with the hormonal changes during it, can affect the blood flow and vessel integrity in the retina. Furthermore, the elevated metabolic demands and the fluctuation in blood pressure may contribute to retinal pathology [10,11,14–16]. It was reported that the rate of progression of diabetic retinopathy was twice as high in pregnant women with diabetes compared non-pregnant women [10]. The Diabetes Control and Complications Trial (DCCT) revealed that the odds of diabetic retinopathy progression in pregnant women were 1.63 in the intensively treated group and 2.48 in the regularly treated group compared to non-pregnant women [17]. Many reports showed that diabetic retinopathy progressed in the first and second trimesters, peaked at the end of the second trimester, and regressed in the third trimester [12,17–19]. The rate of development of diabetic retinopathy in eyes without previous diabetic retinopathy during pregnancy has been reported to be 15% [10,19]. It was higher in type 1 diabetes (15.8%) compared to type 2 diabetes (9.0%). The progression rate from the non-proliferative diabetic retinopathy stage to the proliferative diabetic retinopathy stage was 6.3% and the rate of progression was similar for both type 1 and type 2 diabetes [10,19].

On the other hand, the impact of GDM on the retina is less well understood, primarily because GDM is usually transient and is typically diagnosed later in pregnancy. GDM potentiates the risk of short-term antepartum complications such as preeclampsia and long-term postpartum complications such as dyslipidemia, hypertension, obesity, and type 2 diabetes mellitus, with its subsequent generalized endothelial and small-vessel vasculopathy [20–24]. Type 2 diabetes mellitus is associated with retinal arteriolar narrowing, greater retinal vascular tortuosity, retinal venular widening, and retinal vascular capillary bed reduction [25,26]. Whether these endothelial cell dysfunctions and small-vessel vasculopathy are present in GDM has not been well investigated. Accordingly, Liu and Wang conducted a study evaluating the microvasculature in GDM women compared to non-GDM pregnant women and non-pregnant women utilizing OCT–angiography [27]. They revealed that there was a significant reduction in the vascular density in superficial capillary layer with an increase in the deep capillary layer in the GDM and in the non-GDM pregnant women. However, more capillary "dropout" changes were detected in the GDM group. Unexpectedly, the GDM group revealed the improvement in the central macular thickness thinning and foveal avascular zone enlargement during pregnancy [27]. Li et al. conducted an interesting study regarding the effect of GDM on the retinal microvasculature using retinal photographs with a subsequent computer analyzer [26]. They demonstrated that women with GDM had narrower arteriolar caliber, reduced arteriolar fractal dimension, and larger arteriolar branching angle than women without GDM [26]. Another study conducted by the same investigators aimed to assess the association between the second-trimester retinal microvasculature and the 5-year metabolic syndrome incidence in women with GDM using retinal photographs [28]. Each 10-micron widening of retinal venular caliber was associated with an increased relative risk of 1.6 in the incidence of metabolic syndrome. The retinal venular caliber mildly increased the prediction of 5-year maternal metabolic syndrome by 1.8% [28].

Retinal macular and vascular imaging used to assess the retinal status in women with GDM is now a non-invasive [25,29]. FAF is a non-invasive imaging technique that detects fluorophores, naturally occurring molecules that absorb and emit light of specified wavelengths [30]. There are two main technologies that allow FAF acquisition, the conventional fundus camera and the confocal scanning laser ophthalmoscope [30–32]. As the excitation and emission spectra of retinal fluorophores usually overlay in part, both technologies select certain wavelengths for excitation and emission that avoid the overlay and allow for clear differentiation of the two [32]. The conventional method utilizes barrier filters for excitation and emission to select the required wavelength, and subsequently, the entire fundus is excited at once. This results in a phenomenon called "pseudoautofluorescence", which is defined as scattered light originating from other sources mainly the crystalline lens [31]. Most available conventional devices use excitation wavelengths in the range of 510–580 nm and detection wavelengths in the range of 615–735 nm [31]. In contrast, the confocal scanning laser ophthalmoscope uses a monochromatic laser beam and a point detector that have the same focal plane. Accordingly, the scattered light is minimum [31]. A study by Yoshitake et al. investigated and quantified the signal intensity of FAF and evaluated its association with visual function and OCT findings. They revealed that eyes with diabetic macular edema had lower FAF signal intensity levels in the parafoveal subfields compared with eyes without diabetic macular edema. The FAF intensity in the parafoveal subfields was negatively associated with the visual acuity and the retinal thickness in the corresponding subfields [33]. Another study was conducted by Vujosevic et al. to quantitatively evaluate color FAF in patients with diabetes mellitus and to correlate these data with different stages of retinal disease severity using a 450 nm FAF device. Higher levels of intensity were found in patients affected by diabetes mellitus compared to healthy, non-diabetic subjects, and in patients with diabetic macular edema compared to patients without diabetic macular edema [34]. An interesting study was conducted by Kimura et al. to quantify FAF in laser photocoagulation scars for diabetic retinopathy and to compare the conventional and short-pulse laser. The average luminosity ratio of laser scars at 1, 3, 6, 12, and 18 months was higher for short-pulse laser compared to the conventional laser. These findings suggest that the short-pulse laser displayed delayed hypo-FAF progression [35]. Similar to these retinal imaging studies, we postulate that investigations performed concerning microvascular changes in GDM may provide valuable insights into such pregnancy complications. It is suggested that FAF imaging may be useful for detecting early retinal changes in patients without diabetic retinopathy. As a subclinical indicator for further retinal pathology, the lipofuscin granule in diabetic retinopathy might accumulate in the microglial cells rather than RPE cells, so the increase in FAF macular density might reveal deteriorated function of the neurosensory retina.

Regarding cataract in pregnancy, we have reported a high incidence of cataract (13.2%). GDM has the effect of cataract formation both during and after pregnancy. During pregnancy, high levels of glucose converted into sorbitol can accumulate in the lens and affect the integrity early on, even if the exposure is short [36]. Auger et al. demonstrated that GDM may be an independent risk factor for cataract, even among women who never develop type 2 diabetes, and most of these cases of cataract are mild [36].

Our study is not without limitations and has several limitations. Firstly, the small number of participants enrolled in our study may restrict the generalizability of our findings. Therefore, attention should be paid when extrapolating the results. Secondly, the lack of a control group may limit the comparability of the results with another group, with a subsequent deficit in the generalizability of the findings. Thirdly, many other investigations with interesting findings, such OCT–angiography, were not performed due to the unavailability of these resources at our institution. Lastly, certain confounder factors, such as the variability in the treatment adherence, were not investigated.

In conclusion, certain microvascular changes could reveal the liability of women with GDM for other long-term complications. Poorer control of the GDM, with higher levels at presentation, may be associated with more severe microvascular changes. Certain risk factors, such as a history of miscarriage or the mode of delivery, may warrant further evaluation. Larger studies with more investigations may reveal further findings. Regular ophthalmic screening for women with GDM is warranted at the diagnosis of GDM, antepartum, and after delivery. Women at risk should even be screened more frequently.

Author Contributions: Conceptualization, R.A.-D., O.A. and A.A.; Methodology, R.A.-D., O.A., S.H.A., S.A.S., R.A.-B., I.A. and A.A.; Software, I.A.; Validation, R.A.-D., S.A.S., S.A.B. and A.A.; Formal analysis, A.S., R.A.-B., A.H.A.S. and A.A.; Investigation, R.A.-D., O.A., S.A.S., A.S., I.A., S.A.B. and A.H.A.S.; Resources, R.A.-D., S.A.S., A.S. and I.A.; Data curation, R.A.-D., M.F., S.H.A. and A.A.; Writing—original draft, R.A.-D., M.F., S.H.A., R.A.-B., S.A.B. and A.A.; Writing—review & editing, O.A.; Visualization, R.A.-D., O.A. and A.A.; Supervision, R.A.-D., O.A., S.A.B. and A.A.; Project administration, R.A.-D. and O.A.; Funding acquisition, R.A.-D. and O.A. All authors have read and agreed to the published version of the manuscript.

Funding: The authors would like to acknowledge Jordan University of Science and Technology for supporting the research projects validated by the Deanship of Scientific Research (Funding ID: 20220296).

Institutional Review Board Statement: This study has been performed in accordance with the ethical standards laid down in the 1964 Declaration of Helsinki and its later amendment. We confirm that the privacy of the participants was protected, and the data were anonymized and maintained with confidentiality. Ethical approval was obtained from the Institutional Board Review of Jordan University of Science and Technology (approval ID: 14/147/2021, date of approval: 25.1.2022).

Informed Consent Statement: Written informed consent was obtained from all the patients.

Data Availability Statement: Data generated from this study are available upon request from the corresponding author.

Acknowledgments: We would like to thank Souzan Qutaina and Alaa Alking for their efforts in collecting the OCT and FAF images.

Conflicts of Interest: The authors declare no conflicts of interest.

References

1. McIntyre, H.D.; Catalano, P.; Zhang, C.; Desoye, G.; Mathiesen, E.R.; Damm, P. Gestational diabetes mellitus. *Nat. Rev. Dis. Primers* **2019**, *5*, 47. [CrossRef] [PubMed]
2. Francis, E.C.; Powe, C.E.; Lowe, W.L.; White, S.L.; Scholtens, D.M.; Yang, J.; Zhu, Y.; Zhang, C.; Hivert, M.-F.; Kwak, S.H.; et al. Refining the diagnosis of gestational diabetes mellitus: A systematic review and meta-analysis. *Commun. Med.* **2023**, *3*, 185. [CrossRef] [PubMed]
3. Lee, K.W.; Ching, S.M.; Ramachandran, V.; Yee, A.; Hoo, F.K.; Chia, Y.C.; Sulaiman, W.A.W.; Suppiah, S.; Mohamed, M.H.; Veettil, S.K. Prevalence and risk factors of gestational diabetes mellitus in Asia: A systematic review and meta-analysis. *BMC Pregnancy Childbirth* **2018**, *18*, 494. [CrossRef]
4. Vargas, S.E.V.; Chávez-González, E.L. Obstetric-Neonatal Complications of Gestational Diabetes: A Systematic Review. *Mex. J. Med. Res. ICSA* **2023**, *11*, 1–8. [CrossRef]
5. Alum, E.U.; Ugwu, O.P.; Obeagu, E.I. Beyond Pregnancy: Understanding the Long-Term Implications of Gestational Diabetes Mellitus. *INOSR Sci. Res.* **2024**, *11*, 63–71. [CrossRef]
6. Beharier, O.; Sergienko, R.; Kessous, R.; Szaingurten-Solodkin, I.; Walfisch, A.; Shusterman, E.; Tsumi, E.; Sheiner, E. Gestational diabetes mellitus is a significant risk factor for long-term ophthalmic morbidity. *Arch. Gynecol. Obstet.* **2017**, *295*, 1477–1482. [CrossRef]
7. Madike, R.; Cugati, S.; Qin, Q.; Chen, C.J. Pregnancy and the eye: What do we need to watch out for? A review. *Clin. Exp. Ophthalmol.* **2024**, *52*, 234–247. [CrossRef]
8. Chandrasekaran, P.R.; Madanagopalan, V.G.; Narayanan, R. Diabetic retinopathy in pregnancy—A review. *Indian J. Ophthalmol.* **2021**, *69*, 3015–3025. [CrossRef] [PubMed] [PubMed Central]

9. Angeli, O.; Hajdu, D.; Jeney, A.; Czifra, B.; Nagy, B.V.; Balazs, T.; Nemoda, D.J.; Somfai, G.M.; Nagy, Z.Z.; Peto, T.; et al. Qualitative and quantitative comparison of two semi-manual retinal vascular density analyzing methods on optical coherence tomography angiography images of healthy individuals. *Sci. Rep.* **2023**, *13*, 16981. [CrossRef]
10. Widyaputri, F.; Rogers, S.L.; Kandasamy, R.; Shub, A.; Symons, R.C.A.; Lim, L.L. Global Estimates of Diabetic Retinopathy Prevalence and Progression in Pregnant Women with Preexisting Diabetes: A Systematic Review and Meta-analysis. *JAMA Ophthalmol.* **2022**, *140*, 486–494, Finance Scholarship from the Indonesian Endowment Fund for Education during the conduct of the study. Dr Lim reported receiving grants from Alfred Fenton Trust and Bayer and personal fees from Novartis, Novotech, and Allergan outside the submitted work. No other disclosures were reported. [CrossRef] [PubMed] [PubMed Central]
11. Rosenn, B.; Miodovnik, M.; Kranias, G.; Khoury, J.; Combs, C.A.; Mimouni, F.; Siddiqi, T.A.; Lipman, M.J. Progression of diabetic retinopathy in pregnancy: Association with hypertension in pregnancy. *Am. J. Obstet. Gynecol.* **1992**, *166*, 1214–1218. [CrossRef] [PubMed]
12. Temple, R.C.; Aldridge, V.A.; Sampson, M.J.; Greenwood, R.H.; Heyburn, P.J.; Glenn, A. Impact of pregnancy on the progression of diabetic retinopathy in Type 1 diabetes. *Diabet. Med. A J. Br. Diabet. Assoc.* **2001**, *18*, 573–577. [CrossRef] [PubMed]
13. Moloney, J.B.; Drury, M.I. The effect of pregnancy on the natural course of diabetic retinopathy. *Am. J. Ophthalmol.* **1982**, *93*, 745–756. [CrossRef] [PubMed]
14. Best, R.M.; Chakravarthy, U. Diabetic retinopathy in pregnancy. *Br. J. Ophthalmol.* **1997**, *81*, 249–251. [CrossRef] [PubMed] [PubMed Central]
15. Gupte, S.; Venkataraman, G.; Shah, A.S.; Jamenis, S.; Rao, C.; Jangam, S.M.; Adki, K.M.; Swami, O.C. Prevalence and outcomes of gestational diabetes mellitus in Indian women: Insights from a large real-world study over ten years at tertiary care research institute. *Int. J. Diabetes Dev. Ctries.* **2023**, *43*, 511–516. [CrossRef]
16. Schreiberová, Z.; Chrapek, O.; Šimičák, J. Ocular Complications of Diabetes Mellitus in Pregnancy—Case Report. *Ceska A Slov. Oftalmol. Cas. Ceske Oftalmol. Spol. A Slov. Oftalmol. Spol.* **2020**, *76*, 166–170. [CrossRef] [PubMed]
17. Diabetes Control and Complications Trial Research Group. Effect of pregnancy on microvascular complications in the diabetes control and complications trial. The Diabetes Control and Complications Trial Research Group. *Diabetes Care* **2000**, *23*, 1084–1091. [CrossRef] [PubMed] [PubMed Central]
18. Venkatesh, P.; Makwana, T.; Takkar, B.; Sharma, J.B.; Gupta, Y.; Chawla, R.; Vohra, R.; Kriplani, A.; Tandon, N.; Venkatesh, P.; et al. Prevalence, progression, and outcomes of diabetic retinopathy during pregnancy in Indian scenario. *Indian J. Ophthalmol.* **2018**, *66*, 541–546. [CrossRef] [PubMed] [PubMed Central]
19. Morrison, J.L.; Hodgson, L.A.; Lim, L.L.; Al-Qureshi, S. Diabetic retinopathy in pregnancy: A review. *Clin. Exp. Ophthalmol.* **2016**, *44*, 321–334. [CrossRef] [PubMed]
20. Durnwald, C. Gestational diabetes: Linking epidemiology, excessive gestational weight gain, adverse pregnancy outcomes, and future metabolic syndrome. *Semin. Perinatol.* **2015**, *39*, 254–258. [CrossRef]
21. Feig, D.S.; Zinman, B.; Wang, X.; Hux, J.E. Risk of development of diabetes mellitus after diagnosis of gestational diabetes. *CMAJ* **2008**, *179*, 229–234. [CrossRef] [PubMed]
22. Taylor, R. Type 2 diabetes: Etiology and reversibility. *Diabetes Care* **2013**, *36*, 1047–1055. [CrossRef] [PubMed]
23. Aldhahi, W.; Hamdy, O. Adipokines, inflammation, and the endothelium in diabetes. *Curr. Diab Rep.* **2003**, *3*, 293–298. [CrossRef] [PubMed]
24. Bonetti, P.O.; Lerman, L.O.; Lerman, A. Endothelial dysfunction: A marker of atherosclerotic risk. *Arterioscler. Thromb. Vasc. Biol.* **2003**, *23*, 168–175. [CrossRef] [PubMed]
25. Ikram, M.K.; Cheung, C.Y.; Lorenzi, M.; Klein, R.; Jones, T.L.; Wong, T.Y. Retinal vascular caliber as a biomarker for diabetes microvascular complications. *Diabetes Care* **2013**, *36*, 750–759. [CrossRef]
26. Li, L.-J.; Kramer, M.; Tapp, R.J.; Man, R.E.K.; Lek, N.; Cai, S.; Yap, F.; Gluckman, P.; Tan, K.H.; Chong, Y.S.; et al. Gestational diabetes mellitus and retinal microvasculature. *BMC Ophthalmol.* **2017**, *17*, 4. [CrossRef] [PubMed] [PubMed Central]
27. Liu, G.; Wang, F. Macular vascular changes in pregnant women with gestational diabetes mellitus by optical coherence tomography angiography. *BMC Ophthalmol.* **2021**, *21*, 170. [CrossRef]
28. Li, L.-J.; Tan, K.H.; Aris, I.M.; Man, R.E.K.; Gan, A.T.L.; Chong, Y.S.; Saw, S.M.; Gluckman, P.; Wong, T.Y.; Lamoureux, E. Retinal vasculature and 5-year metabolic syndrome among women with gestational diabetes mellitus. *Metabolism* **2018**, *83*, 216–224. [CrossRef]
29. Benitez-Aguirre, P.Z.; Sasongko, M.B.; Craig, M.E.; Jenkins, A.J.; Cusumano, J.; Cheung, N.; Wong, T.Y.; Donaghue, K.C. Retinal vascular geometry predicts incident renal dysfunction in young people with type 1 diabetes. *Diabetes Care* **2012**, *35*, 599–604. [CrossRef]
30. Yung, M.; Klufas, M.A.; Sarraf, D. Clinical applications of fundus autofluorescence in retinal disease. *Int. J. Retin. Vitr.* **2016**, *2*, 12. [CrossRef]
31. Dumitrescu, O.-M.; Zemba, M.; Brănișteanu, D.C.; Pîrvulescu, R.A.; Radu, M.; Stanca, H.T. Fundus Autofluorescence in Diabetic Retinopathy. *J. Pers. Med.* **2024**, *14*, 793. [CrossRef] [PubMed]
32. Calvo-Maroto, A.M.; Esteve-Taboada, J.J.; Domínguez-Vicent, A.; Pérez-Cambrodí, R.J.; Cerviño, A. Confocal scanning laser ophthalmoscopy versus modified conventional fundus camera for fundus autofluorescence. *Expert Rev. Med. Devices* **2016**, *13*, 965–978. [CrossRef] [PubMed]

33. Yoshitake, S.; Murakami, T.; Uji, A.; Unoki, N.; Dodo, Y.; Horii, T.; Yoshimura, N. Clinical relevance of quantified fundus autofluorescence in diabetic macular oedema. *Eye* **2015**, *29*, 662–669. [CrossRef] [PubMed] [PubMed Central]
34. Vaclavik, V.; Vujosevic, S.; Dandekar, S.S.; Bunce, C.; Peto, T.; Bird, A.C. Autofluorescence imaging in age-related macular degeneration complicated by choroidal neovascularization: A prospective study. *Ophthalmology* **2008**, *115*, 342–346. [CrossRef] [PubMed]
35. Kimura, T.; Ogura, S.; Yasukawa, T.; Nozaki, M. Quantitative Evaluation of Fundus Autofluorescence in Laser Photocoagulation Scars for Diabetic Retinopathy: Conventional vs. Short-Pulse Laser. *Life* **2023**, *13*, 1901. [CrossRef]
36. Auger, N.; Tang, T.; Healy-Profitós, J.; Paradis, G. Gestational diabetes and the long-term risk of cataract surgery: A longitudinal cohort study. *J. Diabetes Complicat.* **2017**, *31*, 1565–1570. [CrossRef]

life

Case Report

Bilateral Fuchs' Superficial Marginal Keratitis Diagnosis and Treatment

Shiori Harada, Yasser Helmy Mohamed *, Mao Kusano, Daisuke Inoue and Masafumi Uematsu

Department of Ophthalmology and Visual Sciences, Graduate School of Biomedical Sciences, Nagasaki University, Nagasaki 852-8501, Japan; haradashiori1211@yahoo.co.jp (S.H.); maok@nagasaki-u.ac.jp (M.K.); d.i.private.3@gmail.com (D.I.); uematsu1124@outlook.jp (M.U.)
* Correspondence: yasserhelmy@nagasaki-u.ac.jp; Tel.: +81-95-819-7345; Fax: +81-95-819-7347

Abstract: In this study, we reported two patients with clinical pictures compatible with the diagnosis of bilateral Fuchs' superficial marginal keratitis (FSMK) treated with surgical treatment and anti-inflammatory drugs. The cases suffered from bilateral photophopia, blurred vision, and pseudopterygium with normal intraocular pressure (IOP). Pseudopterygia extended from temporal and nasal sides and had a gray line between the corneal normal epithelium with no lipid deposits. The first case had a bilateral high mixed astigmatic error and the second had dry eye symptoms. No abnormalities, including systemic inflammatory disease, were found in the laboratory investigations. The first case had bilateral pseudopterygium excision, mitomycin C (MMC) application, and pedicled conjunctival flap transplantation. The patient was followed regularly, and her condition was stable without any recurrence or deterioration in the ocular findings. The second case had conjunctival resection + amniotic membrane transplantation + MMC application six times on the right eye and three times on the left eye during 4 years and suffered recurrences after each operation. Her visual acuity severely decreased with the elevated IOP of both eyes. The patient refused to do any further surgical intervention. Despite its rarity, FSMK should be considered when peripheral corneal infiltration, corneal thinning, and pseudopterygia are observed in both eyes.

Keywords: Fuchs' superficial marginal keratitis; pseudopteryguim; irregular astigmatism; corneal thinning

1. Introduction

Fuchs' superficial marginal keratitis (FSMK) is a rare disorder that was first documented by Von Arlt in 1881 and then described in further detail by Fuchs in 1895 [1].

FSMK is a rare condition marked by episodic ocular inflammation, marginal corneal infiltrates, and the progressive thinning of the corneal stroma. A pseudopterygium may develop over the corneal thinning. In advanced cases, extreme stromal loss may lead to traumatic or even spontaneous perforation [2]. This disease of unknown etiology usually starts as a superficial marginal keratitis that spreads over the cornea in an irregular, nonuniform manner [3,4].

Because the disease is rare, only a few reports in the literature have described it. We report two patients with clinical pictures compatible with a diagnosis of bilateral Fuchs' superficial marginal keratitis treated with surgical treatment and anti-inflammatory drugs. This study was approved by the Institutional Review Board of Nagasaki University Hospital (approval number 24021928) and the patients involved in the study provided informed consent.

2. Case Report

2.1. Case 1

A 47-year-old Japanese woman with no underlying disease was referred to Nagasaki University Hospital in April 2022 by ophthalmology clinic suffering binocular blurred vision and photophobia for the past 6 years. Her best corrected visual acuity (BCVA) at the first visit was 0.2 (decimal correction) in right eye (refraction was +11.0 D sphere, −5.0 D axis 170 cylinder) and 0.4 in the left eye (refraction was +10.0 D sphere, −5.0 D axis 170 cylinder) with normal intraocular pressure (IOP) in both eyes. Both eyes had circumferential corneal infiltrations and pseudopterygia extending from the temporal and nasal sides and had a gray line between the corneal normal epithelium with no lipid deposits (Figure 1A,E). Anterior segment optical coherence tomography (AS-OCT) revealed bilateral pseudopterygium and mild corneal thinning in the same area (Figure 1B,F). Corneal elevation topography revealed binocular irregular astigmatism (Figure 1C,G). No abnormalities, including systemic inflammatory disease, were found in the laboratory investigations. A diagnosis of FSMK was made.

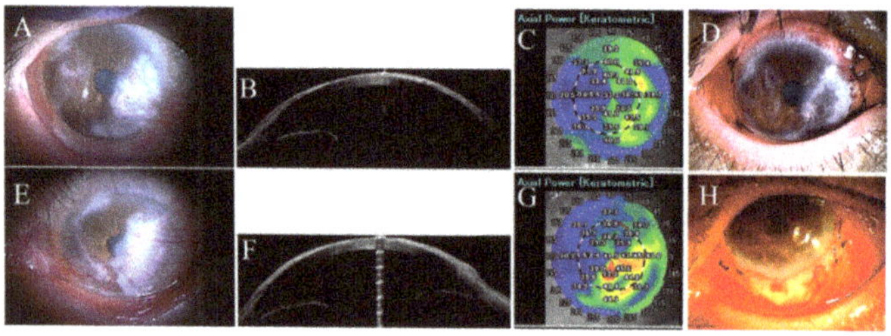

Figure 1. Slit lamp pictures of right (**A**) and left (**E**) eyes of the first case (first visit) showing circumferential corneal infiltrations and pseudopterygia extending from the temporal and nasal sides. Anterior segment optical coherence tomography revealed pseudopterygium and mild corneal thinning in both temporal and nasal sides of right (**B**) and left (**F**) eyes. Corneal elevation topography revealed binocular irregular astigmatism in the right and left eyes ((**C**,**G**) respectively). Slit lamp pictures of right (**D**) and left (**H**) eyes on the first postoperative day.

In June 2022, bilateral pseudopterygium excision, mitomycin C (MMC) application, and pedicled conjunctival flap transplantation were performed (Figure 1D,H). Postoperative treatment includes topical antibiotics and topical steroids for one month (four times/day). Topical antibiotics were discontinued one month after surgery, but weak topical corticosteroids continued to control congestion of the conjunctiva. The oral administration of cyclosporine was started one month after surgery to suppress postoperative inflammation and prevent recurrence to date (Dose = 175 mg/day which control the trough value between 70 and 100 ng/mL).

The patient was followed every 2–3 months, and her condition was stable without any recurrence or deterioration in the ocular findings until her last visit in December 2023. The last follow up picture of her eyes shown in (Figure 2) and her last BCVA was 1.2 in right eye (refraction was +4.0 D sphere, −2.0 D axis 150) and 1.2 in left eye.

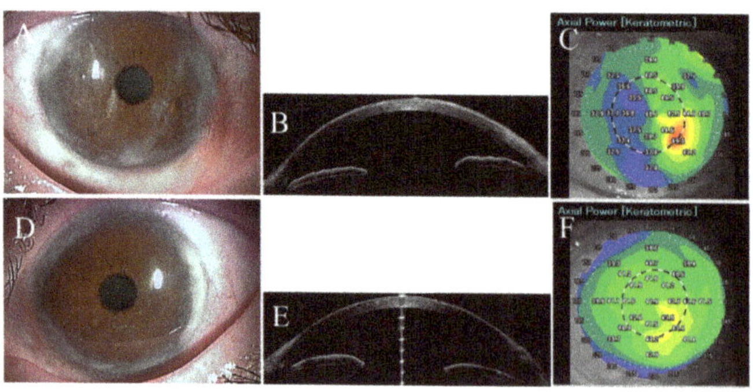

Figure 2. Slit lamp pictures of right (**A**) and left (**D**) eyes of the first case showing the postoperative removal of corneal pseudopterygia from the temporal and nasal sides. Anterior segment optical coherence tomography confirmed the postoperative removal of pseudopterygium of right (**B**) and left (**E**) eyes. Postoperative corneal elevation topography revealed binocular improvement in right and left eyes ((**C**,**F**) respectively).

2.2. Case 2

A 28-year-old female suffered from dryness and photophobia in her both eyes for a few years and was diagnosed with dry eye and pseudopterygium by local ophthalmologist. She was treated with eye drops containing lubricants and topical steroids. When she was 29 years old (November 2011), she was referred to Nagasaki University Hospital for better evaluation and treatment. Her BCVA was 0.6 in right eye (refraction −1.25 D sphere) and 0.9 in left eye with normal IOP in both eyes. There was hyperemia in the bulbar conjunctiva of both palpebral fissures, and the conjunctival epithelium had invaded the cornea circumferentially (Figure 3A,E). She had no conjunctival adhesions. Punctate superficial keratopathy was observed in the lower halves of both corneas, and conjunctival invasion was observed on her nasal and temporal corneas (Figure 3B,F). There were no major abnormalities in corneal elevation topography (Figure 3C,G).

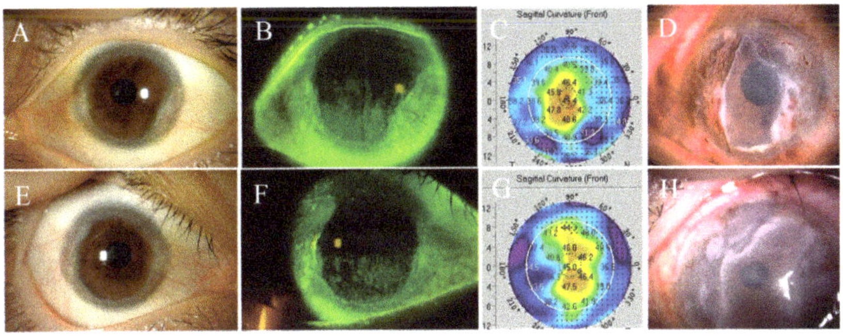

Figure 3. Slit lamp pictures of right (**A**) and left (**E**) eyes of the second case (first visit) showing circumferential corneal infiltrations and pseudopterygia extending from the temporal and nasal sides. Punctate superficial keratopathy was observed in the lower halves of right and left corneas ((**B**,**F**) respectively), and conjunctival invasion was observed on her nasal and temporal corneas. There were no major abnormalities in the corneal elevation topography of the right (**C**) and left (**G**) eyes. Slit lamp pictures of right (**D**) and left (**H**) eyes on the first postoperative day after first operation.

The anterior chambers had normal depth in both eyes with no signs of inflammation, clear lens, and normal fundus of both eyes. Her underlying illnesses included obsessive-compulsive disorder [patient under selective serotonin reuptake inhibitors (SSRIs)], Sjögren's syndrome, and allergic rhinitis. She did not have rheumatoid arthritis.

She was treated with eye drops (lubricants, topical steroids, and tranilast) 4–6 times a day for both eyes with punctal plugs, but the conjunctival invasion gradually worsened. Between 2011 and 2015, the patient was followed every two months. She underwent the first conjunctival resection + MMC + amniotic membrane transplantation in her right and left eyes in June and July 2015, respectively (Figure 3D,H). She started oral prednisolone and cyclosporine postoperatively. Oral prednisolone 20 mg/day was started on the third day after right eye surgery and was tapered after 4 months. Oral prednisolone were used in the same regimen during the second and third perioperative periods. Also, oral cyclosporine 150 mg/day was started two weeks after the first right eye surgery. Cyclosporine is being controlled with a trough value of 70–100 ng/mL). The recurrence of the conjunctival invasion occurred after two months of surgery. The patient underwent conjunctival resection + amniotic membrane transplantation + MMC application (+keratoepithelioplasty on the fourth surgery on right eye) 6 times in the right eye and 3 times in the left eye between the ages of 33 and 37 years (2015–2019) and suffered recurrences after each operation. Both eyes showed progressive conjunctival invasion with repeated peripheral corneal ulcers (Figure 4).

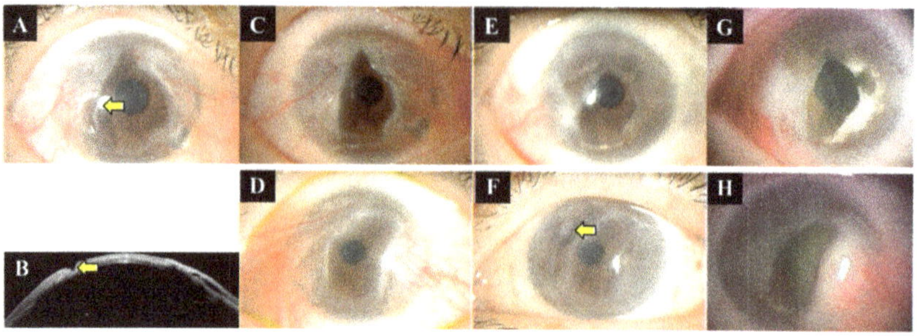

Figure 4. Slit lamp picture (**A**) and ocular coherent tomography (**B**) of the right eye of the second case at age of 32 years showing corneal ulceration and thinning (yellow arrow). Slit lamp pictures of the right (**C**) (after healing of ulceration) and left (**D**) eyes of the second case at the age of 32 years revealing progressive encroachment of psudopterygium on the corneal surface. Slit lamp pictures of right (**E**) and left (**F**) at the age of 34 years. Left corneal ulcer and thinning (yellow arrow) was shown. Slit lamp pictures of right (**G**) and left (**H**) at the age of 37 years.

In February 2019, her visual acuity had decreased to 0.3 in her right eye and 0.07 in her left eye. In addition, elevated IOP was observed both eyes (right = 21 mmHg and left = 26 mmHg), and glaucoma eye drops were prescribed. On her last visit in November 2023 (41 years), her visual acuity further deteriorated to 0.01 in both eyes and intraocular pressure in the right eye was 15 mmHg and 24 mmHg in the left eye with medication. At the last visit, she was using the following eye drops: tacrolimus 2 times a day, tranilast 4 times a day, lubricants 2 times a day, and glaucoma eye drops. Figure 5 shows the patient's corneas on her last visit (November 2023). The patient refused to do any further surgical intervention, and she continued to have the same oral and eye drop treatments.

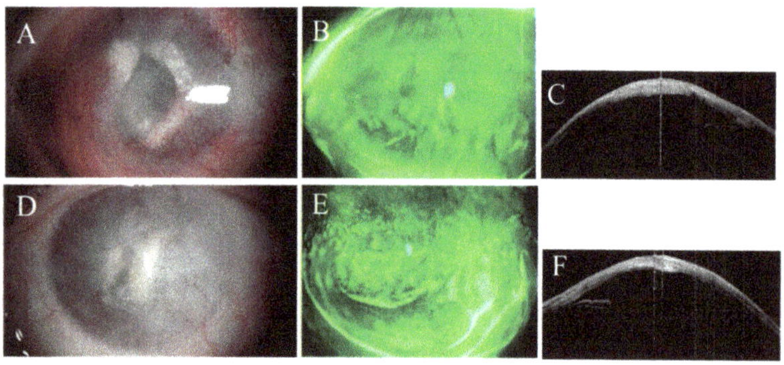

Figure 5. Slit lamp pictures of right (**A**) and left (**D**) eyes of the second patient in November 2023 (41 years) showing extensive encroachment of psudopterygium on the corneal surface. Slit lamp pictures of right (**B**) and left (**E**) eyes of the second patient upon her last visit showing extensive punctate superficial keratopathy. Ocular coherent tomography of right (**C**) and left (**F**) eyes of the second patient at her last visit showing extensive encroachment of psudopterygium on the corneal surface.

3. Discussion

FSMK is a rare entity characterized by episodic ocular inflammation with marginal corneal infiltrates and progressive marginal thinning of the corneal stroma [2]. It most commonly affects young adults between the second and 4th decades of life. It often has a chronic course with recurrent bouts of red eye, pain, and tearing, associated with a marginal stromal thinning, which is typically irregular in its depth and axial extension, delimited by a fine intraepithelial gray line on its advancing edge and without any accompanying lipid deposits [3,5]. The marginal thinning does not have a preferred limbal location and is frequently associated with a pseudopterygium [4,5]. Visual acuity can be compromised in advanced cases secondary to irregular astigmatism [6].

Given the striking similarity in clinical manifestations between our patients and the previously described FSMK cases, FSMK emerged as the most probable diagnosis.

The differential diagnosis of FSMK includes autoimmune peripheral ulcerative keratitis, Mooren's ulcer, Terrien's marginal degeneration (TMD), and limbal stem cell deficiency (LSCD). Autoimmune peripheral ulcerative keratitis was ruled out because various blood tests were negative for collagen disease and systemic inflammation. Mooren's ulcer manifested with painful progressive corneal peripheral ulceration (epithelial defect stained with fluorescein) associated with intense limbal inflammation and swelling, were not identical with our cases.

TMD and FSMK are rare, slowly progressive corneal diseases that affect both eyes and have an unknown cause. They share several clinical signs. TMD is marked by the peripheral thinning of the cornea, typically starting in the upper half but sometimes beginning in the lower half [7]. For FSMK, an early biomicroscopic examination usually reveals peripheral corneal thinning in the lower and lower nasal segments. As a rule, in both diseases, the lesions on the two eyes are asymmetric, but peripheral corneal thinning is the main pathological sign [7]. FSMK is a rare disorder that shares several characteristics with TMD, to the extent that they can be considered a different manifestation of the same degenerative marginal corneal disease whose etiology is unknown [7].

FSMK and TMD are two conditions that primarily affect young and middle aged adults. They both involve paralimbal stromal thinning, typically occurring bilaterally but asymmetrically. While pseudo-pterygium can occur in either disease, it is more classically associated with FSMK. Additionally, both conditions can lead to spontaneous or traumatic corneal perforation [5,8]. Because of these similarities, some authors had suggested that both disorders are manifestations of the same disease [5,7]. FSMK differentiates from TMD in that it affects the limbus at any localization (no preference for superior cornea), presents with accompanying epithelial detects, has an epithelial delimitation gray line, and does not have lipid deposition [3,5].

LSCD can be distinguished from FSMK by its underlying cause, such as mechanical or chemical trauma or other known factors contributing to LSCD [8]. However, because FSMK gradually damages corneal limbal stem cells and causes conjunctivization as it progresses, the possibility that this rare disease is responsible for some LSCDs of unknown cause cannot be ruled out. Determining whether FSMK is a contributing factor to LSCDs will have to wait until more cases accumulate.

Progressive stromal thinning is a risk factor for traumatic and spontaneous perforation [3,9]. It may be difficult to determine the degree of thinning secondary to accompanying pseudopterygium. Care must be taken during surgical intervention because perforation may accidentally occur [9]. The recurrence of the disease has been noted to occur even after lamellar keratoplasty, although this may be peripheral to the border of the graft [2,10].

AS-OCT may be an invaluable preoperative tool as it will allow for the differentiation of the pseudopterygia tissue from the underlying thinned corneal tissue. Although topography may measure the cumulative thickness encompassing both pseudopterygia and corneal tissue, AS-OCT will allow differentiation based on cross-sectional appearance. Cheung et al., observed, that in their FSMK case, the nasal part of the cornea was the thinnest, measuring 34% of the central corneal thickness. However, they suggested that the superonasal quadrant might actually be the thinnest area and the site of the perforation. Interestingly, the AS-OCT images demonstrated thinning to be greatest in the mid-periphery [10]. AS-OCT made it possible to assess the thickness of the cornea more accurately in the affected area, which is important for choosing treatment tactics [7].

The marginal superficial limbal corneal degeneration and ulcers are characteristically demarcated from the central cornea by a curvilinear gray band [3]. The central cornea is generally clear until the late stages of the disease, when visual acuity deteriorates.

This is a chronic disease with periods of remission and relapse accompanied by processive circumferential peripheral corneal thinning that may lead to perforation [9]. Pseudopterygia tend to grow over areas of corneal thinning [4].

Ellis studied two cases of bilateral FSMK and described the histopathology of the disease. One of the eyes showed epithelioid giant cells in the substantia propria of the cornea. Acute inflammatory cells were present most concentrated beneath the ulcerated areas [11]. The degeneration of conjunctival and corneal limbal areas were encountered similar to that of pterygia [11].

The pseudopterygium gradually extends onto the cornea over several years, avoiding the central cornea. Bierly et al. described significant thinning beneath the pseudopterygium in two out of three cases. This resulted in corneal perforation during pseudopterygium excision in one case and following blunt trauma in another. These complications highlight the necessity for special precautions when treating these patients [3].

FSMK treatment depends on its stage. Symptoms' improvement with the use of lubricants [4], topical steroids [4,5], oral doxycycline [5], and vitamin C in the acute phase has been reported [5,6]. The active inflammatory process is well controlled by instillations of corticosteroids, but this group of drugs should be used judiciously, determining the duration and dose. If complaints of severe pain in the eye, severe corneal syndrome, and ineffectiveness of conservative therapy persisted, a perilimbal conjunctivotomy was performed, consisting in the separation of the conjunctiva along the entire circumference of the limbus of the affected eye [7].

Chronic topical corticosteroid treatment may have been effective in limiting the progression of the disease. While FSMK and TMD are usually not treated with long-term anti-inflammatory medications unless there are clinical signs of ocular inflammation, the early use of such therapy might help limit disease progression [5].

In cases of formed reverse astigmatism, it is possible to use scleral contact lenses, which can significantly improve visual acuity. In rare cases, from minimal or even no trauma in patients with TMD and FSMK, perforation is noted, the probability of which is about 15%, as well as the subtotal or total detachment of Descemet's membrane, corneal edema, and the formation of corneoscleral or intracorneal cysts [7].

Cyanoacrylate has transient usefulness in corneal microperforations. There are a few case reports treated with penetrating keratoplasty [3], lamellar keratoplasty [2], amniotic membrane reconstruction [4], superficial keratectomy with conjunctival autograft [4,5], and corneoscleral lamellar patch graft [6].

Keenan et al. highlighted the difficulty in treating slowly progressive peripheral corneal thinning associated with FSMK. They observed progressive thinning despite treating with doxycycline and vitamin C [5]. This approach to treatment had theoretical benefits because in vitro studies have shown that doxycycline inhibits matrix metalloproteinase activity and ascorbate enhances collagen synthesis [12,13].

Pseudopterygia in FSMK may progress to threaten visual acuity. Surgical excision can be safe and can effectively improve vision on the condition that the patients are closely followed in the early postoperative period to notice the corneal infiltrates [7]. Recommended surgical treatment may entail combining superficial keratectomy with a conjunctival autograft or amniotic membrane transplantation to try to retard recurrent pseudopterygia formation through the same mechanism that prevents recurrence after the excision of traditional pterygia [4,14]. Kotecha and Raber noted that this treatment seemed to suppress the flare-ups of marginal keratitis. Given the role that the conjunctiva may play in inflammation, a conjunctival autograft in conjunction with a lamellar patch graft has also been recommended [4].

In severe cases, like our second case, it was difficult to treat even with multiple surgical treatments with long term use of oral cyclosporin. However, in the first case, surgery was performed early in the disease, prior to widespread conjunctival invasion. Oral cyclosporin was administered immediately post-surgery, and no deterioration in the corneal condition was observed for 1.5 years following the procedure. Our cases demonstrated the two extremes of the disease and their responses to treatment, making it difficult to predict treatment outcomes.

It is possible that the progression of FSMK may be suppressed by surgical treatment and strict inflammation control from the early stage of the disease.

4. Conclusions

We encountered two cases where refractory peripheral corneal infiltration and pseudopterygia were present in both eyes, leading to a strong suspicion of FSMK. Despite its rarity, FSMK should be considered when peripheral corneal infiltration, corneal thinning, and pseudopterygia are observed in both eyes. Although treating this condition is challenging, timely surgical and anti-inflammatory interventions may help manage the disease.

Author Contributions: S.H., Y.H.M., M.K., D.I. and M.U. are specialists of the Cornea group in Nagasaki University Hospital whom were responsible for diagnosing, investigating, and treating the patients. M.U. was the surgeon who performed all surgical operations for the patients. S.H., M.K., D.I. and Y.H.M. were collecting the data and writing the draft. M.U. was the supervisor of the whole work. All authors have read and agreed to the published version of the manuscript.

Funding: This research received no external funding.

Institutional Review Board Statement: This study was approved by the Institutional Review Board of Nagasaki University Hospital and approval number is (24021928).

Informed Consent Statement: Institutional Review Board of Nagasaki University Hospital did not require informed consent because the clinical data were collected from medical records and no personal data were revealed.

Data Availability Statement: The datasets used during the current study are available from the corresponding author upon reasonable request.

Conflicts of Interest: The authors declare no conflicts of interest.

References

1. Deluise, V. Peripheral corneal degeneration and tumors. *Int. Ophthalmol. Clin.* **1985**, *26*, 49–61. [CrossRef] [PubMed]
2. Brilakis, H.S.; Nordlund, M.L.; Holland, E.J. Recurrence of Fuchs' marginal keratitis within a lamellar graft. *Cornea* **2004**, *23*, 639–640. [CrossRef]
3. Bierly, J.R.; Dunn, J.P.; Dawson, C.R.; Ostler, H.B.; Wong, I.G. Fuchs superficial marginal keratitis. *Am. J. Ophthalmol.* **1992**, *113*, 541–545. [CrossRef] [PubMed]
4. Kotecha, A.; Raber, I.M. Superficial keratectomy and conjunctival autograft for Fuchs' superficial marginal keratitis. *Cornea* **2001**, *20*, 214–216. [CrossRef] [PubMed]
5. Keenan, J.D.; Mandel, M.R.; Margolis, T.P. Peripheral ulcerative keratitis associated with vasculitis manifesting asymmetrically as Fuchs' superficial marginal keratitis and Terrien's marginal degeneration. *Cornea* **2011**, *30*, 825–827. [CrossRef] [PubMed]
6. Mejía, L.F.; Santamaría, J.P.; Gaviria, A.M.; Rodríguez, A.M. Fuchs' superficial marginal keratitis managed with circumferential marginal corneoscleral lamellar patch graft. *Eur. J. Ophthalmol.* **2013**, *23*, 925–927. [CrossRef] [PubMed]
7. Riks, I.A.; Trufanov, S.V.; Astakhov, Y.S.; Ezugbaya, M. One Disease, but Different Names: Fuchs' Superficial Marginal Keratitis and Terrien Marginal Degeneration. *Ophthalmol. Russ.* **2020**, *17*, 617–624. [CrossRef]
8. Deng, S.X.; Borderie, V.; Chan, C.C.; Dana, R.; Figueiredo, F.C.; Gomes, J.A.; Pellegrini, G.; Shimmura, S.; Kruse, F.E. Global consensus on the definition, classification, diagnosis and staging of limbal stem cell deficiency. *Cornea* **2019**, *38*, 364–375. [CrossRef] [PubMed]
9. Goldberg, M.A.; Lubniewski, A.J.; Williams, J.M.; Smith, M.E.; Pepose, J.S. Cystic hydrops and spontaneous perforation in Fuchs' superficial marginal keratitis. *Am. J. Ophthalmol.* **1996**, *121*, 91–93. [CrossRef] [PubMed]
10. Cheung, A.Y.; Sarnicola, E.; Kurji, K.H.; Genereux, B.M.; Holland, E.J. Three Hundred Sixty-Degree Fuchs Superficial Marginal Keratitis Managed With Annular Lamellar Keratoplasty. *Cornea* **2018**, *37*, 260–262. [CrossRef] [PubMed]
11. Ellis, O.H. Superficial marginal keratitis. *Am. J. Ophthalmol.* **1939**, *22*, 161. [CrossRef]
12. Smith, V.A.; Cook, S.D. Doxycycline-a role in ocular surface repair. *Br. J. Ophthalmol.* **2004**, *88*, 619–625. [CrossRef] [PubMed]

13. Musselmann, K.; Kane, B.; Alexandrou, B.; Hassell, J.R. Stimulation of collagen synthesis by insulin and proteoglycan accumulation by ascorbate in bovine keratocytes in vitro. *Investig. Ophthalmol. Vis. Sci.* **2006**, *47*, 5260–5266. [CrossRef] [PubMed]
14. Tseng, S.C.G.; Prabhaswat, O.; Lee, S.H. Amniotic membrane transplantation for conjunctival surface reconstruction. *Am. J. Ophthalmol.* **1997**, *124*, 765–774. [CrossRef] [PubMed]

life

MDPI

Article

The Prevalence of Accommodative and Binocular Dysfunctions in Children with Reading Difficulties

Ilze Ceple *, Aiga Svede, Evita Serpa, Evita Kassaliete, Liva Volberga, Rita Mikelsone, Asnate Berzina, Angelina Ganebnaya, Linda Krauze and Gunta Krumina

Department of Optometry and Vision Science, Faculty of Science and Technology, University of Latvia, Jelgavas Street 1, LV-1004 Riga, Latvia; aiga.svede@lu.lv (A.S.); evita.serpa@lu.lv (E.S.); evita.kassaliete@lu.lv (E.K.); angelina.ganebnaya@lu.lv (A.G.); linda.krauze@lu.lv (L.K.); gunta.krumina@lu.lv (G.K.)

* Correspondence: ilze.ceple@lu.lv

Abstract: Uncorrected refractive error and unsatisfactory performance on several clinical accommodation and binocular vision tests are more common in children who struggle with reading. The aim of the current study is to explore the prevalence of accommodative and binocular dysfunctions in children with and without reading difficulties. Reading performance was assessed with the Acadience Reading (formerly DIBELS Next) test adjusted and validated for the Latvian language. Children with (N = 39) and without (N = 43) reading difficulties underwent thorough assessment of their subjective refraction, as well as binocular and accommodation functions. The results demonstrate no difference in the prevalence of complaints between children with and without reading difficulties (26% and 23%, respectively). However, children with reading difficulties more frequently present with significant uncorrected refractive errors and/or accommodative and binocular dysfunctions than children without reading difficulties (69% and 47%, respectively). According to the findings, even in cases where a child does not exhibit any ocular or visual complaints, a comprehensive visual function evaluation should be required for any child who struggles with reading.

Keywords: reading difficulties; visual complaints; ocular complaints; refractive error; accommodative dysfunctions; binocular dysfunctions

1. Introduction

The human visual system plays a crucial role in the perception of the surrounding environment. It provides an enormous amount of visual information that we learn to process, integrate, and structure and is therefore involved in the processes of spatial orientation, human–human interaction, and other everyday activities [1–3]. The quality of one's vision can also affect self-reported quality of life and psychological well-being, as well as potentially being related to academic achievement [4–6]. Glewwe et al. [7] demonstrated that by correcting refractive error in rural students, a significant improvement in academic performance could be observed. Similar results were obtained by Ma et al. [8], demonstrating a significant improvement in mathematics test scores as a result of an early vision screening and refraction correction. However, we have to keep in mind that an accurate performance of the visual system does not only rely on the correction of refractive error and good visual acuity, but also on a precise and coordinated performance of the accommodation and vergence systems.

After exploring the visual symptomology associated with refractive, accommodative, and non-strabismic binocular dysfunctions, Cacho-Martínez et al. [9] reported that patients with an uncorrected refractive error usually complained of headache, visual fatigue, blurred

https://doi.org/10.3390/life15010007

vision, eye dryness, sensitivity to light, sore eyes, and ocular pain. Some of the patients even reported avoiding near-vision tasks. Patients with accommodative dysfunctions mainly complain of red and sore eyes, visual fatigue, and difficulties in performing schoolwork [9]. Finally, patients with non-strabismic binocular dysfunctions mainly present with headache, visual fatigue, dry eyes, ocular pain, blurred vision, and lack of concentration. Although there may be some differences in complaints for different vision dysfunctions, in real life the difference is negligible, making it impossible to specify a child's vision problem by looking at the complaints. The results of different questionnaires related to accommodative and non-strabismic binocular dysfunctions have demonstrated that a relatively high proportion of school-age children report subjective symptoms of headache, asthenopia, floating text, and facility problems [10,11]. An even more surprising observation by Junghans et al. [10] is that children referred to as the "emmetropic group" presented with more complaints related to near-vision work activities than children with previously diagnosed binocular vision dysfunctions.

The summary reports of child vision screening in Europe [12,13] indicate that in all EU countries, preschoolers (3–7 years old) are subjected to at least one vision screening, performed mainly by a general practitioner, orthoptist, ophthalmologist, optometrist, optician, nurse, or pediatrician. However, in most of the EU countries, school-age children are not obligated to perform any vision screening, and the management of refractive errors and accommodative and non-strabismic binocular dysfunctions depends on the recognition of different symptoms by the child, parents, teachers, doctors, or other surrounding persons [12]. In some cases, an abnormal head posture might be the only noticeable indicator of visual system dysfunctions [14]. Therefore, if the child is not asked specifically to identify some visual complaints, in some situations, the visual disorder might be unnoticed, and the reduced academic performance might be attributed to disinterest, laziness, or even serious learning problems (e.g., reading difficulties).

Children with reading difficulties are more likely to have an uncorrected refractive error and abnormal performance in different clinical accommodation and binocular vision tests. Two studies by Palomo-Álvarez and Puell [15,16] have demonstrated that children with poor reading skills have lower values of prism fusion range at distance (break and recovery of negative fusional vergence), as well as lower amplitudes of accommodation and reduced accommodative facility performances. Quaid and Simpson [17] demonstrated that children with reading difficulties not only have lower vergence facility results but are also more likely to have under-corrected hyperopia or overcorrected myopia. Furthermore, children with under-corrected hyperopia presented normal values of distance visual acuity, indicating that visual acuity alone is not a sufficient measurement of visual system functioning. Finally, Christian et al. [18] demonstrated that around six percent of children with reading difficulties have some sort of uncorrected refractive error, more than half of the children have distance and/or near fusional vergence results outside of norms, around twenty percent of children have a below-the-norm accommodative performance, and around one-third of children with reading difficulties have near phoria that falls outside of normal values. Uncorrected refractive errors can be linked to the presence of accommodative and binocular dysfunctions, including both non-strabismic and strabismic binocular dysfunctions. Dwyer and Wick [19] demonstrated that prescriptions of small corrections can significantly improve the performance of the accommodative and vergence systems. Furthermore, Scheiman and Wick [20] indicated that in all cases of accommodative, binocular, and ocular motor dysfunctions, the initial management consideration is the full correction of any significant refractive error.

Wilson et al. [21] and Klatte et al. [22] described that an intervention for struggling readers is most effective when involving teamwork between the family, speech and language therapists, teachers, psychologists, and other specialists, since reading difficulties might also be associated with different psychological, physiological, environmental, sociological, and linguistic factors. Furthermore, vision specialists might also play a role in improving a child's academic performance by addressing the functioning of the visual system. While Bush et al. [23] showed a slight improvement in academic performance after vision therapy, the results regarding convergence insufficiency and reading performance pre- and post-therapy were inconclusive. However, the teacher reported a positive impression of vision therapy and its role in academic performance.

The role of optometrists remains unclear, as various studies have yielded inconclusive results regarding which visual functions may deviate from the norm in children with reading difficulties. Additionally, there is a lack of research on whether children with reading difficulties are more likely to exhibit various accommodative and binocular dysfunctions. Therefore, the current research aims to provide a comprehensive evaluation of subjective refraction, accommodation, and binocular functions in school-age children, both with and without reading difficulties, to enhance our understanding of the role of the visual system in academic performance.

2. Materials and Methods

2.1. Participants

Altogether, eighty-two children (6–12 years old, mean age 9.1 ± 1.9 years; 36 girls, 46 boys) from Marupe State Gymnasium participated in the study. All children acquired the general basic education and were not assigned to special education programs. The study was approved by the Life and Medical Sciences Research Ethics Committee of the University of Latvia (13/06/2022). Written informed consent of the parents or legal guardians of each child was obtained prior to the enrolment in the study.

All children were divided into two groups based on their reading performance: the target group (children with reading difficulties, N = 39, mean age 9.1 ± 1.8 years; 16 girls, 23 boys) and the control group (children without reading difficulties, N = 43, mean age 9.3 ± 2.0 years; 20 girls, 23 boys). Reading performance was assessed with the Acadience Reading (formerly DIBELS Next) test, adjusted and validated for the Latvian language [24]. Reading performance was assessed by professional speech therapists who are certified to perform the Acadience Reading test. Children in the target group were those whose Acadience Reading test results were below the 20th quartile, whereas children in the control group had results above the 20th percentile.

2.2. Method

All of the children were examined in the school setting during their school hours from 8:30AM to 2:00PM. Prior to the visual function examination, all children were systematically asked if they had any of the following complaints related to visual system performance: blurry vision at distance or near, diplopia at distance or near, difficulty focusing when switching distances, eyestrain, eye redness, eye pain or pulling sensation, light sensitivity, eye itching, burning, headache, visual fatigue, red or sore eyes [9,20].

After reviewing the case history and complaints, each participant underwent a full visual function examination, including objective refraction without cycloplegia (autorefractometer Huvitz HRK-1), uncorrected visual acuity (VA) at distance, full subjective sphero-cylindrical correction (using the monocular fogging technique for accommodation control [25]), and best corrected visual acuity (BVEA) at distance. In addition, all children were assessed for the following visual functions: near VA, amplitude of accommodation (push-up), dynamic retinoscopy (MEM), positive and negative relative accommodation (PRA and NRA), binocular and monocular accommodative facility (BAF and MAF, respectively; with ±2.00 D), vergence facility (if failed with 12 Δ BI/3 Δ BO, 8 Δ BI/8 Δ BO were applied), stereovision at distance (Osterberg test) and near (TNO test), suppression at distance and near (red filter test), angle of deviation with and without correction at distance and near (modified Thorington test), fusional reserves at distance and near (prism bar), and finally, near point of convergence (push-up method and dot card). Visual functions were determined with full subjective refraction at distance. All examinations (especially subjective refraction) were performed and controlled by certified optometrists. Some visual functions were assessed by 1st and 2nd year master's students in optometry.

Since the management of accommodative and binocular dysfunctions should not be considered isolated from the refractive state, all children were analyzed for the presence of a significant refractive error and/or accommodative or binocular dysfunctions. The children were considered to have a significant refractive error if they demonstrated at least one of the following criteria: uncorrected VA at distance of 0.63 or less in decimal units (considering that the visual acuity demand for distance in modern primary school classrooms is 0.5 in decimal units) [26,27]; astigmatism of 0.75 D or higher; hyperopia level of 1.25 D or above [28,29]; uncorrected near VA lower than with correction. Accommodative and non-strabismic binocular dysfunctions were diagnosed based on the criteria presented by Franco et al. [30] and Scheiman and Wick [20], as well as updated criteria applied in other studies (see Table 1). Children presenting with one of the fundamental signs and at least two complementary signs were considered to have accommodative or non-strabismic binocular dysfunctions. The Cover test is the most useful test for detecting and characterizing strabismus. Since the Cover test allows for differentiation between heterotropia and heterophoria, it was performed on all children to determine whether the binocular dysfunction would be classified as non-strabismic or strabismic [31].

Table 1. Diagnostic criteria for accommodative and non-strabismic binocular dysfunctions (all diagnostic criteria are adapted from Franco et al. [30] and Scheiman and Wick [20]; for some accommodative and non-strabismic binocular dysfunctions, complementary signs were developed, indicated under the dysfunction type).

Dysfunction	Diagnostic Criteria
Accommodative insufficiency [32,33]	*Fundamental signs:* • Reduced AA—at least 2.00 D less than the expected Hofstetter's minimal value of the age and • MAF < 6 cpm (difficulty with −2.00 D flipper) *Complementary signs:* • BAF < 3 cpm (difficulty with −2.00 D flipper) • MEM ≥ +0.75 D • PRA ≤ 1.25 D • PFV < 12/15/4 Δ—blur at near may be reduced
Ill-sustained accommodation	*Fundamental signs:* • MAF < 6 cpm (difficulty with −2.00 D flipper) *Complementary signs:* • BAF < 3 cpm (difficulty with −2.00 D flipper) • MEM ≥ +0.75 D • PRA ≤ 1.25 D • PFV < 12/15/4 Δ—blur at near may be reduced

Table 1. *Cont.*

<table>
<tr><th>Dysfunction</th><th>Diagnostic Criteria</th></tr>
<tr><td>Accommodative excess [9]</td><td>Fundamental signs:
• MAF < 6 cpm (difficulty with +2.00 D flipper)
Complementary signs:
• BAF < 6 cpm (difficulty with +2.00 D flipper)
• MEM ≤ +0.25 D
• NRA ≤ 1.50 D
• NFV < 9/17/8 Δ—blur at near may be reduced</td></tr>
<tr><td>Accommodative infacility [9]</td><td>Fundamental signs:
• MAF < 6 cpm (difficulty with ±2.00 D flipper)
Complementary signs:
• BAF < 3 cpm (difficulty with ±2.00 D flipper)
• PRA ≤ 1.25 D
• NRA ≤ 1.50 D
• PFV < 12/15/4 Δ—blur at near may be reduced
• NFV < 9/17/8 Δ—blur at near may be reduced</td></tr>
<tr><td>Convergence insufficiency [34]</td><td>Fundamental signs:
• Near exophoria at least 4 Δ larger than at distance
Complementary signs:
• NPC > 6 cm
• AC/A ratio < 2:1 (the gradient method)
• PFV < 12/15/4 Δ (reduced finings in at least one of three at near)
• VF < 13 cpm (difficulty with Δ BO)
• BAF < 6 cpm (difficulty with +2.00 D flipper)
• NRA ≤ 1.50 D
• MEM ≤ +0.25 D</td></tr>
<tr><td>Convergence excess [35]</td><td>Fundamental signs:
• Near esophoria at least 2 Δ larger than at distance
Complementary signs:
• NFV < 9/17/8 Δ (reduced findings in at least one of three at near)
• AC/A ratio > 6:1
• MEM ≥ +0.75 D
• PRA ≤ 1.25 D
• VF < 13 cpm (difficulty with Δ BI)
• BAF < 6 cpm (difficulty with −2.00 D flipper)</td></tr>
<tr><td>Fusional vergence dysfunction</td><td>Fundamental signs:
• PFV < 12/15/4 Δ (reduced finings in at least one of three at near)
or
• NFV < 9/17/8 Δ (reduced finings in at least one of three at near)
Complementary signs:
• VF < 13 cpm (difficulty with Δ BO and BI)
• BAF < 6 cpm (difficulty with ±2.00 D flipper)
• PRA ≤ 1.25 D
• NRA ≤ 1.50 D</td></tr>
</table>

Table 1. *Cont.*

Dysfunction	Diagnostic Criteria
Divergence insufficiency [36]	*Fundamental signs:* • Far esophoria at least 4 Δ larger than at near *Complementary signs:* • AC/A ratio < 2:1 • NFV < -/4/2 Δ (reduced finings in at least one of three at distance)
Divergence excess	*Fundamental signs:* • Far exophoria at least 5 Δ larger than at near *Complementary signs:* • AC/A ratio > 6:1 • PFV < 5/11/6 Δ (reduced finings in at least one of three at distance) • NFV < 9/17/8 Δ (reduced finings in at least one of three at near)
Basic exophoria [9]	*Fundamental signs:* • Significant exophoria at distance and near of approximately the same amount (within 5 Δ) *Complementary signs:* • PFV < 5/11/6 Δ (reduced finings in at least one of three at distance) • PFV < 12/15/4 Δ (reduced finings in at least one of three at near) • VF < 13 cpm (difficulty with Δ BO) • BAF < 6 cpm (difficulty with +2.00 D flipper) • NRA ≤ 1.50 D • MEM ≤ +0.25 D
Basic esophoria [35]	*Fundamental signs:* • Significant esophoria at distance and near of approximately the same amount (within 5 Δ) *Complementary signs:* • NFV < -/4/2 Δ (reduced finings in at least one of three at distance) • NFV < 9/17/8 Δ (reduced finings in at least one of three at near) • VF < 13 cpm (difficulty with Δ BI) • BAF < 6 cpm (difficulty with −2.00 D flipper) • PRA ≤ 1.25 D • MEM ≥ +0.75 D

Abbreviations: AA—amplitude of accommodation (monocular); BAF—binocular accommodative facility; MAF—monocular accommodative facility; MEM—monocular estimated method of dynamic retinoscopy; PRA—positive relative accommodation; NRA—negative relative accommodation; PFV—positive fusional vergence; NFV—negative fusional vergence; NPC—near point of convergence; AC/A ratio—accommodative convergence against accommodation ratio; VF—vergence facility; BO—base out; BI—base in; PD—prism dioptres; D—dioptres; cpm—cycles per minute.

2.3. Statistical Analysis

Statistical associations between the reading performance and the amount of complaints as well as refraction, accommodative, and/or binocular vision disorders were determined using the Chi-square test of independence with a significance level of $\alpha = 0.05$. Bar charts and tables depict the summary statistics.

3. Results

The initial analysis of the complaints related to visual system performance demonstrated that 26% of children with reading difficulties and 23% of children without reading difficulties (the control group) presented with visual complaints (see Figure 1). Statistical analyses demonstrated that both groups presented with similar amounts of visual complaints (Chi-square test of independence: χ^2 (1) = 0.063, p = 0.802, Cramer's V/Phi = 0.802).

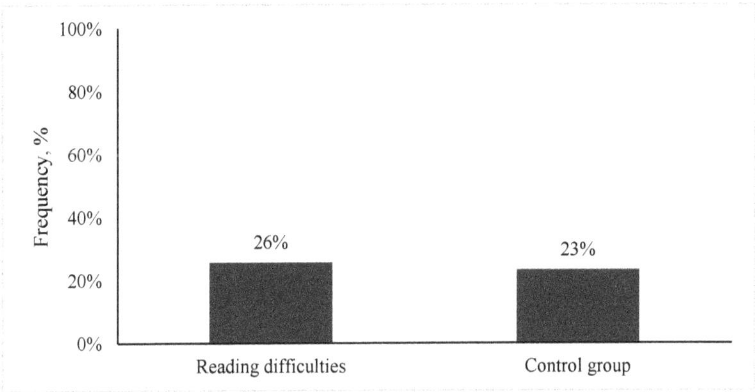

Figure 1. Frequency of visual complaints in children with reading difficulties and without reading difficulties (the control group).

However, both groups presented significant refractive errors and/or accommodative or binocular dysfunctions at least two times more often than visual complaints (see Figure 2), and the prevalence of dysfunctions was significantly higher in children with reading difficulties compared to the control group (Chi-square test of independence: χ^2 (1) = 4.315, p = 0.038, Cramer's V/Phi = 0.038; OR = 2.588, 95% CI 1.045–6.405).

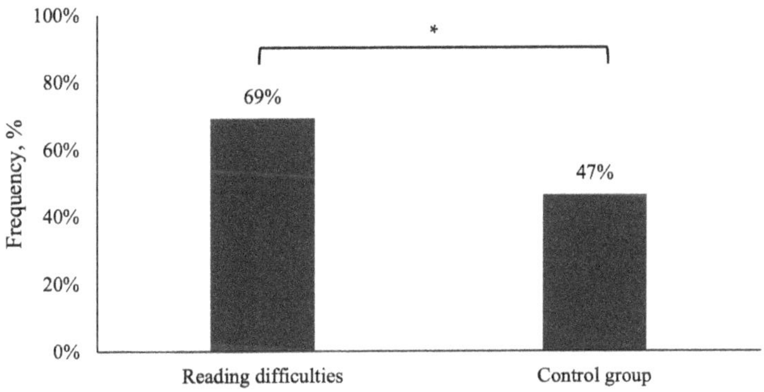

Figure 2. Frequency of significant refractive errors and/or accommodative and binocular dysfunctions in children with reading difficulties and without reading difficulties (the control group). * Statistically significantly difference (Chi-square test of independence $p < 0.05$).

In all children with significant refractive errors and/or accommodative or binocular dysfunctions, accommodative dysfunctions were diagnosed more often than binocular dysfunctions (see Figure 3). When addressed separately, the statistical analysis did not reveal a significant difference in the prevalence of accommodative dysfunctions (χ^2 (1) = 1.567, p = 0.211, Cramer's V/Phi = 0.211) or binocular dysfunctions (χ^2 (1) = 3.375, p = 0.066, Cramer's V/Phi = 0.066) between both groups. However, children with reading difficulties were more likely to present with a significant refractive error compared to the control group (χ^2 (1) = 4.132, p = 0.042, Cramer's V/Phi = 0.224).

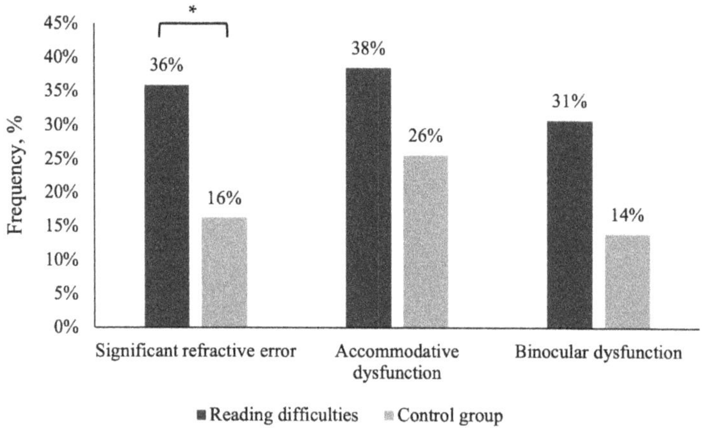

Figure 3. Relative frequency of significant refractive errors and accommodative and binocular dysfunctions in children with reading difficulties and without reading difficulties (the control group). * Statistically significantly difference (Chi-square test of independence $p < 0.05$).

Table 2 presents the relative frequency of the different types of accommodative and binocular dysfunctions (including both strabismic and non-strabismic) in both groups. The most common diagnosis was accommodative excess, which was combined with convergence insufficiency in some patients. The next most common diagnoses in children with reading difficulties were convergence excess and accommodative insufficiency, while ill-sustained accommodation was the next most common form in the control group.

Table 2. The relative frequency (in percentage) of different accommodative and non-strabismic binocular dysfunctions in children with (n = 39) and without reading difficulties (n = 43). Some children had both types of dysfunctions (combination of accommodative and binocular dysfunctions).

Type of Dysfunction	Reading Difficulties N = 39	Control Group N = 43
Accommodative excess	21%	19%
Convergence excess	10%	2%
Convergence insufficiency	8%	7%
Accommodative insufficiency	8%	
Fusional vergence dysfunction	3%	2%
Basic exophoria	3%	2%
Basic esophoria	3%	2%
Ill-sustained accommodation	3%	7%
Accommodative infacility	3%	
Accommodative esotropia	5%	

4. Discussion

The present study explores visual functions in children with and without reading difficulties. The results demonstrate that around every fourth child presented with complaints that might be related to uncorrected refractive error and/or accommodative and non-strabismic binocular dysfunctions. A large amount of children will not complain but will still have an uncorrected refractive error and/or accommodative and binocular dysfunctions, with a significantly higher prevalence in children with reading difficulties.

While one of the limitations of the current study is that a standardized questionary of visual complaints was not applied, all children were systematically asked if they had any of the most common complaints which were previously associated with refractive, accommodative, and binocular vision dysfunctions [9,20].

When delving into the self-perceived health of children, one must consider that there are different psychosocial factors that contribute to the evaluation of the child's health by self-administered questionnaires [37]. Self-perceived health reports can be related to the child's gender and even parental educational levels [38]. Dusek et al. [39] explored whether children with reading and writing difficulties were more likely to experience different visual or ocular complains. While in the study by Dusek et al. [39] children with reading and writing difficulties were more likely to complain of eye burning, tiredness after near-vision work, eye strain when looking at a near target, blurred vision, and diplopia, most of the complaints in this work were still similar in both groups (with and without reading and writing difficulties). The results of the current study only partly coincide with the results by Dusek et al. [39], which is more likely because the symptoms in the current study were not analyzed separately but in a generalized manner—whether there were or were not any complaints at all. Nevertheless, the current study demonstrates that the number of children with uncorrected refractive errors and/or accommodative and binocular dysfunctions was at least two times larger than the number of children with visual complaints, indicating that some of the dysfunctions might go unnoticed or undiagnosed due to the lack of noticeable nonvisual indicators (i.e., complaints). It leads to the question of what the necessary steps for parents, teachers, and primary care specialists are to understand whether the visual system is or is not interfering with a child's daily life and learning process.

Visual complaints associated with uncorrected refractive error in children usually include blurry vision at distance or near, eyestrain, eye pain, watery or dry eyes, ocular pain, difficulty in recognizing faces, headache, glare, and eye irritation [9,40]. Cases of accommodative and binocular dysfunctions may also present with complaints of blurry vision at distance or near as well as diplopia at distance or near, difficulty focusing when changing fixation distances, eyestrain, eye redness, eye pain or pulling sensations, light sensitivity, eye itching, burning, headache, or covering one eye [20]. Teachers and parents have reported that they suspect that children could have uncorrected refractive error when they squeeze their eyes, have difficulties seeing the screen, and struggle copying information from the board, as well as having difficulties in reading or learning [40]. It is worth noting that many of these symptoms are not specific and can be related to other disorders as well, e.g., watery eyes and eye irritation can also be related to allergic reactions [41]; eye dryness, ocular irritation, and blurred vision might be related to dry eye syndrome [42]; and slow thinking, headaches, and reduced school performance might also be related to fatigue or even lack of sleep [43–45]. Therefore, even if a child reports specific complaints or parents and teachers ask specific questions to better understand the problem, the relation to a specific visual problem cannot always be established by evaluating the complaints of the child. Complaints serve as an important primary sign that the child needs a full comprehensive visual function examination by an optometrist.

The current study demonstrates that the prevalence of significant refractive error and/or accommodative and binocular dysfunctions in children without reading difficulties is around 47%, which is slightly higher than the results obtained by Ma et al. [46] and Lara et al. [35], which demonstrated that around 41.2% and 32.3% of children had normal binocular vision, respectively. Furthermore, the current study provides alarming results in children with reading difficulties: around two-thirds of these children presented with a significant uncorrected refractive error and/or accommodative and binocular dysfunctions. In addition, they presented more diversity in accommodative and binocular dysfunctions compared to children without reading difficulties. Since accommodative and binocular dysfunctions are often related to uncorrected refractive error, and different accommodative and binocular dysfunctions often co-exist, the current study aimed to explore the overall performance of the visual system. The data analysis included all of the inter-related factors and therefore led to a higher prevalence of significant refractive errors and/or accommodative and binocular dysfunctions.

As demonstrated by previous studies, children with reading difficulties can present with lower accommodative and vergence system performances, i.e., lower near visual acuity, larger exophoria, as well as lower accommodative facilities. However, the differences in the amplitude of accommodation and vergence facilities and the near point of convergence in children with and without reading difficulties still remain inconclusive [15,16,39,47]. Christian et al. [18] demonstrated that around 30% of children with reading difficulties had a near phoria and near point of convergence outside normal values, approximately 25% of children with reading difficulties had reduced stereoacuity, and 10% of children with reading difficulties had reduced binocular accommodative facilities. Furthermore, around 20% of these children required new spectacle correction. Cacho-Martínez et al. [9] demonstrated that some of the accommodative-system-related complaints could be resolved by correcting refractive error. Thus, all children with reading difficulties (with or without vision-related complaints) should undergo a very thorough assessment of refraction and visual function to ensure that any refractive and/or accommodative and non-strabismic binocular dysfunctions are prevented. Furthermore, even when a child has previously been diagnosed with accommodative or binocular dysfunctions, the child and their parents should be encouraged to perform regular check-ups of the child's visual system performance. The current study revealed that two of the children with reading difficulties presented with previously diagnosed accommodative esotropia, and only one of them used their visual correction on a regular basis.

To solve the observed vision problems in children with reading difficulties, the first and main step is always the optical correction of significant ametropia with spectacles or contact lenses. If an accommodative and/or binocular disorder is still diagnosed, next steps should consider different management options depending on the dysfunction [20], i.e., visual therapy, prism correction, and near additive. However, there is still an insufficient number of studies demonstrating the direct effects of such an approach on children's reading skills. The existing studies also do not provide a clear answer about the importance of such an approach. While some studies only speculate that, from a physiological point of view, such an approach should play a major role in reading disorders, others demonstrate mixed results regarding the effects. Barrett [48] discussed that while accommodative and some non-strabismic binocular dysfunctions respond well to visual therapy, a generalized treatment for dyslexia patients that is not aimed at treating specific accommodative and binocular dysfunctions does not present an unequivocal effect. Handler and Fierson [49] indicated that vision disorders are rarely the primary cause of reading dysfunction and that visual correction or visual therapy only makes reading more comfortable but does not treat the main cause of reading difficulties. Further studies are necessary to explore what is the role of an appropriate visual correction and accommodative and non-strabismic binocular dysfunction management in children with reading difficulties.

Of all the children with reading difficulties involved in the current study, three participants were also diagnosed with unilateral amblyopia: one anisometropic amblyopia, one strabismic amblyopia (with partially accommodative esotropia and high degree hyperopia +6.00 D), and one combined amblyopia (with fully accommodative esotropia). While the binocular and accommodative functions of these children were improved by an appropriate refraction correction, only one of the three participants reported using refraction correction on a daily basis. Studies [50–52] have demonstrated that children with amblyopia can have a slower reading speed, which could be caused by reduced fixation stability and atypical saccadic eye movements [53–55]. Treatment for monocular amblyopia might not only improve vision quality but could also increase reading distance and improve reading speed and efficiency [50,56].

The current study was conducted in Latvia, where, based on the National Health Service guidelines for children's healthcare, all children should have at least three visits at the ophthalmologist at the ages of 1–2, 3–5, and 6–7 years [57]. No other recommendations regarding eye health for older children are given, i.e., school-age children are not obligated to perform any vision screening, and the management of refractive errors and accommodative and binocular dysfunctions depends solely on the recognition of different symptoms by the child, parents, teachers, speech therapists, doctors, or other surrounding persons. While the informative material provided by the Children's Clinical University Hospital in Latvia indicates that all children with reading difficulties should consult with an ophthalmologist in order to rule out any vision disorders, including functional disorders [58], different guidelines for dyslexia management point out that dyslexia is not related to visual system disorders [59]. The results of the current study do not imply that reading difficulties are caused by vision dysfunctions; rather, they suggest that each patient with reading difficulties should have a thorough visual system examination, since accommodative and binocular dysfunctions could potentially add a further hindrance to reading difficulties [60]. While the main limitation of the current study is the sample size, which is smaller than that applied in some other studies addressing the accommodative and binocular system performance in children with reading and learning difficulties [15,16,38], the comprehensive methodology applied in the current study not only allows for comparing the performance of different accommodative and vergence functions but also helps to determine the overall performance of the visual system. Therefore, it is one of only a few studies to explore the prevalence of accommodative and binocular dysfunctions in children with and without reading difficulties.

5. Conclusions

The current study demonstrated that children with reading difficulties are more likely to have either a significant refractive error or an accommodative and/or binocular vision disorder. In addition, children may not feel or even understand typical complaints associated with these disorders. While the observed prevalence of different accommodative and binocular dysfunctions is not the same as in other studies (most likely because different diagnostic criteria were applied), it can be noticed that children with reading difficulties presented with a higher variety of different accommodative and binocular dysfunctions than children without reading difficulties. Therefore, when working with children with reading difficulties, vision specialists should perform a full visual function examination even if the child does not present with any ocular or visual complaints. Additionally, even though reading is a multifactorial process and reading difficulties have been linked to different psychological, physiological, environmental, sociological, and linguistic factors, the improvement of the visual quality might also make at least a small contribution to facilitating the reading process by taking out at least one hindering factor and allowing the focus to be directed to other factors that might be contributing to the reduced reading performance.

Author Contributions: Conceptualization, I.C., A.S., E.K. and G.K.; methodology, I.C., A.S., E.K. and G.K.; software, I.C.; validation, A.S., E.K. and G.K.; formal analysis, I.C. and A.S.; investigation, A.S., E.S., E.K., L.V., R.M. and A.B.; resources, I.C., E.K. and G.K.; data curation, I.C. and A.G.; writing—original draft preparation, I.C.; writing—review and editing, I.C., A.S., E.S., A.G. and

L.K.; visualization, I.C.; supervision, I.C., A.S., E.K. and G.K.; project administration, I.C. and G.K.; funding acquisition, I.C. and G.K. All authors have read and agreed to the published version of the manuscript.

Funding: This research was funded by the Latvian Council of Science (project no. lzp-2021/1-0219), the University of Latvia (project no. Y5-AZ77-ZF-N-100), and SIA Mikrotikls and the University 522 of Latvia Foundation (project no. 2260).

Institutional Review Board Statement: The study was conducted in accordance with the Declaration of Helsinki and approved by the UL Life and Medical Sciences Research Ethics Committee (No. 13/06/2022, 13 June 2022).

Informed Consent Statement: Informed consent was obtained from all legal guardians of the subjects involved in the study.

Data Availability Statement: The data presented in this study are available on request from the corresponding author. The data are not publicly available due to privacy reasons.

Acknowledgments: We would like to express our gratitude to the school that participated in the study (Marupe State Gymnasium, Marupe Elementary School, Riga Cultures Secondary School, and Kuldiga Center Secondary School), as well as the speech therapists J. Hanzovska, L. Meiersone, M. Vorza, I. Petuhova, S. Depa, and S. Jirgensone.

Conflicts of Interest: The authors declare no conflicts of interest.

References

1. Chokron, S.; Colliot, P.; Bartolomeo, P. The role of vision in spatial representation. *Cortex* **2004**, *40*, 281–290. [CrossRef] [PubMed]
2. Papeo, L.; Abassi, E. Seeing social events: The visual specialization for dyadic human–human interactions. *J. Exp. Psychol. Hum. Percept. Perform.* **2019**, *45*, 877. [CrossRef]
3. Lateiner, J.E.; Sainburg, R.L. Differential contributions of vision and proprioception to movement accuracy. *Exp. Brain Res.* **2003**, *151*, 446–454. [CrossRef] [PubMed]
4. Misajon, R.; Hawthorne, G.; Richardson, J.; Barton, J.; Peacock, S.; Iezzi, A.; Keeffe, J. Vision and quality of life: The development of a utility measure. *Investig. Ophthalmol. Vis. Sci.* **2005**, *46*, 4007–4015. [CrossRef]
5. Garcia, G.A.; Khoshnevis, M.; Gale, J.; Frousiakis, S.E.; Hwang, T.J.; Poincenot, L.; Karanjia, R.; Baron, D.; Sadun, A.A. Profound vision loss impairs psychological well-being in young and middle-aged individuals. *Clin. Ophthalmol.* **2017**, *2017*, 417–427. [CrossRef]
6. Shin, H.S.; Park, S.C.; Park, C.M. Relationship between accommodative and vergence dysfunctions and academic achievement for primary school children. *Ophthalmic Physiol. Opt.* **2009**, *29*, 615–624. [CrossRef]
7. Glewwe, P.; Park, A.; Zhao, M. A better vision for development: Eyeglasses and academic performance in rural primary schools in China. *J. Dev. Econ.* **2016**, *122*, 170–182. [CrossRef]
8. Ma, Y.; Congdon, N.; Shi, Y.; Hogg, R.; Medina, A.; Boswell, M.; Rozelle, S.; Iyer, M. Effect of a local vision care center on eyeglasses use and school performance in rural China: A cluster randomized clinical trial. *JAMA Ophthalmol.* **2018**, *136*, 731–737. [CrossRef]
9. Cacho-Martínez, P.; Cantó-Cerdán, M.; Carbonell-Bonete, S.; García-Muñoz, Á. Characterization of visual symptomatology associated with refractive, accommodative, and binocular anomalies. *J. Ophthalmol.* **2015**, *2015*, 895803. [CrossRef]
10. Junghans, B.M.; Azizoglu, S.; Crewther, S.G. Unexpectedly high prevalence of asthenopia in Australian school children identified by the CISS survey tool. *BMC Ophthalmol.* **2020**, *20*, 408. [CrossRef]
11. Sterner, B.; Gellerstedt, M.; Sjöström, A. Accommodation and the relationship to subjective symptoms with near work for young school children. *Ophthalmic Physiol. Opt.* **2006**, *26*, 148–155. [CrossRef] [PubMed]
12. Griffiths, H.; Carlton, J.; Mazzone, P. *Summary Report: Childhood Vision Screening in Europe*; University of Sheffield: Sheffield, UK; UScreen: Sheffield, UK, 2019.
13. Carlton, J.; Griffiths, H.J.; Mazzone, P.; Horwood, A.M.; Sloot, F.; Euroscreen Study Consortium. A comprehensive overview of vision screening programmes across 46 countries. *Br. Ir. Orthopt. J.* **2022**, *18*, 27–47. [CrossRef] [PubMed]
14. Zhang, D.; Zhang, W.H.; Dai, S.Z.; Peng, H.Y.; Wang, L.Y. Binocular vision and abnormal head posture in children when watching television. *Int. J. Ophthalmol.* **2016**, *9*, 746–749. [CrossRef] [PubMed]
15. Palomo-Álvarez, C.; Puell, M.C. Accommodative function in school children with reading difficulties. *Graefes Arch. Clin. Exp. Ophthalmol.* **2008**, *246*, 1769–1774. [CrossRef] [PubMed]

16. Palomo-Álvarez, C.; Puell, M.C. Binocular function in school children with reading difficulties. *Graefe's Arch. Clin. Exp. Ophthalmol.* **2010**, *248*, 885–892. [CrossRef] [PubMed]
17. Quaid, P.; Simpson, T. Association between reading speed, cycloplegic refractive error, and oculomotor function in reading disabled children versus controls. *Graefe's Arch. Clin. Exp. Ophthalmol.* **2013**, *251*, 169–187. [CrossRef] [PubMed]
18. Christian, L.W.; Nandakumar, K.; Hrynchak, P.K.; Irving, E.L. Visual and binocular status in elementary school children with a reading problem. *J. Optom.* **2018**, *11*, 160–166. [CrossRef]
19. Dwyer, P.; Wick, B. The influence of refractive correction upon disorders of vergence and accommodation. *Optom. Vis. Sci.* **1995**, *72*, 224–232. [CrossRef] [PubMed]
20. Scheiman, M.; Wick, B. *Clinical Management of Binocular Vision: Heterophoric, Accommodative, and Eye Movement Disorders*; Lippincott Williams & Wilkins: Philadelphia, PA, USA, 2008.
21. Wilson, G.; Nash, M.; Earl, G. Supporting students with language learning difficulties in secondary schools through collaboration: The use of concept maps to investigate the impact on teachers' knowledge of vocabulary teaching. *Child Lang. Teach. Ther.* **2010**, *26*, 163–179. [CrossRef]
22. Klatte, I.S.; Lyons, R.; Davies, K.; Harding, S.; Marshall, J.; McKean, C.; Roulstone, S. Collaboration between parents and SLTs produces optimal outcomes for children attending speech and language therapy: Gathering the evidence. *Int. J. Lang. Commun. Disord.* **2020**, *55*, 618–628. [CrossRef] [PubMed]
23. Bush, S.; Hinkley, S.; Jenerou, A.; Damari, D.; Buckingham, R.; Geneva, C.; Reger, M. The impact of binocular vision and tracking intervention on academic performance: An in-school vision therapy pilot program. *Optom. Vis. Perform.* **2019**, *7*, 9–21.
24. Rascevska, M.; Orlovska, M.; Griskevica, I.; Vabale, A.; Ozola, E.; Legzdins, P. *Agrīnās Lasītprasmes Attīstības Rādītāju DIBELS Next Latviešu Valodas Versija*; McĀbols: Rīga, Latvia, 2013.
25. Benjamin, W.J. *Borish's Clinical Refraction-E-Book: Borish's Clinical Refraction*; Elsevier Health Sciences: Amsterdam, The Netherlands, 2006.
26. Leone, J.F.; Mitchell, P.; Morgan, I.G.; Kifley, A.; Rose, K.A. Use of visual acuity to screen for significant refractive errors in adolescents: Is it reliable? *Arch. Ophthalmol.* **2010**, *128*, 894–899. [CrossRef]
27. Narayanasamy, S.; Vincent, S.J.; Sampson, G.P.; Wood, J.M. Visual demands in modern Australian primary school classrooms. *Clin. Exp. Optom.* **2016**, *99*, 233–240. [CrossRef]
28. Leat, S.J. To prescribe or not to prescribe? Guidelines for spectacle prescribing in infants and children. *Clin. Exp. Optom.* **2011**, *94*, 514–527. [CrossRef] [PubMed]
29. Leat, S.J.; Mittelstaedt, A.; McIntosh, S.; Machan, C.M.; Hrynchak, P.K.; Irving, E.L. Prescribing for hyperopia in childhood and teenage by academic optometrists. *Optom. Vis. Sci.* **2011**, *88*, 1333–1342. [CrossRef] [PubMed]
30. Franco, S.; Moreira, A.; Fernandes, A.; Baptista, A. Accommodative and binocular vision dysfunctions in a Portuguese clinical population. *J. Optom.* **2022**, *15*, 271–277. [CrossRef] [PubMed]
31. Ticho, B.H. Strabismus. *Pediatr. Clin. N. Am.* **2003**, *50*, 173–188. [CrossRef] [PubMed]
32. Hussaindeen, J.R.; Murali, A. Accommodative Insufficiency: Prevalence, Impact and Treatment Options. *Clin. Optom.* **2020**, *12*, 135–149. [CrossRef] [PubMed]
33. Cacho, P.; García, A.; Lara, F.; Seguí, M. Diagnostic signs of accommodative insufficiency. *Optom. Vis. Sci.* **2002**, *79*, 614–620. [CrossRef] [PubMed]
34. Gantz, L.; Stiebel-Kalish, H. Convergence insufficiency: Review of clinical diagnostic signs. *J. Optom.* **2022**, *15*, 256–270. [CrossRef]
35. Lara, F.; Cacho, P.; García, Á.; Megías, R. General binocular disorders: Prevalence in a clinic population. *Ophthalmic Physiol. Opt.* **2001**, *21*, 70–74. [CrossRef]
36. Jacobson, D.M. Divergence insufficiency revisited: Natural history of idiopathic cases and neurologic associations. *Arch. Ophthalmol.* **2000**, *118*, 1237–1241. [CrossRef]
37. Piko, B.F.; Keresztes, N. Self-perceived health among early adolescents: Role of psychosocial factors. *Pediatr. Int.* **2007**, *49*, 577–583. [CrossRef]
38. Padilla-Moledo, C.; Ruiz, J.R.; Castro-Piñero, J. Parental educational level and psychological positive health and health complaints in Spanish children and adolescents. *Child Care Health Dev.* **2016**, *42*, 534–543. [CrossRef]
39. Dusek, W.; Pierscionek, B.K.; McClelland, J.F. A survey of visual function in an Austrian population of school-age children with reading and writing difficulties. *BMC Ophthalmol.* **2010**, *10*, 16. [CrossRef]
40. Kumaran, S.E.; Balasubramaniam, S.M.; Kumar, D.S.; Ramani, K.K. Refractive error and vision-related quality of life in South Indian children. *Optom. Vis. Sci.* **2015**, *92*, 272–278. [CrossRef]
41. Leonardi, A.; Motterle, L.; Bortolotti, M. Allergy and the eye. *Clin. Exp. Immunol.* **2008**, *153*, 17–21. [CrossRef]
42. Barabino, S.; Labetoulle, M.; Rolando, M.; Messmer, E.M. Understanding symptoms and quality of life in patients with dry eye syndrome. *Ocul. Surf.* **2016**, *14*, 365–376. [CrossRef]
43. Fisk, J.D.; Ritvo, P.G.; Ross, L.; Haase, D.A.; Marrie, T.J.; Schlech, W.F. Measuring the functional impact of fatigue: Initial validation of the fatigue impact scale. *Clin. Infect. Dis.* **1994**, *18*, 79–83. [CrossRef]

44. Neu, D.; Linkowski, P.; Le Bon, O. Clinical complaints of daytime sleepiness and fatigue: How to distinguish and treat them, especially when they become 'excessive' or 'chronic'? *Acta Neurol. Belg.* **2020**, *110*, 15–25.
45. Viner, R.; Christie, D. Fatigue and somatic symptoms. *BMJ* **2005**, *330*, 1012–1015. [CrossRef]
46. Ma, M.M.L.; Yeo, A.C.H.; Scheiman, M.; Chen, X. Vergence and accommodative dysfunctions in emmetropic and myopic Chinese young adults. *J. Ophthalmol.* **2019**, *2019*, 5904903. [CrossRef] [PubMed]
47. Niechwiej-Szwedo, E.; Alramis, F.; Christian, L.W. Association between fine motor skills and binocular visual function in children with reading difficulties. *Hum. Mov. Sci.* **2017**, *56*, 1–10. [CrossRef]
48. Barrett, B.T. A critical evaluation of the evidence supporting the practice of behavioural vision therapy. *Ophthalmic Physiol. Opt.* **2009**, *29*, 4–25. [CrossRef] [PubMed]
49. Handler, S.M.; Fierson, W.M. Reading difficulties and the pediatric ophthalmologist. *J. AAPOS* **2017**, *21*, 436–442. [CrossRef]
50. Kelly, K.R.; Jost, R.M.; De La Cruz, A.; Birch, E.E. Amblyopic children read more slowly than controls under natural, binocular reading conditions. *J. AAPOS* **2015**, *19*, 515–520. [CrossRef] [PubMed]
51. Stifter, E.; Burggasser, G.; Hirmann, E.; Thaler, A.; Radner, W. Monocular and binocular reading performance in children with microstrabismic amblyopia. *Br. J. Ophthalmol.* **2005**, *89*, 1324–1329. [CrossRef]
52. Webber, A.L. The functional impact of amblyopia. *Clin. Exp. Optom.* **2018**, *101*, 443–450. [CrossRef]
53. Chung, S.T.; Kumar, G.; Li, R.W.; Levi, D.M. Characteristics of fixational eye movements in amblyopia: Limitations on fixation stability and acuity? *Vis. Res.* **2015**, *114*, 87–99. [CrossRef]
54. Subramanian, V.; Jost, R.M.; Birch, E.E. A quantitative study of fixation stability in amblyopia. *Investig. Ophthalmol. Vis. Sci.* **2013**, *54*, 1998–2003. [CrossRef] [PubMed]
55. Niechwiej-Szwedo, E.; Goltz, H.C.; Chandrakumar, M.; Hirji, Z.A.; Wong, A.M. Effects of anisometropic amblyopia on visuomotor behavior, I: Saccadic eye movements. *Investig. Ophthalmol. Vis. Sci.* **2010**, *51*, 6348–6354. [CrossRef]
56. Rosa, H.A.; Adrián, A.C.; Beatriz, I.S.; María-José, L.C.; Miguel-Ángel, S. Psychomotor, psychosocial and reading skills in children with amblyopia and the effect of different treatments. *J. Mot. Behav.* **2021**, *53*, 176–184. [CrossRef]
57. National Health Service of the Republic of Latvia. Children. Available online: https://www.vmnvd.gov.lv/lv/berniem?utm_source=https:// (accessed on 2 August 2023).
58. Children's Clinical University Hospital in Latvia. Dyslexia. Available online: https://www.veselapasaule.lv/lv/enciklopedija/diagnoze/disleksija#celoni (accessed on 11 September 2024).
59. Latvian Dyslexia Association. 2015. Empowering Parents for Support of Their Children with Dyslexia. Available online: https://www.32pii.daugavpils.lv/wp-content/uploads/2019/03/rokasgraamata-latvisk_berna_disleksija.pdf (accessed on 10 December 2024).
60. Hussaindeen, J.R.; Shah, P.; Ramani, K.K.; Ramanujan, L. Efficacy of vision therapy in children with learning disability and associated binocular vision anomalies. *J. Optom.* **2018**, *11*, 40–48. [CrossRef]

life

MDPI

Article

Simultaneous Color Contrast Increments with Complexity and Identity of the Target Stimulus

Paolo A. Grasso [1,2,*], Federico Tommasi [1], Rebecca Franconi [1], Elisabetta Baldanzi [1,2], Alessandro Farini [1,2] and Massimo Gurioli [1]

1 Department of Physics and Astronomy, University of Florence, 50019 Florence, Italy; federico.tommasi@unifi.it (F.T.); rebecca.franconi@edu.unifi.it (R.F.); elisabetta.baldanzi@unifi.it (E.B.); alessandro.farini@unifi.it (A.F.); massimo.gurioli@unifi.it (M.G.)
2 National Research Council, National Institute of Optics, 50125 Florence, Italy
* Correspondence: paolo.grasso@unifi.it

Abstract: Simultaneous color contrast is a perceptual phenomenon in which a target stimulus appears to change its hue due to color induction from the surrounding background. In this study, we investigated whether this phenomenon is influenced by the structural complexity and identity of the stimuli used. In Experiment 1, we created two sets of stimuli varying in structural complexity and asked participants to perform a color-matching task on the achromatic target. Low-complexity targets consisted of simple squares, while high-complexity targets were stylized cars. The results showed that high-complexity stimuli triggered stronger color induction from the background and exhibited greater interindividual variation in perceived color saturation. Conversely, low-complexity stimuli were predominantly perceived as achromatic across all participants. In Experiment 2, we further explored whether these effects were influenced by differences in the stimuli's topology and identity. Topological factors were controlled by ensuring similar organizations of stimulus elements across conditions, while the role of stimulus identity was examined by including a condition in which the high-complexity stimuli from Experiment 1 were presented in a scrambled arrangement, preventing recognition. The results demonstrated that color contrast increased with the complexity of the stimuli but also highlighted the role of identity, as the condition where the car was recognizable elicited the strongest color induction. We conclude that simultaneous color contrast is strengthened by factors that pertain to both the complexity of the stimuli used and their identity.

Keywords: simultaneous color contrast; structural complexity; identity

1. Introduction

Colors are an integral part of our daily lives, playing a crucial role in the rapid detection and categorization of objects and significantly influencing perceptual judgments [1–4]. Our experience of color is based on the ability to discriminate wavelengths of light reflected by surfaces. This ability is mediated by the activation of cone photoreceptors, which transduce light into neural signals. These signals are then combined to produce opponent responses that are transmitted to the brain [5,6].

However, this description does not fully account for a range of perceptual phenomena related to color appearance. One of the most striking examples is simultaneous color contrast, where a target appears to change its hue due to interactions with its surrounding background [7,8]. The origins of this phenomenon are still debated, but numerous studies have sought to understand variations in its strength under different methodological conditions [9]. For example, the vividness of chromatic induction has been shown to depend on the saturation of the background, with more saturated backgrounds inducing more intense color experiences [10]. Furthermore, the magnitude of simultaneous color contrast has been found to decrease with increasing target-surround contrast. A low-contrast target in a uniform background appears more saturated than the same target in a variegated background, although this difference diminishes as the target's contrast increases [11,12]. Moreover, some authors proposed that simultaneous contrast involves separate "fast" and "slow" mechanisms, with stronger induction effects for fast mechanisms than slow ones [13–15]. In line with this, recent research has suggested that simultaneous color contrast may be linked to the perception of transparency, which tends to be stronger for low-contrast stimuli [16].

Despite these findings, it remains unclear whether higher-order factors such as stimulus identity and structural complexity influence the phenomenon. This study aimed to address this question by creating purpose-built stimuli designed to induce chromatic effects from the background while differing in complexity and identity. The stimuli were carefully balanced for low-level visual properties but systematically varied in terms of structural complexity and the presence or absence of recognizable identity.

2. Methods

2.1. Participants

Thirty participants took part in Experiment 1 (mean age: 22.7 years, SD: 2.56 years; 18 females; age range: 18–30 years) and thirteen participants took part in Experiment 2 (mean age: 22 years, SD: 1.51 years; 9 females; age range: 20–25 years). All participants had normal or corrected-to-normal visual acuity and normal color vision as assessed by the Ishihara Test.

2.2. Assessment of Simultaneous Color Contrast

The magnitude of simultaneous color contrast was measured using a matching procedure. Participants were instructed to match the perceived color of a series of achromatic stimuli (hue: 0°; saturation: 0; value: 0.74) embedded within various chromatic backgrounds (see Figures 1–3 for examples of stimuli employed).

2.2.1. Experiment 1

In Experiment 1, we designed two conditions to investigate the role of structural complexity in the magnitude of color induction. Structural complexity was broadly defined as the level of detail or intricacy within an image [17] with perceived complexity positively correlating with the variety present in a picture [18]. In the first condition, structural complexity was kept "low" (low-complexity condition), where the stimulus to be matched was a simple gray square surrounded by a dark frame and a light frame. In the second condition, structural complexity was relatively "high" (high-complexity condition), where the stimulus to be matched was the body of a car, featuring sketch-like details such as rear-view mirrors, a rear window, rear lights, and a license plate. Importantly, the two stimuli (i.e., the square and the car) were comparable in terms of low-level visual characteristics. The car's body shared the same gray tone and area as the square, while the car's details (e.g., rear-view mirrors, rear window, and rear lights) matched the cumulative area and colors of the two frames surrounding the square in the low-complexity condition. Thus, the primary difference between the two conditions was the level of structural complexity provided (Figure 1).

However, it is worth noting that in the low-complexity condition, the target stimulus was consistently surrounded by a dark frame, whereas in the high-complexity condition, the car's contours directly bordered the background in most areas. To control the potential influence of this difference, we included a control condition in which the stimuli from the low-complexity condition were presented directly bordering the background (Figure 2). In each condition of Experiment 1, participants were shown eight distinct images, each with a different background hue designed to induce varying levels of color in the target stimulus (see Figures 1 and 2).

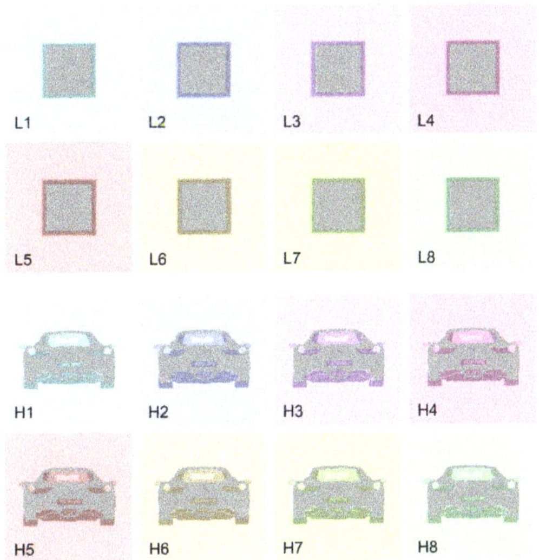

Figure 1. Stimuli employed in Experiment 1. L1 to L8 depict stimuli employed in the low-complexity condition, while H1 to H8 depict stimuli employed in the high-complexity condition.

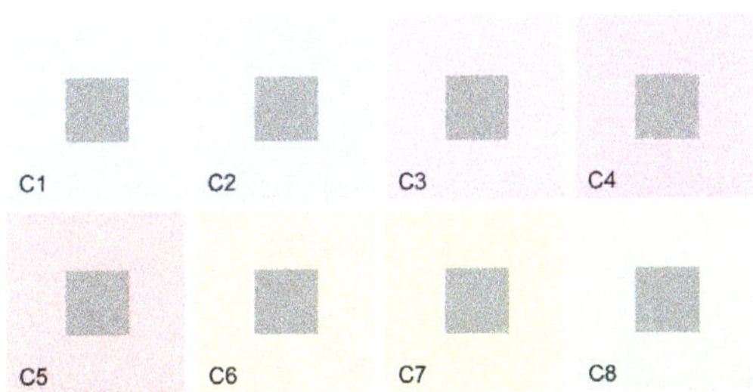

Figure 2. C1 to C8 depict stimuli employed in the control condition in Experiment 1.

2.2.2. Experiment 2

However, we acknowledge that the stimuli used in the two conditions (i.e., low and high complexity) also differed in several other respects. For example, high-complexity stimuli were associated with an "identity", the recognition of the object as a sketched car, while the low-complexity stimuli did not evoke any familiar object beyond a simple geometric shape. Additionally, the high-complexity stimuli included colored details, not only around the contours of the car but also within its body. To control the potential effects of these differences, in Experiment 2, we explored simultaneous color contrast in four new conditions, with a different set of participants.

The first condition mirrored the low-complexity condition from Experiment 1, featuring a simple low-complexity arrangement and the absence of any identifiable stimulus (LC-NoID). The second condition involved a medium-complexity arrangement, incorporating colored details within the achromatic surface but still lacking identity (MC-NoID). The third condition involved a scrambled version of the car image (from the high-complexity condition in Experiment 1), creating a high-complexity arrangement without identity (HC-NoID). Finally, the fourth condition replicated the high-complexity condition from Experiment 1, featuring both high complexity and an identifiable stimulus (HC-ID). These manipulations enabled a thorough examination of the effects of complexity, topological factors related to color arrangements, and identity. Consistent with Experiment 1, the cumulative area covered by the different colors was comparable across all four conditions.

In each condition of Experiment 2, participants were presented with two distinct images, each with a different background hue designed to induce a varying color experience in the target stimulus (see Figure 3).

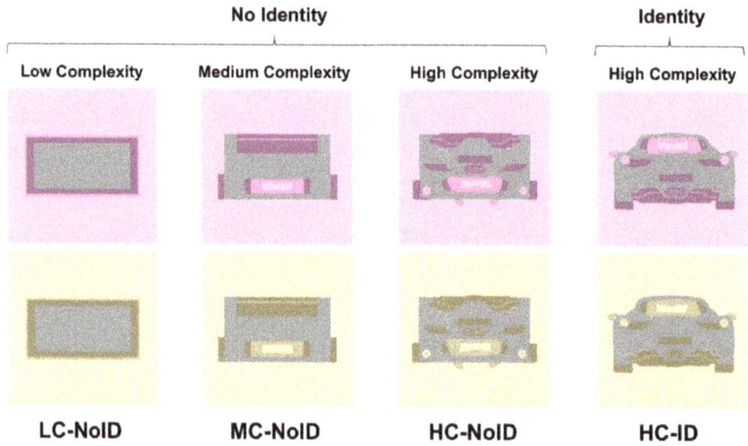

Figure 3. Stimuli employed in Experiment 2. Condition LC-NoID depicted stimuli with a low-complexity arrangement of elements and lack of identity. Condition MC-NoID depicted stimuli with a medium-complexity arrangement and lack of identity. Condition HC-NoID depicted stimuli with a high-complexity arrangement and lack of identity. Condition HC-ID depicted stimuli with a high-complexity arrangement and a clear identity.

2.3. General Procedure and Equipment Details

Stimuli were presented on a linearized and calibrated LED monitor. Participants had to navigate a cursor on a fixed-luminance color-space diagram to change the color of a nearby rectangle (see Figure 4) and were instructed to select the combination of hue (horizontal shift) and saturation (vertical shift) that better matched the target stimulus (color matching). Afterwards, they were asked to classify their perceptual experience by selecting the closest match within a predetermined set of color names (color classification). Each image was displayed three times, and the order of stimuli was randomized.

This procedure generated an RGB triplet corresponding to the response provided to each image. Each RGB triplet was transformed into HSV coordinates using the in-built Matlab function rgb2hsv [19] and, afterwards, hue and saturation values corresponding to the same image were averaged across different trials. The experiment was run using a custom script built in Matlab 2021b (The Mathworks, Inc., Natick, MA, USA) with stimuli being presented using PsychToolbox 3 routines [20].

The calibration and characterization of the display (24 inches, refresh rate: 60 Hz, 1920 $\times$ 1080-pixel resolution) were made using the approach described by Westland and collaborators [21]. We used a Konica Minolta CS-1000 (Chiyoda, Tokyo, Japan) spectrophotometer measuring spectra and colorimetric quantities. With this procedure, we were able to link RGB values with CIE 1931 XYZ values using gogvals and M retrievable in Tables 1 and 2.

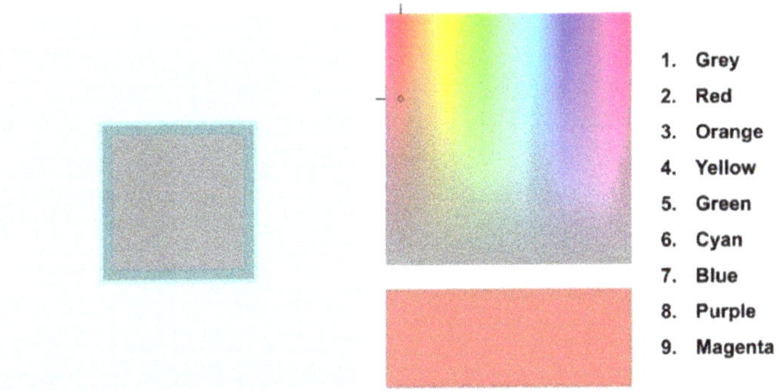

Figure 4. An example of a trial. Participants navigated a cursor (black circle) through a fixed-luminance color-space diagram to find the combination of hue and saturation that better matched the individual perception of the color of the target stimulus (color matching). The rectangle below changed its color according to the position of the cursor. Afterwards, they had to classify their perceptual experience by selecting the closest match within a set of predetermined color names (color classification).

Table 1. Gamma and gain values for the three channels' RGB for the display used in the task.

Gogvals	
2.24	0.91
2.25	0.92
2.21	0.92

Table 2. Transformation matrix from RGB to XYZ for the display used in the task.

	M	
82.8	37.7	29.5
37.8	102.9	13.8
2.3	16.3	150.5

2.4. Statistical Analyses

Analyses were performed using JASP 0.14.1.0 (University of Amsterdam, Amsterdam, The Netherlands). Repeated measures ANOVAs and paired sample *t*-tests were used to compare different experimental conditions. To compensate for violations of sphericity, Greenhouse–Geisser corrections were applied whenever appropriate [22] and corrected *p*-values (but uncorrected degrees of freedom) are reported. Post hoc comparisons were performed using Bonferroni correction.

3. Results

3.1. Experiment 1

The first experiment was designed to test the role played by complexity, defined as the level of detail or intricacy within an image [17]. To contrast differences in saturation responses between low and high complexity from Experiment 1 conditions, we performed a 2 × 8 within-factor ANOVA with complexity (low and high) and color (1 to 8) as factors. Results revealed a highly significant main effect of complexity ($F_{(1,29)}$ = 32.41; $p < 0.001$; $\eta_p{}^2 = 0.52$) explained by higher saturation responses in the high-complexity condition (mean: 0.14) compared to the low-complexity condition (mean: 0.03; $p < 0.001$). Also, a main effect of color emerged ($F_{(7,203)}$ = 15.85; $p < 0.001$; $\eta_p{}^2 = 0.35$) suggesting that the eight background colors elicited different amounts of simultaneous color contrast regardless of complexity. Finally, an interaction between complexity and color emerged ($F_{(7,203)} = 10.57$; $p < 0.001$; $\eta_p^2 = 0.26$), which has to be mainly attributable to differences in the amount of chromatic induction between stimuli selectively evident in the high-complexity condition, rather than representing a lack of difference between low and high complexity for some specific set of stimuli. Indeed, all direct comparisons between low- and high-complexity conditions among the same set of stimuli (e.g., L1 vs. H1, L2 vs. H2, etc.) were highly significant (all $p < 0.001$).

Importantly, the increased saturation responses for the high-complexity condition were evident across almost all the participants as 93.3% of participants reported larger saturation in the high-complexity condition compared to the low-complexity condition. Furthermore, Figure 5 also shows that the two conditions were characterized by a clear difference in terms of variability of responses as in the high-complexity condition, saturation responses varied a lot, spanning from close to 0 to more than 0.5, while in the low complexity, saturation responses were condensed in the range between 0 and 0.08.

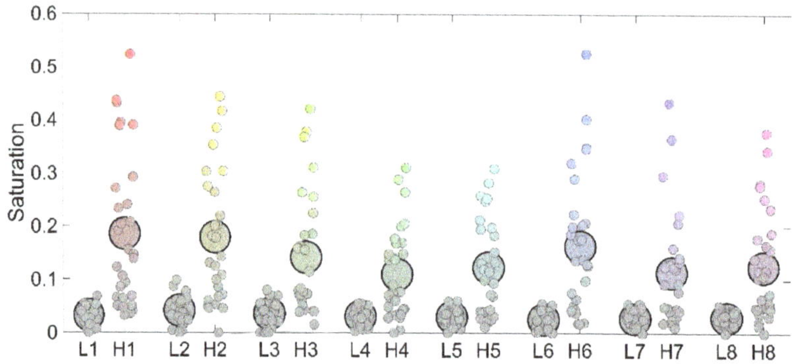

Figure 5. Individual (small dots) and average (large dots) responses to the eight stimuli employed in terms of saturation. The color assigned represents the combination of hue and saturation that each participant chose to best represent the perceived color of the target stimulus. For each image, left-sided dots represent responses in the low-complexity condition while right-sided dots represent responses in the high-complexity condition.

However, one may be convinced that the difference reported between high- and low-complexity conditions could be due to the fact that in the low-complexity condition, a dark frame was continuously interposed between the target stimulus and the background and this was not the same in the high-complexity condition where the body of the car was mostly directly bordering the background. To control the potential role played by this difference, we assessed simultaneous color contrast in an additional control condition in which no frame was interposed between the central gray square and the background. Results made evident that this condition produced results in close agreement with those reported in the low-complexity condition, thus ruling out the possibility that the weak color contrast found in such a condition could be ascribed to the larger amount of interposed dark regions between the target and the background (Figure 6).

These results made evident that the high-complexity condition led to a much larger chromatic induction compared to both the low-complexity and the control condition. This was also evident from the classification task. The percentage of times participants perceived the stimulus as achromatic drastically dropped in the high-complexity condition (Figure 8A). This was evident across all eight stimuli employed, although some variations were present as, for instance, stimuli 3 and 4 had a greater chance to be classified as gray even in the high-complexity condition.

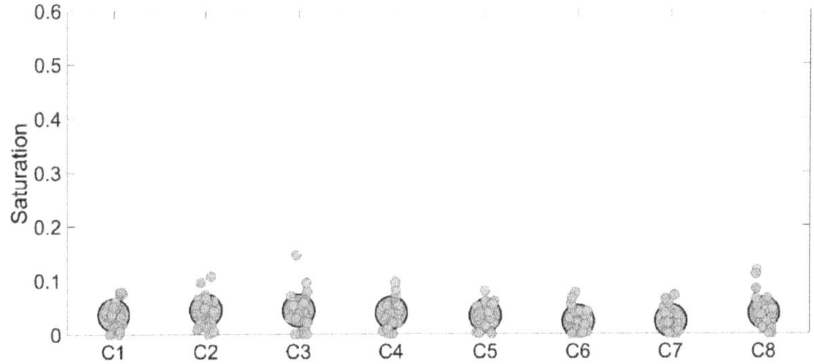

Figure 6. Individual (small dots) and average (large dots) responses to the eight stimuli employed in the control condition in terms of saturation. The color assigned represents the combination of hue and saturation that each participant chose to best represent the perceived color of the target stimulus.

3.2. Experiment 2

In the second experiment, we aimed at stepping further in the direction of results obtained in our first experiment. Indeed, data obtained from Experiment 1 cannot rule out that the increase in the high-complexity condition could be due to other differences between the two conditions such as the presence of colored elements inside the gray area in the high-complexity condition but not in the low-complexity one, or the fact that the high-complexity condition was characterized by a clear stimulus identity (i.e., being a car). Experiment 2 aimed at disentangling such points. Participants were presented with four types of stimuli. The first was identical to the one used in the low-complexity condition of Experiment 1, featuring low complexity and no identifiable shape (LC-NoID). The second had a medium level of complexity, with additional elements distributed within the target stimulus but no identity (MC-NoID). The third had high complexity, created by scrambling elements from the high-complexity stimuli in Experiment 1 to prevent recognition (HC-NoID). The fourth category consisted of the original high-complexity stimuli from Experiment 1, which maintained both high complexity and a recognizable identity (HC-ID).

A 4 × 2 within-factor ANOVA with condition (LC-NoID, MD-NoID, HC-NoID, HC-ID) and color (two levels) as factors was performed. Results revealed a main effect of condition ($F_{(3,36)} = 21.16$; $p < 0.001$; $\eta_p^2 = 0.64$), which was explained by the HC-ID condition producing significantly higher saturation estimates compared to each of the other three conditions (all $p < 0.002$). Also, a condition x color interaction emerged ($F_{(3,36)} = 6.43$; $p = 0.001$; $\eta_p^2 = 0.35$), which was mainly explained by a differential increase in saturation as a function of complexity between the two colors used (see Figure 7). More specifically, the HC-ID condition showed higher saturation estimates compared to all the other conditions for stimuli with a yellow background (Figure 7, right panel), while it showed higher saturation estimates compared to LC-NoID and MC-NoID for stimuli with a magenta background (Figure 7, left panel).

Taken together, the results from Experiment 2 confirm that a complex arrangement of elements within a target stimulus leads to a significantly stronger chromatic induction. Furthermore, these findings highlight the role of stimulus identity in generating color contrast, as the condition using a recognizable stimulus produced the largest chromatic induction. This effect was also evident in the classification task, where the likelihood of participants perceiving the stimulus as achromatic decreased as stimulus complexity and identity increased (Figure 8B).

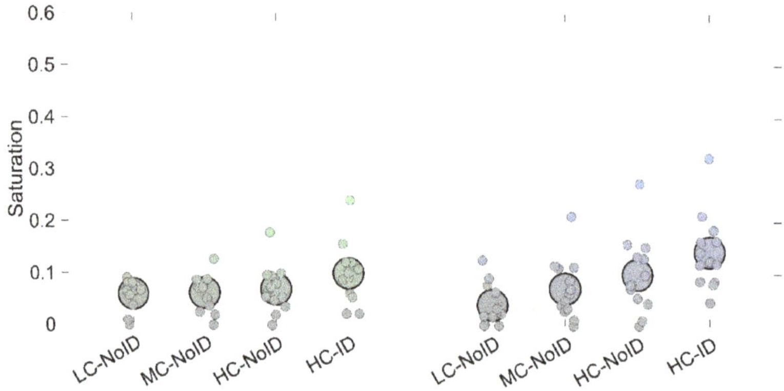

Figure 7. Saturation estimates obtained in the four conditions employed in Experiment 2. The left side depicts stimuli with a magenta background; right-side stimuli had a yellow background. Small dots depict individual while large dots depict average responses.

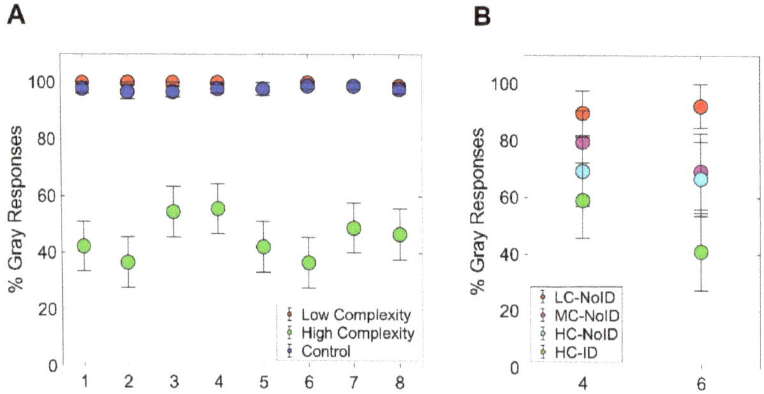

Figure 8. (**A**) Percentages of gray responses obtained in the low-complexity, high-complexity, and control conditions of Experiment 1 for each of the eight stimuli employed. Error bars represent standard errors of the mean. (**B**): Percentages of gray responses obtained in the four conditions employed in Experiment 2 (LC-NoID, MC-NoID, HC-NoID, HC-ID) for each of the two stimuli employed. Error bars represent standard errors of the mean.

4. Discussion

In this study, we further investigated the factors influencing simultaneous color contrast, a phenomenon in which a target stimulus appears to shift its hue as a consequence of the background in which it is embedded [23]. Specifically, the target stimulus tends to shift its hue toward the complementary color of the background. This "illusory" perceptual experience demonstrates that color perception is a global process, influenced by high-order mechanisms. Here, we examined whether factors such as the structural complexity and/or identity of a stimulus play a role in this phenomenon. Participants were asked to match the color of a central achromatic target stimulus embedded in various colored backgrounds by moving a cursor on a fixed-luminance color-space diagram. In Experiment 1, stimuli varied in complexity: low-complexity stimuli consisted of simple squares, while high-complexity stimuli were stylized cars. Our findings support the notion that complexity enhances chromatic induction, as strong chromatic effects were observed exclusively for the high-complexity stimuli. To control low-level differences between the two categories, both low- and high-complexity stimuli were designed to display identical colors, with the cumulative area covered by each color being roughly equivalent. Thus, the primary distinction between the two categories was the degree of structural complexity. Results revealed a pronounced simultaneous color contrast effect for high-complexity stimuli, whereas low-complexity stimuli induced only a faint color hue in the achromatic target.

Additionally, the high-complexity condition exhibited greater interindividual variability in saturation responses compared to the low-complexity condition, in which responses were more uniform. However, one might argue that differences in contour transitions between the target and background could have contributed to these results, as previous research has shown that contours influence the strength of simultaneous color contrast [24]. To address this concern, we included a condition with gray squares embedded in colored backgrounds but without any surrounding frame. The results for this condition closely resembled those of the low-complexity condition, suggesting that contour differences were unlikely to account for the observed effects.

Since the two stimulus categories also differed in other aspects, such as the topographical arrangement of colored elements and stimulus identity, Experiment 2 was designed to control for these confounds. In this experiment, we introduced two additional conditions to disentangle the roles of stimulus identity and topological complexity. Results showed that saturation estimates increased with stimulus complexity. Notably, the condition featuring a recognizable car (HC-ID) elicited significantly stronger saturation estimates compared to both simpler stimuli and the condition with a scrambled car (HC-NoID). This finding suggests that the stronger saturation effects observed in the high-complexity condition of Experiment 1 were not solely driven by structural complexity but also by the identity of the stimulus. Our results align with previous evidence on the relationship between transparency perception and simultaneous color contrast, which suggests that a more realistic perception of transparency enhances color contrast [16]. One possibility is that increasing the complexity and topological distribution of colored elements within the target stimulus helps observers estimate the filter's transmittance, resulting in a more vivid color illusion. A similar effect may apply to identity: when the target is a recognizable object, it may strengthen the impression of viewing a real image through a transparent filter.

In summary, our findings suggest that the structural components of an image contribute to the strength of chromatic induction. Specifically, more "realistic" images appear to elicit a more vivid illusion of color. We speculate that this may be due to higher-order cognitive processes related to the identity of the stimulus, which are bound to its structural complexity.

Author Contributions: P.A.G., M.G. and A.F. conceived the experiments. P.A.G. performed the experiments and analyzed data. R.F. collected data. P.A.G., F.T., R.F., E.B., A.F. and M.G. contributed to interpreting data, and writing and revising the manuscript. All authors have read and agreed to the published version of the manuscript.

Funding: This research received no external funding.

Institutional Review Board Statement: The study was conducted in accordance with the Declaration of Helsinki and approved by the local ethics committee ("Commissione per l'Etica e l'Integrità nella Ricerca", CNR, 5 September 2024, Prot. n. 0306205).

Informed Consent Statement: Informed consent was obtained from all participants involved in the study.

Data Availability Statement: The raw data were deposited in the Zenodo repository and are publicly available at the following link: https://zenodo.org/records/14541019 (accessed on 3 February 2025).

Acknowledgments: The study was conducted with the contribution of the researcher Paolo Antonino Grasso with a research contract co-funded by the European Union—PON Research and Innovation 2014–2020—in accordance with Article 24, paragraph 3a, of Law No. 240 of 30 December 2010, as amended, and Ministerial Decree No. 1062 of 10 August 2021.

Conflicts of Interest: The authors declare no competing interests.

References

1. D'Zmura, M. Color in Visual Search. *Vision Res.* **1991**, *31*, 951–966. [CrossRef]
2. Grasso, P.A.; Anobile, G.; Arrighi, R.; Burr, D.C.; Cicchini, G.M. Numerosity Perception Is Tuned to Salient Environmental Features. *iScience* **2022**, *25*, 104104. [CrossRef] [PubMed]
3. Hansen, T.; Olkkonen, M.; Walter, S.; Gegenfurtner, K.R. Memory Modulates Color Appearance. *Nat. Neurosci.* **2006**, *9*, 1367–1368. [CrossRef] [PubMed]
4. Caponi, C.; Castaldi, E.; Grasso, P.A.; Arrighi, R. Feature-Selective Adaptation of Numerosity Perception. *Proc. B* **2025**, *292*, 1841. [CrossRef]
5. Gegenfurtner, K.R. Cortical Mechanisms of Colour Vision. *Nat. Rev. Neurosci.* **2003**, *4*, 563–572. [CrossRef]
6. Stockman, A.; Sharpe, L.T. The Spectral Sensitivities of the Middle- and Long-Wavelength-Sensitive Cones Derived from Measurements in Observers of Known Genotype. *Vision Res.* **2000**, *40*, 1711–1737. [CrossRef] [PubMed]
7. Hurlbert, A.; Wolf, K. Color Contrast: A Contributory Mechanism to Color Constancy. *Prog. Brain Res.* **2004**, *144*, 145–160.
8. Lotto, R.B.; Purves, D. An Empirical Explanation of Color Contrast. *Proc. Natl. Acad. Sci. USA* **2000**, *97*, 12834–12839. [CrossRef] [PubMed]
9. Ratnasingam, S.; Anderson, B.L. What Predicts the Strength of Simultaneous Color Contrast. *J. Vis.* **2017**, *17*, 13. [CrossRef] [PubMed]
10. Bosten, J.M.; Mollon, J.D. Kirschmann's Fourth Law. *Vision Res.* **2012**, *53*, 40–46. [CrossRef] [PubMed]
11. Ekroll, V.; Faul, F. A Simple Model Describes Large Individual Differences in Simultaneous Colour Contrast. *Vision Res.* **2009**, *49*, 2261–2272. [CrossRef]
12. Ekroll, V.; Faul, F.; Wendt, G. The Strengths of Simultaneous Colour Contrast and the Gamut Expansion Effect Correlate across Observers: Evidence for a Common Mechanism. *Vision Res.* **2011**, *51*, 311–322. [CrossRef] [PubMed]
13. Kaneko, S.; Murakami, I.; Kuriki, I.; Peterzell, D.H. Individual Variability in Simultaneous Contrast for Color and Brightness: Small Sample Factor Analyses Reveal Separate Induction Processes for Short and Long Flashes. *Iperception* **2018**, *9*, 1–22. [CrossRef] [PubMed]
14. Kaneko, S.; Murakami, I. Flashed Stimulation Produces Strong Simultaneous Brightness and Color Contrast. *J. Vis.* **2012**, *12*, 1. [CrossRef]
15. Kaneko, S.; Anstis, S.; Kuriki, I. Brief Presentation Enhances Various Simultaneous Contrast Effects. *J. Vis.* **2017**, *17*, 7. [CrossRef] [PubMed]
16. Ekroll, V.; Faul, F. Transparency Perception: The Key to Understanding Simultaneous Color Contrast. *J. Opt. Soc. Am. A* **2013**, *30*, 342–352. [CrossRef] [PubMed]
17. Snodgrass, J.G.; Vanderwart, M. A Standardized Set of 260 Pictures: Norms for Name Agreement, Image Agreement, Familiarity, and Visual Complexity. *J. Exp. Psychol. Hum. Learn. Mem.* **1980**, *6*, 174–215. [CrossRef] [PubMed]
18. Heylighen, F. The Growth of Structural and Functional Complexity During Evolution. *Evol. Complex.* **1999**, *8*, 17–44.
19. Smith, A.R. Color Gamut Transform Pairs. In *Proceedings of the 5th Annual Conference on Computer Graphics and Interactive Techniques*; SIGGRAPH: New York, NY, USA, 1978.
20. Kleiner, M.; Brainard, D.H.; Pelli, D.G.; Broussard, C.; Wolf, T.; Niehorster, D. What's New in Psychtoolbox-3? *Perception* **2007**, *36*, 1–16.
21. Westland, S.; Ripamonti, C.; Cheung, V. *Computational Colour Science Using MATLAB®*, 2nd ed.; John Wiley & Sons: Hoboken, NJ, USA, 2012.
22. Greenhouse, S.W.; Geisser, S. On Methods in the Analysis of Profile Data. *Psychometrika* **1959**, *24*, 95–112. [CrossRef]
23. Soranzo, A. Simultaneous Contrast, Simultaneous Brightness Contrast, Simultaneous Color. In *Encyclopedia of Color Science and Technology*; Springer: New York, NY, USA, 2015.
24. Kanematsu, T.; Koida, K. Large Enhancement of Simultaneous Color Contrast by White Flanking Contours. *Sci. Rep.* **2020**, *10*, 20136. [CrossRef] [PubMed]

life

MDPI

Article

Evaluation of Static and Dynamic Pupil and Light Sensitivity to a Single Drop of Various Concentrations of Low-Dose Atropine (0.01%, 0.025%, and 0.05%)

Muteb K. Alanazi [1,*], Abdulmalik Almansour [1], Sarah S. Almutairi [1], Ahmad Alharbi [1], Mohammed S. Alhazmi [1], Ali Almustanyir [1], Basal H. Altoaimi [1], Meznah S. Almutairi [1], Mona M. Alamri [1] and Maria Liu [2]

[1] Optometry Department, College of Applied Medical Sciences, King Saud University, Riyadh 11362, Saudi Arabia; 441100366@student.ksu.edu.sa (A.A.); 441200446@student.ksu.edu.sa (S.S.A.); ahmaalharbi@ksu.edu.sa (A.A.); malhazmyi@ksu.edu.sa (M.S.A.); aalmustanyir@ksu.edu.sa (A.A.); baltoaimi@ksu.edu.sa (B.H.A.); mzalmutairi@ksu.edu.sa (M.S.A.); malamrie@ksu.edu.sa (M.M.A.)

[2] School of Optometry, University of California, Berkeley, CA 94720, USA; marialiu@berkeley.edu

* Correspondence: mkalanazi@ksu.edu.sa; Tel.: +966-118063613

Abstract: This study aimed to evaluate the static and dynamic pupil changes, and light sensitivity following a single dose of low-dose atropine at concentrations of 0.01%, 0.025%, and 0.05% over a 24 h period. Healthy young adults (20–22 years; n = 25) participated in this randomized, double-blind study. Each participant received one of three atropine concentrations in a masked fashion. Baseline mesopic and dynamic pupil sizes were measured at various post-instillation intervals (5 min, 30 min, 1 h, 2 h, 4 h, and 24 h). A minimum 48 h washout period was observed between treatments. Subjective light sensitivity was assessed using the Visual Light Sensitivity Questionnaire (VLSQ-8) at 24 h. All atropine concentrations caused significant pupil dilation ($p < 0.001$), with the 0.05% concentration producing the greatest dilation (peak mesopic size: 7.4 mm, $p < 0.001$) and the slowest recovery at 24 h (6.4 mm, $p < 0.001$). The dynamic pupil constriction range was most restricted with 0.05% (1.7 mm, $p < 0.05$), compared to 0.025% (2.2 mm) and 0.01% (2.6 mm). Subjective symptoms, including light sensitivity and glare, followed a dose-dependent pattern ($p < 0.05$). In 60% participants, 0.05% caused the most symptoms, while in 70% participants, 0.01% caused the least. Despite significant pupil dilation, the pupil center coordinates did not shift significantly along the horizontal or vertical axes ($p > 0.05$). Low-dose atropine induced dose-dependent pupil dilation and light sensitivity; 0.05% atropine caused the most pronounced effects. These findings underscore the importance of tailoring the atropine dosage to balance its efficacy and tolerability. Further studies are needed to explore the long-term impact of repeated dosing on pupillary behavior and subjective symptoms.

Keywords: low-dose atropine; pupil; light sensitivity; dynamic pupil

1. Introduction

Currently, approximately one-third of the world's population is myopic, a prevalence projected to reach 50% by 2050, affecting nearly five billion people worldwide [1]. This alarming rise in myopia prevalence represents more than a refractive inconvenience; it is a significant public health concern that could lead to substantial vision loss. The risks of vision-threatening conditions, including myopic maculopathy, cataracts, retinal detachment, and glaucoma [2] have been associated with myopia [3].

These complications are particularly pronounced in individuals with moderate (spherical equivalent ≤−3.0 to >−6.0 D) and high myopia (spherical equivalent ≤−6.0 D). The earlier the onset of myopia in childhood, the greater the likelihood of progression to severe forms, thereby increasing the lifetime risk of vision loss and economic burden [4,5]. Thus, early and effective management of myopia progression is crucial.

Several myopia control strategies have been investigated, demonstrating effectiveness rates ranging from 10 to 77%, depending on patient-specific factors, such as age, baseline refractive error, and treatment adherence. Myopia management approaches generally fall into two categories: optical treatments (e.g., overnight orthokeratology, peripheral defocus spectacle lenses, and soft multifocal contact lenses) and pharmaceutical interventions (e.g., atropine eye drops). Atropine eye drops are among the most widely studied and used options due to their effectiveness in slowing axial elongation and refractive error progression. However, higher concentrations of atropine (1% and 0.5%) are associated with significant side effects, including photophobia, near-vision blurring, and a higher risk of myopic rebound upon cessation. These disadvantages have shifted the focus toward low-dose atropine (≤0.05%), which still offers clinically meaningful efficacy with fewer side effects [6–9].

Low-dose atropine concentrations, particularly 0.01% and 0.025%, have gained widespread acceptance due to their ability to minimize pupil dilation and accommodation impairment compared to higher doses. Studies suggest that atropine concentrations of up to 0.02% cause negligible photophobia and blurring. Atropine at 0.01% remains the preferred starting concentration because of its excellent tolerability [10], though its myopia control efficacy is lower compared to 0.025% and 0.05% concentrations [11]. Despite these advantages, limited research has investigated the effects of low-dose atropine on static and dynamic pupillary behavior and light sensitivity across different concentrations. Understanding these effects is critical, as pupil size and responsiveness to light directly influence visual comfort, functional vision, and treatment adherence. Additionally, while higher concentrations of atropine are known to cause more pronounced physiological effects, there are limited data on pupil dynamics and subjective light sensitivity symptoms at low-dose concentrations of atropine. This information is essential for optimizing dosing strategies and balancing tolerability with clinical efficacy.

This study aimed to evaluate static and dynamic pupil changes and subjective light sensitivity over a 24 h period following a single application of low-dose atropine at concentrations of 0.01%, 0.025%, and 0.05% in healthy young adults. By investigating the physiological and subjective effects of these low-dose atropine concentrations, the findings contribute to tailoring atropine use to individual patient needs; this addresses tolerability concerns in myopia control and other clinical applications.

2. Materials and Methods

This randomized, blinded study enrolled 25 healthy young adults (15 males and 10 females) aged 20–22 years, all with no history of ocular or systemic diseases. Participants were screened for normal ocular health through comprehensive eye examinations, including best-corrected visual acuity (BCVA), slit-lamp biomicroscopy, and dilated fundus examination.

Participants were randomly assigned to receive a single drop of either 0.05%, 0.025%, or 0.01% atropine in both eyes. Both participants and examiners were masked to the assigned concentrations. Baseline static and dynamic pupil size measurements were taken before drop instillation. Mesopic and dynamic pupil responses were measured in an environment with an ambient light level of 20 lux using a MYAH (Topcon Healthcare Inc., Tokyo, Japan) at specific intervals: immediately after atropine instillation, and at 5 min, 30 min, 1 h, 2 h, 4 h, and 24 h. To control for diurnal variations, all baseline pupil measurements and atropine drop instillations for the three doses were conducted between 8:00 a.m. and 10:00 a.m.

Self-reported light sensitivity associated with pupil dilation was assessed at the 24 h time point for each concentration using the validated Visual Light Sensitivity Questionnaire (VLSQ-8) [12]. A 48 h washout period was implemented between doses to minimize carryover effects. This period starts 24 h after the drop instillation of the previous dose, ensuring a minimum of 36 h between atropine administrations. Previous studies on low-dose atropine, including 0.01%, have indicated that significant pupil changes and symptoms generally resolve within 18–24 h, supporting the adequacy of this interval for eliminating any residual effects [13].

This study was conducted in accordance with the guidelines of the Declaration of Helsinki and received approval from the Institutional Review Board of the College of Medicine, King Saud University (E-22-6783). Informed consent was obtained from all participants after the nature and purpose of the study were described.

Preservative-free atropine sulfate eye drops (0.01%, 0.025%, and 0.05%) were aseptically compounded by ImprimisRx (Irvine, CA, USA) and provided in single-dose vials. Each vial contained 5 mL of solution, which was stable for 6 months and stored at room temperature.

Statistical analysis included a summary of demographic and ocular characteristics, such as age, spherical equivalent (SE), axial length, best-corrected visual acuity, pupil size, and amplitude (Table 1). Continuous measurements were presented as mean ± standard deviation.

Table 1. Demographic and ocular characteristics of the study participants (N = 25).

	Mean ± SD	Range
Age (years)	21.1 ± 0.7	20–22
Best-corrected visual acuity (LogMAR)	0.013 ± 0.05	−0.1–+0.1
Spherical equivalent (D)	−1.3 ± 2.2	−6.7–+2.1
Axial length (mm)	24.2 ± 1.2	22.05–26.9

Repeated-measures analysis of variance (ANOVA) was employed to evaluate changes in mesopic and dynamic pupil sizes over the 24 h period. In this design, atropine concentrations (0.01%, 0.025%, and 0.05%) and eye (left or right) were considered within-subject factors, meaning that each participant was exposed to all three atropine concentrations, and pupil measurements were collected for both eyes of the same individual, allowing the direct comparison of effects across the different concentrations and between eyes within the same participant. Additionally, interactions between atropine concentration and eye were analyzed to determine whether the effects of atropine concentration differed significantly between the two eyes. Group comparisons were also performed using repeated-measures ANOVA, with post hoc multiple comparisons adjusted using the Bonferroni correction to control for Type I errors. Statistical significance level was set at 5% ($p < 0.05$). All statistical analyses were conducted using IBM SPSS Statistics version 29 (IBM Corp., Armonk, NY, USA).

3. Results

The pupil size data were collected from both eyes. No significant interocular differences were found between the two eyes ($p > 0.05$) for the main and interaction effects in the static and dynamic pupil size measurements. Thus, only data from the right eye were reported. The study demonstrated significant pupil dilation across all concentrations of low-dose atropine, with effects varying based on the dose. At baseline, the average mesopic pupil sizes were similar across concentrations, measuring 5.34 ± 0.8 mm, 5.35 ± 0.8 mm, and 5.43 ± 0.8 mm for 0.01%, 0.025%, and 0.05%, respectively. At 30 min post-instillation, mesopic pupil sizes increased to 6.2 mm, 6.4 mm, and 6.7 mm for 0.01%, 0.025%, and 0.05%, respectively. Peak dilation occurred at 4 h, with mean pupil sizes reaching 7.4 ± 0.6 mm, 7.1 ± 0.5 mm, and 6.7 ± 0.5 mm for 0.05%, 0.025%, and 0.01%, respectively. Partial recovery was observed by 24 h; however, mean pupil sizes remained elevated compared to baseline, measuring 6.4 mm, 6.3 mm, and 6.0 mm, respectively (Figure 1).

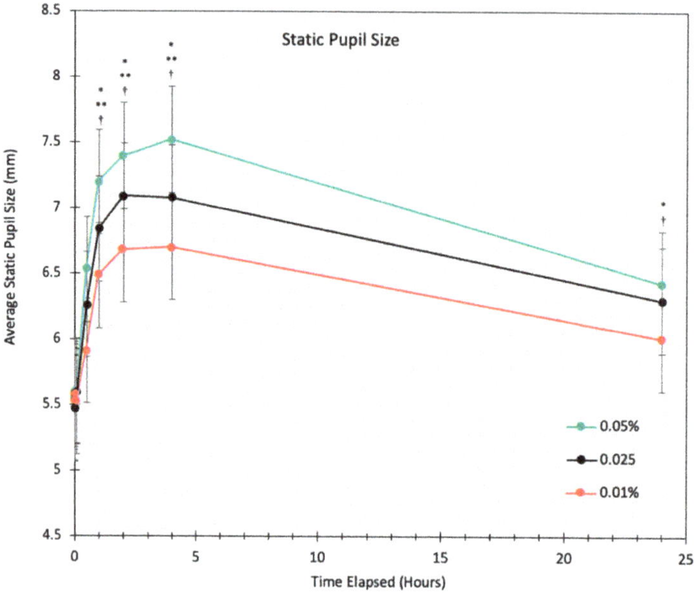

Figure 1. The static mesopic pupil size (mm) over a 24 h period for 0.01%, 0.025%, and 0.05% atropine concentrations. Error bars represent the standard error of the mean (SEM). An asterisk (*) indicates a significant difference in pupil size with 0.05% compared to 0.01% ($p < 0.05$) with adjustment for multiple comparisons (Bonferroni). A double asterisk (**) indicates a significant difference in pupil size with 0.05% compared to 0.025% ($p < 0.05$) with adjustment for multiple comparisons (Bonferroni). A dagger (†) indicates a significant difference in pupil size with 0.025% compared to 0.01% ($p < 0.05$) with adjustment for multiple comparisons (Bonferroni).

Dynamic pupil responses, measured as the difference between maximum and minimum pupil sizes, revealed a dose-dependent reduction in the constriction range. The smallest dynamic pupil range was observed with 0.05% atropine (1.7 mm), compared to 2.2 mm for 0.025% and 2.6 mm for 0.01% (Figure 2). The analysis also revealed that there were no significant differences between male and female participants in static pupil size, minimum dynamic pupil size, or maximum dynamic pupil size, either as a main effect or in interaction with atropine concentration (all $p > 0.05$).

At baseline, the pupil center was displaced approximately 0.24 ± 0.014 mm nasally and 0.1 ± 0.09 mm inferiorly. Following the instillation of all three low-dose atropine concentrations, the pupil center remained consistently displaced nasally and inferiorly over the 24 h period. No significant shift in the pupil center was observed over time or when the three atropine concentrations were compared ($p > 0.05$).

Subjective light sensitivity scores collected using the Visual Light Sensitivity Questionnaire (VLSQ-8), demonstrated a clear dose-dependent trend. Participants reported significantly higher overall symptom scores for 0.05% atropine (20.7 ± 5.9) compared to 0.025% (16.8 ± 5.5) and 0.01% (13.2 ± 4.7). Specific symptoms, such as glare, blurred vision, and outdoor daylight sensitivity, were most pronounced with 0.05% atropine (Table 2).

Participants were also asked to guess the concentration that caused the most and least symptoms after trying all three doses. Despite being blinded to the atropine concentration, 63% (15 participants) correctly identified 0.05% as causing the most symptoms, and 71% (17 participants) correctly identified 0.01% as causing the least symptoms, further supporting the subjective nature of dose-dependent symptom perception (Table 3).

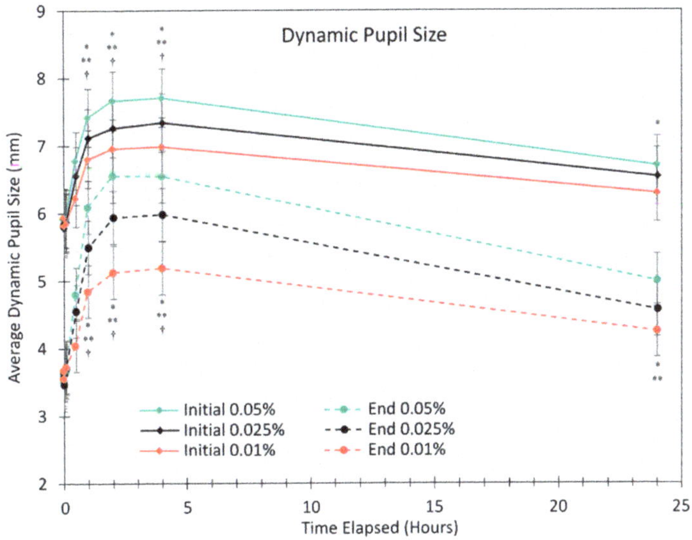

Figure 2. The initial (constriction to a light flash) and end (maximum re-dilation after a light flash) pupil size (mm) over a 24 h period for 0.01%, 0.025%, and 0.05% atropine concentrations. Error bars represent the standard error of the mean (SEM). An asterisk (*) indicates a significant difference in pupil size between 0.05% and 0.01% ($p < 0.05$), adjusted for multiple comparisons (Bonferroni). A double asterisk (**) indicates a significant difference in pupil size between 0.05% and 0.025% ($p < 0.05$), adjusted for multiple comparisons (Bonferroni). A dagger (†) indicates a significant difference in pupil size between 0.025% and 0.01% ($p < 0.05$), adjusted for multiple comparisons (Bonferroni).

Table 2. Visual Light Sensitivity Questionnaire (VLSQ-8) scores for individual items across atropine concentrations (0.01%, 0.025%, and 0.05%). Data are presented as mean ± standard deviation (SD).

Questionnaire Item	0.01% Mean ± SD	0.025% Mean ± SD	0.05% Mean ± SD
Outdoor Daylight	1.9 ± 1	2.7 ± 1.5 *	3.2 ± 1.1 *
Glare	1.5 ± 0.8	2 ± 1.1	2.6 ± 1.4 *
Flickering lights	1.6 ± 0.8	2.2 ± 1.2	2.6 ± 1.3 *
Severity	1.7 ± 0.8	2.2 ± 1	2.9 ± 1 *†
Headache	1.5 ± 0.9	1.6 ± 0.8	2 ± 0.8
Blur vision	1.7 ± 0.9	2.5 ± 1.1 *	2.9 ± 1.4 *
limitations	1.7 ± 0.9	2.1 ± 1.2	2.2 ± 1.2
Dark glasses	1.8 ± 1.4	1.7 ± 1.2	2.4 ± 1.5
Overall Score	13.2 ± 4.7	16.8 ± 5.5 *	20.7 ± 5.9 *†

An asterisk (*) indicates a significant difference compared to 0.01% ($p < 0.05$), and a dagger (†) indicates a significant difference compared to 0.025% ($p < 0.05$), both adjusted for multiple comparisons using the Bonferroni method.

A significant negative correlation was found between the overall symptom scores and the magnitude of change in dynamic pupil size at 1, 2, and 4 h post-instillation, with Pearson correlation coefficients of −0.298, −0.345, and −0.280, respectively (all $p < 0.05$). These associations indicate that larger dynamic pupil changes are associated with lower symptom scores, suggesting an inverse relationship between pupil adaptability and symptom severity.

Table 3. The number of participants who identified the atropine concentration based on experienced symptoms.

	Guessed Atropine Concentration Correctly	Guessed Atropine Concentration Incorrectly	Unable to Differentiate
Least symptoms (0.01% Atropine)	17	5	3
Most symptoms (0.05% Atropine)	15	8	2

4. Discussion

This study highlights the concentration-dependent effects of low-dose atropine on pupillary behavior, light sensitivity, and subjective visual symptoms. The significant pupil dilation observed at all concentrations aligns with atropine's pharmacological inhibition of parasympathetic activity. Despite substantial changes in pupil size, the lack of significant shifts in pupil center coordinates along the horizontal (X) and vertical (Y) axes suggests that atropine-induced dilation does not alter the spatial alignment of the pupil. This finding is clinically relevant, as significant displacement of the pupil center could affect higher-order optical aberrations and visual function.

Dynamic pupil behavior demonstrated a dose-dependent reduction in the constriction range, with 0.05% atropine causing the most pronounced impairment. This suggests that higher concentrations not only prolong dilation, but also hinder the pupil's ability to respond dynamically to changing light conditions. While this effect was less pronounced at lower concentrations, it underscores the need for caution when prescribing higher doses, particularly in patients requiring good photopic vision.

Subjective light sensitivity data revealed that higher atropine concentrations resulted in more pronounced visual symptoms, such as glare and discomfort. Interestingly, participants were able to accurately identify the concentration causing the most symptoms (0.05%) and the least symptoms (0.01%) in most cases despite being blinded to the concentrations. This finding reinforces the subjective impact of dose-dependent side effects and highlights the importance of patient education regarding potential symptoms during atropine therapy. While higher concentrations may offer greater efficacy for myopia control, the associated symptoms could reduce adherence, particularly in pediatric populations.

In addition to directly antagonizing muscarinic receptors, atropine's effects on pupil dynamics and light sensitivity are affected by other pharmacological factors. The interaction of atropine with melanin in the iris can modulate its duration of action, as dark-brown irises with high melanin content bind more atropine molecules, potentially delaying its release into intraocular tissues. This can result in a slower onset but prolonged duration of action. Conversely, lighter-colored irises with lower melanin content may allow faster atropine penetration but shorter drug retention, resulting in a quicker yet shorter-lived effect. Furthermore, the transcorneal absorption and systemic clearance of atropine contribute to individual variability in its pharmacodynamic profile. These factors show the complexity of atropine's effects and highlight the importance of considering both pharmacological mechanisms and individual characteristics when designing personalized atropine regimens [14,15].

This study's findings align with those of Tran et al. (2024), who tested the daily administration of three low-dose atropine concentrations (0.01%, 0.02%, and 0.03%) in children for 2 weeks. Their results demonstrated a dose-dependent increase in pupil dilation with low-dose atropine, with higher concentrations inducing greater dilation, and more eyes experiencing pupil dilation exceeding 3 mm [16]. In contrast, the current study found that a single drop of low-dose atropine caused pupillary dilation lasting up to 24 h. Specifically, the proportion of eyes showing at least a 1 mm increase in mesopic pupil size 24 h after post-instillation was 16%, 68%, and 76% for 0.01%, 0.025%, and 0.05% concentrations, respectively. Notably, no eyes in this study exhibited pupil dilation exceeding 3 mm at the 24 h time point, suggesting that the greater pupil dilation observed in Tran et al.'s study is likely due to the cumulative effect associated with repeated daily doses over a 2-week period.

Kaymak et al. demonstrated significant pupil dilation under both photopic and mesopic conditions after a single drop of lower-concentration atropine (0.01%, 0.005%, and 0.001%). Similar to the current study, the effect of pupil dilation in Kaymak et al.'s study persisted for at least 24 h, with partial recovery observed during this period, even at much lower concentrations [17]. Additionally, Kaymak et al. reported increased variability in pupil size following a single drop, potentially influenced by iris pigmentation or atropine penetration variability. In contrast, the current study did not show any significantly increased variability, likely because all participants were Middle Eastern with dark brown irises. This homogenous population may have reduced variability and allowed for clearer correlations between pupil dynamics and subjective symptoms.

The significant correlation observed between the total symptom scores and the magnitude of dynamic pupil size changes at 1, 2, and 4 h post-instillation can be attributed to the critical role of dynamic pupil behavior in adapting to varying light conditions. Dynamic pupil size changes reflect the pupil's ability to respond to light stimuli, regulating retinal light exposure, and consequently mitigating photosensitivity symptoms. This relationship highlights the functional importance of dynamic pupil adaptability in maintaining visual comfort, particularly in the context of atropine-induced dilation.

No significant correlation was observed at earlier time points (before 1 h), likely because the drops had not yet induced maximal dilation. Similarly, no significant correlation was observed at the 24 h mark, as the drops' effects on pupil size had begun to wear off, reducing its impact on the photosensitivity symptom score. These findings align with the physiological timeline of atropine's pharmacodynamics, where the most significant dilation typically begins approximately 1 h post-instillation and peaks at approximately 4 h under both mesopic and dynamic conditions.

The data further demonstrated that low-dose atropine affected both mesopic and dynamic pupil behavior, with the largest dilation occurring between 1 and 4 h post-administration. This highlights a critical period where patients are most likely to experience photosensitivity symptoms, correlating directly with the magnitude of dynamic pupillary changes. These results emphasize the need to address dynamic pupil effects when designing more tolerable atropine regimens, as reducing dynamic changes could help alleviate symptoms and improve adherence. These findings align with those of Cooper et al., who identified 0.02% atropine as the maximum concentration at which no significant symptoms were produced [10].

The myopia inhibition mechanisms of atropine remain unclear, and accommodation-related effects have been ruled out [18]. Atropine mimics light stimulation by enhancing nitric oxide and dopamine release and increasing contrast sensitivity at intermediate spatial frequencies [19–22]. Atropine likely does not act through muscarinic receptors, as the concentrations required for myopia suppression exceed those needed to saturate these receptors. Atropine also binds to alpha-adrenergic receptors, which may contribute to its effects. A 0.01% atropine drop is estimated to produce vitreal concentrations exceeding the M4 receptor half-saturation threshold, while lower doses (0.005% or 0.001%) approach this threshold. Although daily atropine use may lead to accumulation due to its prolonged effects on pupil size, this is less likely at lower doses. Further studies are needed to confirm whether accumulation occurs and its impact on pupillary behavior during prolonged application.

This study had some limitations. First, the sample size was small and limited to only young adults, which may limit the generalizability of the findings. While the randomized crossover design lessened variability by allowing each participant to serve as their own control, larger sample sizes are needed in future studies to validate these results and strengthen the conclusions drawn. Future studies should investigate pediatric populations with larger sample sizes. Second, all participants were Middle Eastern with dark-brown irises. Iris pigmentation may influence interocular absorption and the duration of action of low-dose atropine. Dark-colored irises with high melanin content bind more atropine molecules than light-colored irises, potentially delaying drug release into intraocular tissues [23,24]. This may be associated with a more gradual onset of action, but may have an advantage in prolonging the effect of the drug because atropine is gradually released from melanin stores. In contrast, lighter-colored irises containing less melanin may allow quicker atropine penetration and shorter drug retention, thereby producing a quicker but probably shorter duration of action. This variability could explain individual differences in pupil size changes and symptom duration following low-dose atropine, depending on iris pigmentation. These findings could have important implications for optimizing atropine regimens, especially among different populations. Expanding the study to include participants with diverse iris colors, particularly lighter-colored irises, would provide a broader understanding of how pigmentation influences atropine's effects, including pupil dynamics and symptom variability. Third, the accommodative response following a single low dose of atropine was not measured in this study, which limits our ability to fully understand the functional impact of atropine on near vision and how it may contribute to subjective symptoms like blurred vision. Lastly, a formal statistical power calculation was not performed before the study, possibly affecting the generalizability of the findings. While significant results were found, future studies with larger sample sizes and pre-calculated power analyses are needed to validate and build upon these findings.

These results also emphasize the need for individualized treatment strategies. Lower concentrations, such as 0.01%, may provide a more tolerable option for patients prioritizing visual comfort, whereas higher doses may be reserved for those requiring maximal myopia control efficacy. Clinicians should also consider alternative strategies, such as alternate-day dosing, to minimize side effects. Future research should investigate the long-term effects of daily low-dose atropine on pupil dynamics and subjective symptoms. Additionally, studies assessing the impact of repeated dosing on static and dynamic pupil changes would provide further insights into atropine-induced dilation and the associated light sensitivity symptoms.

5. Conclusions

This study demonstrated the dose-dependent effects of low-dose atropine (0.01%, 0.025%, and 0.05%) on static and dynamic pupil behavior, as well as subjective light sensitivity, in a controlled cohort of young adults. Significant pupil dilation was observed across all concentrations, with the 0.05% dose producing the most pronounced and sustained effects. Dynamic pupil responses revealed a dose-dependent reduction in constriction range, suggesting that higher atropine concentrations impair the pupil's ability to adapt to changing light conditions. Subjective symptoms, including glare and light sensitivity, followed a similar dose-dependent pattern, underscoring the trade-off between therapeutic efficacy and tolerability.

These findings highlight the need for individualized atropine dosing strategies that balance efficacy with minimizing adverse effects, particularly for long-term use in myopia control. While higher concentrations demonstrate greater physiological effects, they are associated with increased visual symptoms, which may impact treatment adherence, especially in pediatric populations. The study establishes foundational data on short-term of a single drop of low dose atropine concentrations, providing a foundation for future research exploring its use in pediatric populations and long-term treatment to improve both clinical outcomes and patient comfort.

Author Contributions: Conceptualization, M.K.A. and M.L.; Methodology, formal analysis, investigation, and data curation, A.A. (Abdulmalik Almansour), S.S.A., A.A. (Ahmad Alharbi) and M.M.A.; Manuscript writing, M.K.A., B.H.A., M.S.A. (Meznah S. Almutairi), A.A. (Ali Almustanyir), and M.S.A. (Mohammed S. Alhazmi); Writing, review, and editing, M.K.A., M.L., B.H.A., M.S.A. (Meznah S. Almutairi), A.A. (Ali Almustanyir), M.M.A. and M.S.A. (Mohammed S. Alhazmi). All authors have read and agreed to the published version of the manuscript.

Funding: This project was funded by the Researcher Supporting Project (RSPD2024R882) of King Saud University, Riyadh, Saudi Arabia.

Institutional Review Board Statement: This study was conducted according to the guidelines of the Declaration of Helsinki and approved by the Institutional Review Board of the College of Medicine, King Saud University (E-25-9722).

Informed Consent Statement: Informed consent was obtained from all subjects involved in the study after the nature and purpose of the study were described.

Data Availability Statement: Data were collected and analyzed as part of this study to assess the effects of low-dose atropine on static and dynamic pupil behavior and light sensitivity. The data are available upon reasonable request.

Acknowledgments: The authors thank King Saud University—Researcher Supporting Project (RSPD2024R882) for funding this project.

Conflicts of Interest: The authors declare no conflict of interest. The funders had no role in the design of the study; in the collection, analyses, or interpretation of data; in the writing of the manuscript; or in the decision to publish the results.

Abbreviations

The following abbreviations are used in this manuscript:

BCVA	best-corrected visual acuity
VLSQ-8	Visual Light Sensitivity Questionnaire
ANOVA	analysis of variance
SEM	standard error of the mean

References

1. Holden, B.A.; Fricke, T.R.; Wilson, D.A.; Jong, M.; Naidoo, K.S.; Sankaridurg, P.; Wong, T.Y.; Naduvilath, T.J.; Resnikoff, S. Global Prevalence of Myopia and High Myopia and Temporal Trends from 2000 through 2050. *Ophthalmology* **2016**, *123*, 1036–1042. [CrossRef] [PubMed]
2. Ha, A.; Kim, C.Y.; Shim, S.R.; Chang, I.B.; Kim, Y.K. Degree of myopia and glaucoma risk: A dose-response meta-analysis. *Am. J. Ophthalmol.* **2022**, *236*, 107–119. [CrossRef] [PubMed]
3. Saw, S.M.; Gazzard, G.; Shih-Yen, E.C.; Chua, W.H. Myopia and associated pathological complications. *Ophthalmic Physiol. Opt.* **2005**, *25*, 381–391. [CrossRef] [PubMed]

4. Holden, B.; Sankaridurg, P.; Smith, E.; Aller, T.; Jong, M.; He, M. Myopia, an underrated global challenge to vision: Where the current data takes us on myopia control. *Eye* **2014**, *28*, 142–146. [CrossRef]
5. Chen, Y.X.; Liao, C.M.; Tan, Z.; He, M.G. Who needs myopia control? *Int. J. Ophthalmol.* **2021**, *14*, 1297–1301. [CrossRef]
6. Chia, A.; Chua, W.H.; Cheung, Y.B.; Wong, W.L.; Lingham, A.; Fong, A.; Tan, D. Atropine for the treatment of childhood myopia: Safety and efficacy of 0.5%, 0.1%, and 0.01% doses (Atropine for the Treatment of Myopia 2). *Ophthalmology* **2012**, *119*, 347–354. [CrossRef]
7. Yam, J.C.; Jiang, Y.; Tang, S.M.; Law, A.K.P.; Chan, J.J.; Wong, E.; Ko, S.T.; Young, A.L.; Tham, C.C.; Chen, L.J.; et al. Low-Concentration Atropine for Myopia Progression (LAMP) Study: A Randomized, Double-Blinded, Placebo-Controlled Trial of 0.05%, 0.025%, and 0.01% Atropine Eye Drops in Myopia Control. *Ophthalmology* **2019**, *126*, 113–124. [CrossRef]
8. Yam, J.C.; Li, F.F.; Zhang, X.; Tang, S.M.; Yip, B.H.K.; Kam, K.W.; Ko, S.T.; Young, A.L.; Tham, C.C.; Chen, L.J.; et al. Two-Year Clinical Trial of the Low-Concentration Atropine for Myopia Progression (LAMP) Study: Phase 2 Report. *Ophthalmology* **2020**, *127*, 910–919. [CrossRef]
9. Yam, J.C.; Zhang, X.J.; Zhang, Y.; Wang, Y.M.; Tang, S.M.; Li, F.F.; Kam, K.W.; Ko, S.T.; Yip, B.H.K.; Young, A.L.; et al. Three-Year Clinical Trial of Low-Concentration Atropine for Myopia Progression (LAMP) Study: Continued Versus Washout: Phase 3 Report. *Ophthalmology* **2022**, *129*, 308–321. [CrossRef]
10. Cooper, J.; Eisenberg, N.; Schulman, E.; Wang, F.M. Maximum atropine dose without clinical signs or symptoms. *Optom. Vis. Sci.* **2013**, *90*, 1467–1472. [CrossRef]
11. Khanal, S.; Phillips, J.R. Which low-dose atropine for myopia control? *Clin. Exp. Optom.* **2020**, *103*, 230–232. [CrossRef] [PubMed]
12. Verriotto, J.D.; Gonzalez, A.; Aguilar, M.C.; Parel, J.M.A.; Feuer, W.J.; Smith, A.R.; Lam, B.L. New Methods for Quantification of Visual Photosensitivity Threshold and Symptoms. *Transl. Vis. Sci. Technol.* **2017**, *6*, 18. [CrossRef] [PubMed]
13. Li, M.; Chen, Y.; Chen, J.; Qin, G.; Li, L.; He, W.; Yu, S.; He, X.; Pazo, E.E.; Xu, L. Short-term effects of ophthalmic topical 0.01% atropine on the ocular surface, pupil size, and subsequent subjective quality of vision in young myopic Chinese adults. *Front. Med.* **2024**, *11*, 1436551. [CrossRef] [PubMed]
14. Salazar, M.; Shimada, K.; Patil, P.N. Iris pigmentation and atropine mydriasis. *J. Pharmacol. Exp. Ther.* **1976**, *197*, 79–88. [CrossRef]
15. Ji, Y.; Wang, Y.; Zhang, H.; Chen, X.; Zhao, K. Thermosensitive chitosan-based hydrogel as a topical ocular drug delivery system for atropine. *Biomaterials* **2012**, *33*, 7001–7010.
16. Tran, H.D.M.; Ha, T.T.X.; Tran, Y.H.; Coroneo, M.; Tran, T.D.; Truong, T.U.; Sankaridurg, P. Impact of Various Concentrations of Low-Dose Atropine on Pupillary Diameter and Accommodative Amplitude in Children with Myopia. *J. Ocul. Pharmacol. Ther.* **2024**, *40*, 232–239. [CrossRef]
17. Kaymak, H.; Fricke, A.; Mauritz, Y.; Löwinger, A.; Klabe, K.; Breyer, D.; Langenbucher, A.; Seitz, B.; Schaeffel, F. Short-term effects of low-concentration atropine eye drops on pupil size and accommodation in young adult subjects. *Graefes Arch. Clin. Exp. Ophthalmol.* **2018**, *256*, 2211–2217. [CrossRef]
18. McBrien, N.A.; Moghaddam, H.O.; Reeder, A.P. Atropine reduces experimental myopia and eye enlargement via a nonaccommodative mechanism. *Investig. Ophthalmol. Vis. Sci.* **1993**, *34*, 205–215.
19. Carr, B.J.; Stell, W.K. Nitric oxide (NO) mediates the inhibition of form-deprivation myopia by atropine in chicks. *Sci. Rep.* **2016**, *6*, 9. [CrossRef]
20. Diether, S.; Schaeffel, F. Local Changes in Eye Growth induced by Imposed Local Refractive Error despite Active Accommodation. *Vision. Res.* **1997**, *37*, 659–668. [CrossRef]
21. Schmucker, C.; Schaeffel, F. Contrast sensitivity of wildtype mice wearing diffusers or spectacle lenses, and the effect of atropine. *Vision. Res.* **2006**, *46*, 678–687. [CrossRef]
22. Diether, S.; Schaeffel, F.; Lambrou, G.N.; Fritsch, C.; Trendelenburg, A.U. Effects of intravitreally and intraperitonally injected atropine on two types of experimental myopia in chicken. *Exp. Eye Res.* **2007**, *84*, 266–274. [CrossRef]
23. Salazar, M.; Patil, P.N. An explanation for the long duration of mydriatic effect of atropine in eye. *Investig. Ophthalmol.* **1976**, *15*, 671–673.
24. Del Amo, E.M.; Rimpelä, A.K.; Heikkinen, E.; Kari, O.K.; Ramsay, E.; Lajunen, T.; Schmitt, M.; Pelkonen, L.; Bhattacharya, M.; Richardson, D.; et al. Pharmacokinetic aspects of retinal drug delivery. *Prog. Retin. Eye Res.* **2017**, *57*, 134–185. [CrossRef]

life

MDPI

Case Report

Case Report of Schnyder Corneal Dystrophy—A Rare Lipid Metabolic Disorder of the Cornea

Nina Stoyanova [1], Abdulrahman Imran [2], Zain Ul Hassan [2], Krasimir Kraev [3,*], Yordanka Basheva-Kraeva [1], Maria Kraeva [4], Petar Uchikov [5], Plamena Novakova [6], Veselin Vasilev [7], Ivaylo Minev [8], Bozhidar Hristov [9], Desislava Koleva-Georgieva [1], Petko Petrov [10], Luboslav Dimov [11], Svetlan Dermendzhiev [12] and Marin Atanassov [1]

1 Department of Ophthalmology, Faculty of Medicine, Medical University of Plovdiv, 4002 Plovdiv, Bulgaria; nina.st.st@abv.bg (N.S.); dannybasheva@gmail.com (Y.B.-K.); desislava.koleva@mu-plovdiv.bg (D.K.-G.); marin_aa@abv.bg (M.A.)
2 Faculty of Medicine, Medical University of Plovdiv, 4000 Plovdiv, Bulgaria; imran.ar057@gmail.com (A.I.); zulhassan2002@gmail.com (Z.U.H.)
3 Department of Propedeutics of Internal Diseases, Medical Faculty, Medical University of Plovdiv, 4002 Plovdiv, Bulgaria
4 Department of Otorhinolaryngology, Medical Faculty, Medical University of Plovdiv, 4002 Plovdiv, Bulgaria; kraevamaria93@gmail.com
5 Department of Special Surgery, Medical Faculty, Medical University of Plovdiv, 4002 Plovdiv, Bulgaria; puchikov@yahoo.com
6 Department of Allergy, Medical Faculty, Medical University of Sofia, 1000 Sofia, Bulgaria; nplamena@yahoo.com
7 Department of Physiology, Medical Faculty, Medical University of Plovdiv, 4002 Plovdiv, Bulgaria; veselin.vasilev@mu-plovdiv.bg
8 Department of Anaesthesiology, Emergency and Intensive Care Medicine, Medical Faculty, Medical University of Plovdiv, 4000 Plovdiv, Bulgaria; ivaylo.minev@mu-plovdiv.bg
9 Second Department of Internal Diseases, Section "Gastroenterology", Medical Faculty, Medical University of Plovdiv, 4002 Plovdiv, Bulgaria; hristov.bozhidar@abv.bg
10 Department of Maxillofacial Surgery, Faculty of Dental Medicine, Medical University of Plovdiv, 4000 Plovdiv, Bulgaria; petkogpetrov0@gmail.com
11 Department of Endocrinology, Medical Faculty, Medical University of Plovdiv, 4000 Plovdiv, Bulgaria; lyuboslav.dimov@phd.mu-plovdiv.bg
12 Department of Occupational Diseases and Toxicology, Medical Faculty, Medical University of Plovdiv, 4000 Plovdiv, Bulgaria; svetlan_d@yahoo.com
* Correspondence: kkraev@hotmail.com

Abstract: Background: Schnyder corneal dystrophy (SCD) is a rare autosomal dominant disorder characterized by bilateral corneal opacification due to abnormal cholesterol and phospholipid deposition. Mutations in the UBIAD1 gene, identified as causative in 2007, underline the condition, although its exact pathogenesis remains unclear. Case Presentation: A 55-year-old female presented with persistent photophobia, blepharospasm, and corneal discomfort. She also reported joint pain related to rheumatoid arthritis (RA), managed with Ro-Actemra (tocilizumab). The ophthalmological evaluation revealed bilateral corneal stromal deposits resembling snowflakes, with visual acuities of 0.8 (right eye) and 0.7 (left eye). Multimodal imaging confirmed stromal hyperreflective deposits. Based on the clinical findings, SCD was diagnosed, although no genetic testing was performed. Symptomatic management with artificial tears was initiated. Discussion: This case illustrates the diagnostic challenges of SCD, particularly in the absence of corneal crystals, a hallmark feature that is not universally present. Advanced imaging techniques aided diagnosis, and the coexistence of SCD and RA highlights the need for multidisciplinary care. Treatment options remain limited, although emerging therapies targeting oxidative stress and lipid metabolism show promise. Conclusions: This case highlights the importance of integrating ophthalmological and systemic care in SCD management and underscores the need for further research to expand diagnostic and therapeutic strategies for this rare disorder.

 https://doi.org/10.3390/life15030409

Keywords: Schnyder corneal dystrophy; lipid metabolism; tocilizumab-induced dyslipidemia

1. Introduction

Schnyder corneal dystrophy (SCD) is a rare, progressive autosomal dominant disorder that was first described by the Swiss ophthalmologist Franz Schnyder in 1924 [1–3]. It has a prevalence estimated at less than 1 in 1,000,000 individuals. It is characterized by bilateral opacification of the cornea due to abnormal accumulation of lipids, primarily cholesterol and phospholipids, within the corneal stroma (Figure 1) [4]. This lipid deposition leads to progressive corneal clouding and visual impairment, often beginning in early adulthood and advancing with age [5]. Clinically, SCD is notable for its variable presentation, ranging from subtle stromal haze to conspicuous crystalline deposits, depending on the stage and severity of the disease [6,7].

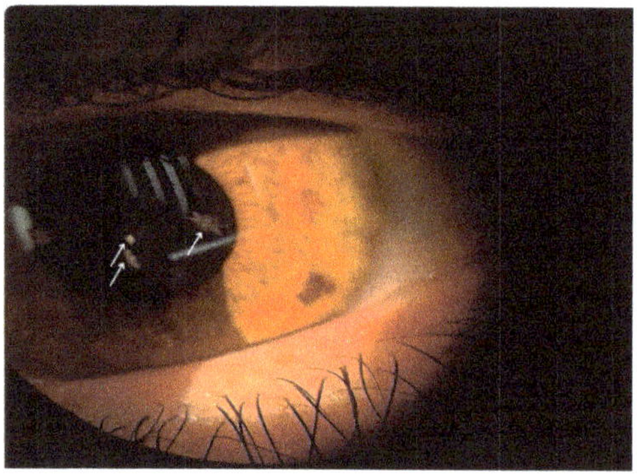

Figure 1. Crystalline corneal deposits in SCD, reflecting abnormal lipid accumulation and disease progression.

The genetic basis of SCD was elucidated in 2007, with the identification of mutations in the UBIAD1 gene as the primary causative factor. UBIAD1 encodes a key enzyme that is involved in cholesterol metabolism and vitamin K2 biosynthesis, underscoring the metabolic underpinnings of the disease [8]. However, the exact molecular mechanisms linking UBIAD1 mutations to corneal lipid accumulation remain poorly understood. Dysregulated lipid metabolism is thought to impair corneal transparency, leading to progressive visual decline [9–11].

While traditionally considered a corneal disorder, SCD is increasingly recognized for its potential systemic implications, including dyslipidemia. Advances in imaging modalities, such as optical coherence tomography (OCT) and confocal microscopy, have enhanced the diagnostic accuracy, particularly in cases lacking visible corneal crystals. Despite these advancements, treatment options remain limited, with penetrating keratoplasty being reserved for advanced cases [11–15].

This case underscores the importance of recognizing rare corneal dystrophies such as SCD, particularly in patients with systemic comorbidities or atypical corneal findings. Enhanced clinical awareness and improved diagnostic strategies could facilitate earlier diagnosis, timely management, and better visual outcomes for affected individuals.

2. Case Presentation

2.1. Patient History

A 55-year-old female presented with persistent ophthalmic complaints, including pain and photophobia, necessitating the frequent use of sunglasses. She also reported joint pain in the hands, specifically involving the metacarpophalangeal (MCP), proximal interphalangeal (PIP), and distal interphalangeal (DIP) joints, as well as in the right knee. Her medical history was significant for rheumatoid arthritis, managed with RoActemra (tocilizumab).

2.2. Clinical Findings

An ophthalmological examination revealed bilateral corneal stromal deposits resembling snowflakes (Figure 2), a characteristic finding of Schnyder corneal dystrophy (SCD). The visual acuity of the right eye was 0.8 (VOD), with an intraocular pressure of 17.5 mmHg (TOD). The left eye had a visual acuity of 0.7/0.8 (VOS) and an intraocular pressure of 14.1 mmHg (TOS). Both eyes exhibited the following:

- Blepharospasm;
- A calm conjunctiva;
- A clear and normally deep anterior segment;
- A round and centered pupil that reacted to light;
- A transparent lens.

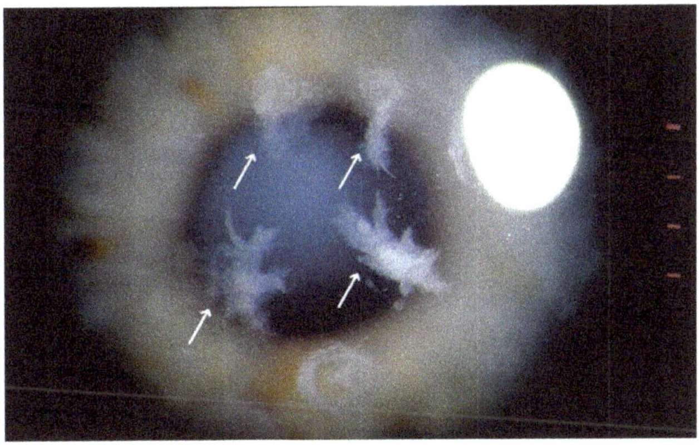

Figure 2. Bilateral corneal stromal deposits with a snowflake-like pattern, characteristic of Schnyder corneal dystrophy (SCD), resulting from abnormal lipid accumulation and contributing to corneal clouding and visual impairment.

2.3. Diagnostic Assessment

The diagnosis of Schnyder corneal dystrophy was established based on the clinical findings of bilateral corneal stromal deposits and the patient's ophthalmic symptoms. No genetic testing was performed, but the characteristic corneal features supported the diagnosis. Additionally, laboratory tests revealed elevated serum cholesterol (7.1 mmol/L) and triglyceride levels (4.8 mmol/L), further supporting the metabolic nature of the disease.

2.4. Therapeutic Interventions

The patient was managed with artificial tears for symptomatic relief of her ocular discomfort and photophobia. Her ongoing treatment with Ro-Actemra for rheumatoid arthritis was continued to manage systemic symptoms. A multidisciplinary approach was emphasized to address the coexistence of SCD and rheumatoid arthritis.

3. Discussion

3.1. Clinical Presentation and Diagnostic Challenges

The clinical presentation of SCD has evolved in its understanding over time. Weiss et al. [1] conducted a cohort study of 115 patients and revealed that corneal crystals, long considered a hallmark of SCD, are present in only 54% of cases. This finding challenges traditional diagnostic perceptions, underscoring the need to consider SCD even in the absence of visible crystals.

This case illustrates the diagnostic complexity of Schnyder corneal dystrophy (SCD), particularly in the absence of visible corneal crystals. While the characteristic snowflake-like stromal deposits that were observed in this patient aligned with descriptions of SCD in advanced stages, corneal crystals—a traditionally defining feature—were not universally present, aligning with Weiss et al.'s findings. The patient's additional symptoms, such as photophobia and blepharospasm, underscore the broader impact of SCD on patients' quality of life, beyond vision impairment. These findings emphasize the need for a comprehensive clinical evaluation and the importance of recognizing atypical presentations. In atypical cases, additional tools must be employed to aid in diagnosis, such as OCT imaging and pachymetry (Figures 3 and 4).

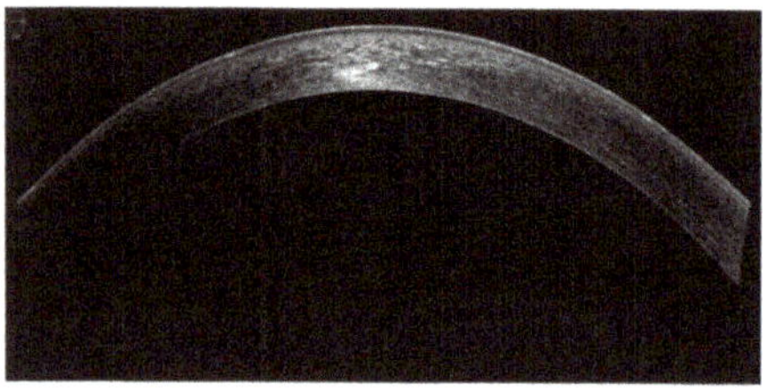

Figure 3. Optical coherence tomography (OCT) image of the cornea, demonstrating stromal hyperreflective deposits. The corneal architecture remains intact, with no evidence of significant thinning or scarring.

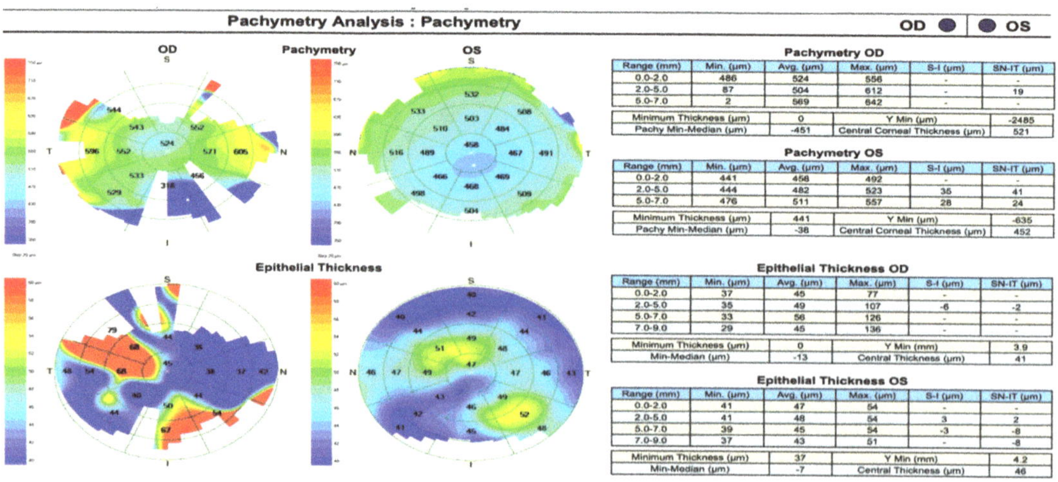

Figure 4. Pachymetry and epithelial thickness maps of both eyes. The right eye (OD) exhibits focal epithelial thickening, while the left eye (OS) demonstrates mild central thinning, consistent with lipid deposition affecting corneal structure.

Making a diagnosis can be challenging in SCD due to the variability in presentation and incomplete penetrance of crystallization in the cornea. The early presentation can be in the form of corneal haze without specificity and can be mistaken for corneal dystrophies or degeneration. The lack of family history in some cases and overlap with lipid corneal deposition in systemic dyslipidemia can be complicating factors. The use of a slit-lamp alone may be insufficient for identifying mild stromal abnormalities, and hence, supportive imaging tools like OCT and confocal microscopy are required.

3.2. Differential Diagnoses

The differential diagnoses of corneal lipid deposition must include a range of conditions beyond SCD. These include systemic lipid metabolism disorders such as hyperlipidemia, corneal arcus secondary to dyslipidemia, and certain lysosomal storage diseases like Fabry disease. A key consideration in this case was the potential impact of the patient's ongoing treatment with Ro-Actemra (tocilizumab) for rheumatoid arthritis. Tocilizumab, an IL-6 receptor antagonist, has been associated with alterations in lipid profiles, including elevated cholesterol and triglyceride levels. While the exact contribution of Ro-Actemra to the corneal findings is unclear, it raises the possibility that lipid dysregulation induced by the medication may have exacerbated or contributed to the lipid accumulation in this patient's cornea. In this case, a serum lipid assessment confirmed elevated cholesterol and triglyceride levels, reinforcing the metabolic component of SCD. This finding further supports the need for regular lipid monitoring in patients with SCD, particularly those receiving IL-6 inhibitors such as tocilizumab, which has been linked to dyslipidemia. This underscores the need for a thorough systemic and pharmacological history in patients presenting with atypical corneal findings.

3.3. Systemic Implications

The systemic dimensions of SCD remain a critical yet underexplored area. Dyslipidemia, which has a well-documented association with SCD, was not explicitly evaluated in this patient. Kurtul et al. [4] described a 34-year-old male with SCD and dyslipidemia, highlighting the importance of systemic co-management. Similarly, our patient presented with joint pain and was undergoing treatment for rheumatoid arthritis with RoActemra, emphasizing the need for a multidisciplinary approach. While no direct link has been established in the literature, the coexistence of these conditions suggests a need for further investigation into their potential interplay.

3.4. Advances in Molecular Understanding

The genetic and molecular underpinnings of SCD, particularly the role of UBIAD1 mutations, have been thoroughly established in the literature. Nowinska et al. [2] identified a novel mutation (I245N) and confirmed a known mutation (N102S) in a Polish cohort. Their use of advanced imaging techniques like optical coherence tomography (OCT) provided detailed morphological insights, similar to the multimodal imaging that was utilized in the diagnosis of our patient. However, the lack of genetic testing in our case represents a limitation, as identifying specific mutations could provide insights into the disease progression and prognosis.

3.5. Potential Treatment Approaches and Future Directions

The current treatment landscape for SCD remains limited, with penetrating keratoplasty being the primary option for advanced cases. Weiss et al. [1,11,15–18] suggested its effectiveness for patients with photopic vision loss who are over 50 years old, but the risk of disease recurrence in the donor cornea remains a concern. In this case, the use of artificial tears provided symptomatic relief, reflecting the constrained options that are available for early or less severe diseases.

Recent research has explored novel therapeutic approaches that target the underlying pathophysiology of SCD:

- Topical Statins: Given the lipid metabolism dysfunction in SCD, statins such as atorvastatin and simvastatin have been investigated for their ability to reduce corneal cholesterol deposition. Preliminary studies suggest that they may slow disease progression by modulating lipid homeostasis.
- Antioxidants and Autophagy Modulators: Kim et al. [7] explored parallels between SCD and Granular Corneal Dystrophy type 2, proposing treatments targeting oxidative damage and autophagy, such as rapamycin and melatonin. These approaches could provide novel avenues for managing SCD in the future, although clinical trials are essential for validation. Nanotechnology-based ocular drug delivery offers a promising approach for SCD management. Gold nano-urchins significantly enhance corneal drug retention, improving tear production, reducing IL-6 expression, suppressing angiogenesis, and promoting nerve regeneration in preclinical models [19]. These innovations may help address oxidative stress, inflammation, and neurodegeneration in SCD.
- Gene Therapy: With the identification of UBIAD1 mutations as the primary genetic driver of SCD, gene therapy targeting cholesterol metabolism pathways is a promising yet undeveloped frontier. Advances in CRISPR-based gene editing may enable future correction of pathogenic mutations, offering a potential cure.
- Lipid-Lowering Agents: Systemic lipid-lowering medications, such as ezetimibe or fibrates, may be explored in select patients with concomitant hyperlipidemia, although their role in preventing corneal lipid accumulation remains uncertain.

For our patient, continued follow-up is necessary to monitor her disease progression and evaluate emerging therapeutic options. Future research should focus on refining these interventions and assessing their long-term efficacy in clinical settings.

3.6. Implications for Multidisciplinary Care

This case underscores the importance of a multidisciplinary approach in managing SCD. Collaboration between ophthalmologists, geneticists, and systemic specialists, such as rheumatologists and cardiologists, is critical for addressing the complex interplay between ocular and systemic health. Future research should aim to better elucidate the relationship between systemic diseases, such as rheumatoid arthritis, and SCD, as well as explore novel therapeutic strategies targeting the disease's molecular and genetic basis.

Establishing a registry for Schnyder corneal dystrophy and other rare ocular disorders would be valuable in offering information about the disease course, genotype–phenotype correlations, and outcomes after treatments. National rare disease registries in France, the United States, and Nordic nations are established and are used for research, trial enrollment, and guideline generation. A European or global SCD registry would enhance awareness and direct the generation of guidelines based on evidence for treating SCD.

4. Conclusions

This case of Schnyder corneal dystrophy highlights the complex interplay between ocular and systemic health in rare corneal disorders. The patient's presentation, characterized by bilateral stromal deposits, photophobia, and systemic comorbidities, underscores the diagnostic and management challenges associated with SCD. While advances in understanding the genetic and molecular basis of the disease, particularly the role of UBIAD1 mutations, have provided valuable insights, the absence of universally accessible genetic testing and limited therapeutic options remain significant barriers to optimal care.

This case reinforces the importance of a multidisciplinary approach, integrating ophthalmological, systemic, and genetic evaluations to address the full spectrum of SCD manifestations. Emerging therapeutic strategies, such as targeting oxidative stress and vitamin K metabolism, offer promise but require further research and clinical validation. Future studies should focus on expanding diagnostic tools, exploring genotype–phenotype correlations, and developing non-invasive treatments to improve outcomes for patients with SCD. This case contributes to the growing body of research, emphasizing the need for individualized and collaborative care in managing this rare disorder.

Author Contributions: Conceptualization: P.N. and P.P.; Methodology: N.S., M.A. and K.K.; Validation: P.P., P.N. and D.K.-G.; Formal Analysis: M.K., Y.B.-K. and P.U.; Investigation: M.K., Y.B.-K. and B.H.; Resources: P.U., B.H. and L.D.; Writing—Original draft preparation: K.K., N.S. and A.I.; Writing-review and editing: Z.U.H. and A.I.; Data curation: V.V. and S.D.; Visualization: I.M., V.V. and L.D.; Supervision: M.A., D.K.-G. and S.D.; Project administration: Z.U.H. and I.M. All authors have read and agreed to the published version of the manuscript.

Funding: This research received no external funding.

Institutional Review Board Statement: Ethical review and approval were waived for this study due to the fact that the patient did not undergo any invasive interventions.

Informed Consent Statement: Written informed consent has been obtained from the patients to publish this paper.

Data Availability Statement: Data are contained within the article.

Conflicts of Interest: The authors declare no conflicts of interest.

References

1. Weiss, J.S. Schnyder corneal dystrophy. *Curr. Opin. Ophthalmol.* **2009**, *20*, 292–298. [CrossRef] [PubMed]
2. Nowinska, A.K.; Wylegala, E.; Teper, S.; Lyssek-Boron, A.; Aragona, P.; Roszkowska, A.M.; Micali, A.; Pisani, A.; Puzzolo, D. Phenotype–genotype correlation in patients with Schnyder corneal dystrophy. *Cornea* **2014**, *33*, 497–503. [CrossRef] [PubMed]
3. Weiss, J.S.; Khemichian, A.J. Differential diagnosis of Schnyder corneal dystrophy. *Dev. Ophthalmol.* **2011**, *48*, 67–96. [CrossRef] [PubMed]
4. Kurtul, B.E.; Elbeyli, A.; Ozarslan Ozcan, D.; Ozcan, S.C.; Karaaslan, A. Schnyder corneal dystrophy: A rare case report. *Nepal. J. Ophthalmol.* **2020**, *12*, 110–113. [CrossRef] [PubMed]
5. Sarosiak, A.; Oziębło, D.; Udziela, M.; Vermeer, C.; Malejczyk, J.; Szaflik, J.P.; Ołdak, M. High expression of matrix GLA protein in Schnyder corneal dystrophy patients points to an active role of Vitamin K in corneal health. *Acta Ophthalmol.* **2020**, *99*, E171–E177. [CrossRef] [PubMed]
6. Ghazal, W.; Georgeon, C.; Grieve, K.; Bouheraoua, N.; Borderie, V. Multimodal imaging features of Schnyder corneal dystrophy. *J. Ophthalmol.* **2020**, *2020*, 6701816. [CrossRef] [PubMed]
7. Kim, E.K.; Lee, H.; Choi, S. Molecular pathogenesis of corneal dystrophies. *Prog. Mol. Biol. Transl. Sci.* **2015**, *134*, 99–115. [CrossRef] [PubMed]
8. Khan, A.; Al-Ghadeer, H.; Mohamed, J. Schnyder corneal dystrophy in a Saudi Arabian family with heterozygous UBIAD1 mutation (p.L121F). *Middle East. Afr. J. Ophthalmol.* **2011**, *18*, 61. [CrossRef]
9. Jun, D.-J.; Schumacher, M.M.; Hwang, S.; Kinch, L.N.; Grishin, N.V.; DeBose-Boyd, R.A. Schnyder corneal dystrophy-associated UBIAD1 is defective in MK-4 synthesis and resists autophagy-mediated degradation. *J. Lipid Res.* **2020**, *61*, 746–757. [CrossRef] [PubMed]
10. Gatzioufas, Z.; Charalambous, P.; Loew, U.; Kozobolis, V.; Schirra, F.; Krause, M.; Seitz, B. Evidence of oxidative stress in Schnyder corneal dystrophy. *Br. J. Ophthalmol.* **2010**, *94*, 1262–1264. [CrossRef] [PubMed]
11. Nickels, T.J.; Roderick, M.; Dupps, W.J. Schnyder corneal dystrophy: A review and update on the clinical, genetic, and therapeutic aspects. *Eye Contact Lens* **2021**, *47*, 303–311. [CrossRef]

12. Orr, A.; Dubé, M.P.; Marcadier, J.; Jiang, H.; Federico, A.; George, S.; Seamone, C.; Andrews, D.; Dubord, P.; Holland, S.; et al. Mutations in the UBIAD1 gene on chromosome 1p36 cause Schnyder crystalline corneal dystrophy. *PLoS ONE* **2007**, *2*, e685. [CrossRef] [PubMed]
13. Aldave, A.J.; Sonmez, B. The genetics of corneal dystrophies. *Dev. Ophthalmol.* **2011**, *48*, 51–66. [CrossRef] [PubMed]
14. Evans, C.J.; Dudakova, L.; Skalicka, P.; Mahelkova, G.; Horinek, A.; Hardcastle, A.J.; Tuft, S.J.; Liskova, P. Schnyder corneal dystrophy and associated phenotypes caused by novel and recurrent mutations in the UBIAD1 gene. *BMC Ophthalmol.* **2018**, *18*, 250. [CrossRef] [PubMed]
15. Weiss, J.S. Visual morbidity in thirty-four families with Schnyder crystalline corneal dystrophy (an American Ophthalmological Society thesis). *Trans. Am. Ophthalmol. Soc.* **2007**, *105*, 616–648. [PubMed]
16. Weiss, J.S.; Moller, H.U.; Aldave, A.J.; Seitz, B.; Bredrup, C.; Kivela, T.; Munier, F.L.; Rapuano, C.J.; Nischal, K.K.M.; Kim, E.K.; et al. IC3D classification of corneal dystrophies—Edition 2. *Cornea* **2015**, *34*, 117–159. [CrossRef] [PubMed]
17. Weiss, J.S.; Waring, G.O., 3rd; Krachmer, J.H.; Holland, E.J. The clinical diagnosis of Schnyder's crystalline dystrophy. *Am. J. Ophthalmol.* **1992**, *113*, 629–634.
18. Weiss, J.S.; Kruth, H.S.; Kuivaniemi, H.; Tromp, G.; White, P.S.; Winters, R.S.; Karkera, J.; Mahurkar, S.; Lisch, W.; Dupps, W.J., Jr.; et al. Genetic analysis of 14 families with Schnyder crystalline corneal dystrophy reveals clues to UBIAD1 protein function. *Am. J. Med. Genet. A* **2008**, *146*, 2711.
19. Ghosh, S.; Su, Y.-H.; Yang, C.-J.; Lai, J.-Y. Design of Highly Adhesive Urchin-Like Gold Nanostructures for Effective Topical Drug Administration and Symptomatic Relief of Corneal Dryness. *Small Struct.* **2025**, *6*, 2400484. [CrossRef]

life

MDPI

Article

Segmental Scleral Buckle: A Novel Strategy for Addressing Early Recurrent Inferior Retinal Detachment in Silicone Oil-Filled Eyes

Luca Ventre [1], Antonio Valastro [1], Erik Mus [1], Fabio Maradei [1], Giulia Pintore [1] and Gabriella De Salvo [2,3,*]

[1] Ophthalmology Department, Beauregard Hospital, Azienda USL della Valle d'Aosta, Via L. Vaccari 5, 11100 Aosta, Italy
[2] Southampton Eye Unit, University Hospital Southampton Foundation Trust, Southampton SO16 6YD, UK
[3] University of Southampton, Southampton SO16 6YD, UK
* Correspondence: gabrielladesalvo@gmail.com

Abstract: Recurrence of retinal detachment (RD) following pars plana vitrectomy (PPV) with silicone oil tamponade is a surgical challenge. This study proposes a novel approach utilizing segmental scleral buckle to manage early recurrences, especially in inferior quadrants. A retrospective case series of four patients with early recurrent inferior RD post-PPV with silicone oil tamponade was conducted. The segmental scleral buckle technique, with or without subretinal fluid drainage, was employed. Clinical and surgical data were collected, including visual outcomes and complications. No intraoperative or postoperative complications were observed during the 6-month follow-up period. Visual acuity remained stable, and retinal reattachment was achieved in 100% of cases after silicone oil removal. Segmental scleral buckle emerges as a promising technique for managing early recurrent inferior RD in silicone oil-filled eyes. The technique demonstrates favorable outcomes, including retinal reattachment and visual acuity stability, without significant complications. Further studies are warranted to validate its efficacy and establish standardized protocols.

Keywords: pars plana vitrectomy; recurrent retinal detachment; retinal detachment; segmental scleral buckle; silicone oil tamponade

1. Introduction

Rhegmatogenous retinal detachment (RRD) is one of the leading causes of vision loss, with an incidence of approximately 1 in 10,000 [1,2].

RRD occurs when a break in the retina, often caused by posterior vitreous detachment or trauma, allows liquefied vitreous to pass into the subretinal space, leading to detachment of the neurosensory retina from the retinal pigment epithelium [3].

Treatment of rhegmatogenous retinal detachment involves identifying and closing all retinal breaks using techniques such as laser retinopexy, pneumatic retinopexy, scleral buckling, or pars plana vitrectomy (PPV) [4].

Pars plana vitrectomy involves the removal of the vitreous body to eliminate all tractional forces on the retina, followed by flattening of the detached retina and treatment of all identified retinal breaks with laser photocoagulation or cryotherapy. At the end of the procedure, a tamponade agent—air, gas, or silicone oil (SiO)—is introduced into the vitreous cavity to stabilize the retina and promote reattachment [4].

Recurrence of retinal detachment (RD) may develop at different postoperative times following PPV for RRD. When the retinal detachment recurrences occur within the first

6 weeks post-primary PPV, we refer to those as "early recurrences"; when they occur after the first 6 weeks from primary surgery, they are referred to as "late recurrences" [5,6].

In this study, we focus specifically on early recurrences of retinal detachment in eyes filled with silicone oil tamponade.

Several factors contribute to early re-detachment in SiO–filled eyes, including underfilling the vitreous chamber with silicone oil, incomplete release of vitreoretinal tractions at the edge of the break, the buoyancy characteristics of silicone oil itself, and the development of early (immature) proliferative vitreoretinopathy. Inadequate SiO filling can result in a meniscus of residual fluid accumulating inferiorly, reducing the tamponade effect on the lower retina [6]. Additionally, residual vitreoretinal tractions at the edge of the break may lead to detachment in the lower quadrants of the retina, particularly when the silicone oil tamponade is insufficient [6].

Conventional surgical interventions to address these recurrences involve a re-do vitrectomy (revitrectomy) or a 360-degree scleral buckle [6,7].

Revitrectomy typically involves the removal of silicone oil, revision of the vitrectomy to release any remaining vitreoretinal tractions, reflattening of the retina using air or perfluorocarbon liquids, and possibly revisiting the endolaser performed during the previous surgery, either to reinforce treatment of pre-existing breaks or to address any new breaks that may have formed or been missed during primary surgery. In most cases, silicone oil is then added [6].

The 360-degree scleral buckle procedure involves performing a 360-degree peritomy, isolating the four rectus muscles (superior, medial, lateral, and inferior), placing a silicone band around the globe (beneath the previously isolated rectus muscles), optionally performing a transscleral drainage puncture to evacuate subretinal fluid, tightening the band to achieve the desired indentation, and applying cryotherapy (or, alternatively, laser treatment in the postoperative period) to retinal breaks. The procedure is completed by closing the conjunctiva [8].

However, scleral buckle has drawbacks, such as prolonged surgical time, increased refractive error, and a higher risk of complications like diplopia and anterior segment ischemia [9]. On the other hand, revitrectomy carries the risk of repeating previous errors, such as inadequate filling of silicone oil or failure to fully address residual tractional forces from remaining membranes, which may compromise the success of the procedure.

Current guidelines for managing recurrent RD in silicone oil-filled eyes are limited [6], and the choice of surgical approach, and associated outcomes have not been thoroughly defined.

Thus, the aim of this study is to present an alternative surgical approach for treating early inferior retinal detachment in silicone oil-filled eyes, avoiding the need for further pars plana vitrectomy and/or a 360-scleral buckle. We propose the use of an inferior, segmental (circumferential) scleral buckle, with or without external drainage of subretinal fluid (depending on the amount of subretinal fluid present). In cases of shallow or "flat" detachments, we opted not to drain the subretinal fluid and instead placed the buckle alone to avoid potential iatrogenic retinal damage from the drainage puncture. However, in cases with a significant amount of subretinal fluid, drainage was performed, as the risk of iatrogenic damage from the puncture was lower, to enhance the inferior tamponade effect. By applying pressure to the eye wall, the sponge pushes the retina into contact with the silicone oil but also helps to counteract tractional forces. At the same time, the silicone oil provides a counterpressure against the retina, effectively stabilizing its position. This dual action also eliminates the meniscus of residual fluid that may persist due to accidental underfilling, thereby enhancing the overall success of the procedure.

2. Materials and Methods

This retrospective analysis of a series of cases was conducted at Beauregard Hospital, Aosta between November 2021 and July 2023. All surgeries were performed by an experienced vitreoretinal surgeon (L.V.). The study was conducted in adherence to Italian bioethical guidelines and the Declaration of Helsinki. All patients received detailed information and were provided with informed consent regarding the type of surgical procedure performed.

To be enrolled in the study, the four consecutive patients had to meet the following eligibility criteria: (1) recurrent inferior retinal detachment occurring within one month after primary surgery or "early recurrence" (inferior RD defines a RD localized in the quadrants comprising the inferior six clock hours of the retinal clock—3 o'clock to 9 o'clock); (2) silicone oil used as tamponade in primary surgery; (3) recurrence of inferior RD did not involve the macular region (early inferior recurrence with macula-on RD). Exclusion criteria included the following: (1) relaxing retinectomies during the initial surgery; (2) scleral buckling procedure during the primary vitreoretinal surgery; (3) recurrence of macula-off RD.

All patients underwent a thorough ocular assessment, including best-corrected visual acuity (BCVA) assessment, anterior segment examination, intraocular pressure (IOP) measurement, fundus examination, fundus photography (Cobra+, CSO, Florence, Italy), and spectral-domain optical coherence tomography (SD-OCT) (Spectralis Heidelberg Engineering, Heidelberg, Germany). These examinations were performed before the primary surgery, within one month of primary surgery, and then at one week, one month, three months, and six months after segmental scleral buckle surgery.

Further data regarding age, gender, pre-reoperation BCVA, timeframe between primary PPV and reoperation, extent of retinal detachment, recurrence factors, location of retinal breaks, surgical procedures undertaken, retinal reattachment rate, final visual outcome, postoperative intraocular pressure (IOP), and intra- and postoperative complications were collected.

The surgical technique used in all four patients was inferior segmental scleral buckle with (or without) drainage of subretinal fluid; the latter was performed in two out of four patients.

The steps of the surgery are described in detail below:

2.1. STEP 1–Identification and Isolation of the Inferior, Medial, and Lateral Rectus Muscles

The procedure begins with a 180-degree lower conjunctival peritomy to gain access to the underlying scleral area. The conjunctiva and Tenon's capsule are carefully dissected using Westcott scissors, isolating the sub-Tenon space and exposing the sclera beneath. Following this, the inferior, medial, and lateral rectus muscles are identified and isolated individually using a fenestrated muscle hook. This step facilitates the placement of a reverse-mounted suture (2/0 silk suture) around the belly of each muscle to secure and maneuver them as needed during the subsequent stages of surgery. This careful preparation ensures optimal exposure and access to the surgical site (Figure 1A).

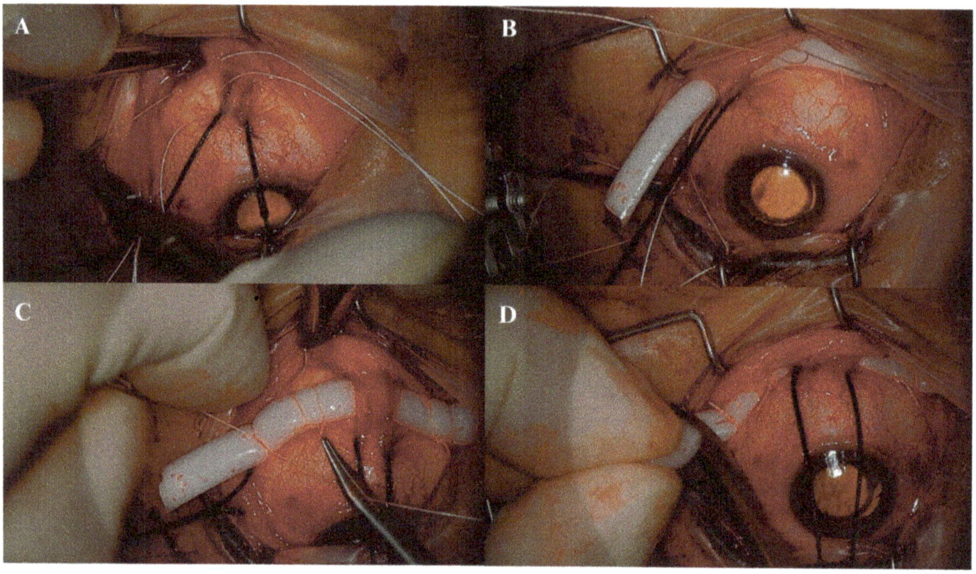

Figure 1. Intraoperative view of the surgical steps of an inferior segmental scleral buckle. (**A**): Placement of 5/0 Tycron scleral horizontal mattress sutures in the inferotemporal quadrant; (**B**): positioning of the 5 mm × 3 mm silicone sponge beneath the rectus muscles and under the previously placed horizontal mattress sutures; (**C**): tightening of the four horizontal mattress sutures to achieve the desired indentation; (**D**): trimming of the excess portion of the silicone sponge.

2.2. STEP 2–Placement of Horizontal Mattress Sutures

Once the surgical field has been prepared, scleral marking is performed at a distance of 12 mm from the limbus to guide the correct placement of sutures. Two horizontal mattress sutures are then placed in each lower quadrant using a 5/0 Tycron suture (Figure 1B). These sutures serve as the primary anchors for securing the scleral buckle and ensuring proper indentation. Accurate placement of these sutures is critical for achieving the desired tamponade effect in the affected retinal areas.

2.3. STEP 3–Positioning of the Scleral Buckle

The scleral buckle, consisting of a 5 mm × 3 mm sponge, is positioned beneath the horizontal mattress sutures that were previously placed in the inferior retinal quadrants, typically spanning the 3 to 6 o'clock positions (Figure 1C). If subretinal fluid drainage is performed, it is performed at this stage to facilitate retinal reattachment.

The horizontal mattress sutures are then tightened properly to induce the desired level of indentation in the inferior retinal quadrants (Figure 1C). Excess sponge material is carefully cut to avoid unnecessary bulk or interference with the surrounding ocular structures (Figure 1D). Finally, the conjunctiva is sutured.

3. Results

This series includes four pseudophakic eyes of four patients (three females and one male) with early inferior recurrent retinal detachment, three of whom initially presented with primary macula-off rhegmatogenous retinal detachment, while in one case, the macula remained attached during the primary retinal detachment (macula-on) (Table 1).

Table 1. Clinical and surgical data for patients with early recurrent inferior retinal detachment. Summary of retinal detachment characteristics and postoperative outcomes. RD = Retinal Detachment; VTC = Vitrectomy; sSB = segmental Scleral Buckle; SiO = Silicone Oil.

	OCT-Based Stage of Primary RD (Melo et al. [10])	Intraop./Postop. Complications	BCVA Pre-VTC	BCVA 1-Week Post-VTC	BCVA 1-Week Post-sSB	BCVA 6-Months Post-SiO Removal
Patient 1	2	No	20/30	20/25	20/25	20/20
Patient 2	4	No	HM	20/70	20/70	20/40
Patient 3	3A	No	CF 1 m	20/50	20/50	20/30
Patient 4	3A	No	CF 3 m	20/40	20/40	20/25

Primary surgery consisted of PPV with silicone oil as tamponade in all four patients: Patient 1 was an 80-year-old male who presented with a macula-on (Stage 2 according to the OCT-based classification of Melo et al. [10]) retinal detachment accompanied by a giant retinal tear located in the superior quadrants, extending from 10 o'clock to 2 o'clock. Patient 2 was a 63-year-old female who presented with a longstanding subtotal retinal detachment (Stage 4 according to the OCT-based classification of Melo et al. [10]), characterized by advanced proliferative vitreoretinopathy (PVR) of grade C; two star folds—one at 5 o'clock and one at 7 o'clock—located posterior to the equator were present. According to the Machemer classification [11], the proliferative vitreoretinopathy was graded as PVR C3; these star folds were peeled using a monomanual technique employing ILM forceps without the use of staining; the detachment was associated with multiple retinal breaks extending circumferentially around the retina, spanning a full 360 degrees. Patient 3 was a female with a longstanding macula-off retinal detachment (Stage 3A according to the OCT-based classification of Melo et al. [10]); the detachment was associated with a retinal horseshoe tear located at 5 o'clock, which was observed in the context of lattice degeneration. Patient 4 was also a female who presented with a longstanding macula-off retinal detachment (Stage 3A according to the OCT-based classification of Melo et al. [10]); in her case, the detachment was linked to a retinal horseshoe tear at 11 o'clock, similarly occurring in an area of lattice degeneration. During primary PPV, the surgeon confirmed the presence of the posterior hyaloid by injecting triamcinolone acetonide (0.1–0.3 mL at a concentration of 40 mg/mL). In all four cases, a PVD was already present. In the last two patients, the decision to use silicone oil as a tamponade was influenced by the high altitudes of their place of residence, with both living at elevations exceeding 2000 m above sea level. At such altitudes, the use of gas tamponade would have been contraindicated due to the significant risk of gas expansion caused by reduced atmospheric pressure, which could lead to postoperative complications, including elevated intraocular pressure (ocular hypertension).

In all four cases, varying degrees of hypofilling of the vitreous cavity by silicone oil were observed. In Patient 2, previously undetected (or newly formed) microholes were identified in the inferior quadrants, which likely contributed to the early recurrence of the detachment. In Patient 3, early (immature) PVR was noted, along with inferior microholes; in combination with the incomplete filling of the vitreous cavity by silicone oil, these factors likely led to an early inferior re-detachment.

Neither intraoperative nor postoperative complications were observed during the follow-up examinations at 1 week, 1 month, 3 months, and 6 months after the segmented scleral buckle procedure (Table 1). As indicated in Table 1, visual acuity exhibited stability throughout the 6-month follow-up period. Axial length remained unchanged after segmental scleral buckle. Furthermore, the reattachment rate achieved was 100% during the

6-month follow-up period after the removal of silicone oil, a procedure conducted within 3 months of the primary surgery.

4. Discussion

The success rate in addressing complex rhegmatogenous retinal detachment (RRD) has significantly improved due to the adoption of advanced pars plana vitrectomy (PPV) techniques and the application of silicone oils as tamponade. These advancements have provided better retinal stabilization and facilitated the management of even the most challenging cases. However, despite these technical improvements, the recurrence rate of retinal detachment can reach up to 10% of cases [12].

Recurrences of retinal detachment can occur at different times following primary surgery and are typically categorized as either "early recurrences", which occur within the first 6 weeks, or "late recurrences", which manifest more than 6 weeks after the initial procedure [5,13]. Understanding the distinction between these types of recurrences is essential as the underlying causes and management strategies differ significantly.

Early recurrences usually impact the lower retinal quadrants, and several factors contribute to their occurrence, many of which are related to technical aspects of the primary surgery. One common issue is inadequate filling of the vitreous cavity with silicone oil during the initial surgery. Silicone oil, being lighter than water, rises to the superior part of the vitreous cavity when the patient is in an upright position. This buoyancy provides an effective tamponade for the upper retinal quadrants but leaves the inferior sectors less protected. As a result, recurrences of retinal detachment in eyes with silicone oil tamponade often occur in the inferior retinal sectors.

This issue is further exacerbated when the vitreous cavity is underfilled with silicone oil, leading to the formation of a meniscus of water in the inferior quadrants [14]. The rounded shape of the silicone oil bubble compounds the problem as part of its volume is utilized to form this meniscus rather than maintaining direct contact with the retina [15]. This lack of tamponade efficiency, particularly in the lower quadrants, increases the likelihood of recurrent detachment [16]. Another significant factor is the presence of undetected retinal breaks or microholes during the primary surgery. These lesions may go unnoticed during primary surgery and remain untreated. Due to the buoyant nature of silicone oil, these breaks are less effectively tamponaded when localized in the inferior retina, allowing SRF to seep through and contributing to the recurrence of RD.

Additionally, early recurrences may result from an incomplete release of vitreoretinal tractions at the edge of breaks during the primary surgery. Residual tractions can exert pulling forces on the retinal surface, particularly in the inferior quadrants where the tamponade effect of silicone oil is less. This mechanical stress can lead to new tears or exacerbate existing ones, resulting in recurrent detachment.

Another possible cause of early re-detachment could be the development of early (immature) proliferative vitreoretinopathy.

The combination of these factors—insufficient silicone oil filling, undetected retinal breaks, unrelieved vitreoretinal tractions, and immature PVR—can act independently or synergistically to cause early recurrences. Each of these issues is particularly problematic in the inferior retinal quadrants, where silicone oil provides less reliable support.

On the contrary, late recurrences of retinal detachment are primarily attributed to the development of mature PVR, which is a complex process characterized by the proliferation, migration, and contraction of retinal pigment epithelial (RPE) cells, inflammatory cells, and fibroblasts [17]. This pathological response can lead to the formation of fibrotic membranes that exert traction on the retina, causing the development of new retinal breaks or reopening previously treated ones. Additionally, the contraction of these membranes often results in a progressive shortening and distortion of the retinal tissue, further complicating the anatomical and functional outcomes of retinal reattachment procedures [18].

The surgical approach to managing recurrent RD in silicone oil-filled eyes necessitates a comprehensive evaluation of the underlying causes of the initial surgical failure. Surgeons must carefully assess the extent and location of PVR, residual tractional forces, undetected or new retinal breaks, and the effectiveness of the tamponade. In certain cases, reoperations can be performed without removing the silicone oil, focusing on peeling PVR membranes and reinforcing the retinal attachment using endolaser or cryotherapy [19]. However, in more complex cases, the procedure involves the removal of the silicone oil to allow better access to the retina for a more thorough intervention. This often includes performing extensive PVR peeling to relieve traction, reflattening the retina using perfluorocarbon liquids, addressing any new or preexisting retinal breaks, and ensuring adequate tamponade. Depending on the severity and location of the detachment, tamponading agents such as silicone oil (for long-term support) or gas (for temporary but effective tamponade) are used to stabilize the retina [20].

The success of these reoperations relies heavily on meticulous surgical planning, careful intraoperative handling of delicate retinal tissue, and the ability to adapt the surgical approach based on the extent of PVR and other contributing factors to the recurrent detachment.

A different surgical approach in cases of RD recurrence is external. In this case, scleral buckling (SB) enhances the tamponade effect of silicone oil (SiO) on the inferior retina by establishing contact between the peripheral retina and the silicone oil bubble, reducing traction on the retina circumferentially and providing support to the retinal breaks [16].

Segmental scleral buckle represents a straightforward, time-efficient, and cost-effective surgical technique that, despite its simplicity, proves to be highly effective in managing and addressing retinal detachments [21].

Typically utilized for the treatment of primary rhegmatogenous retinal detachments involving a single retinal break, this technique offers localized support specifically at the site of the break [21]. By focusing on the affected area, it eliminates the need for a more extensive 360-degree buckle procedure, reducing surgical time and minimizing potential complications while still ensuring effective retinal reattachment and stabilization [22].

In early recurrent inferior retinal detachments, as previously mentioned, detachment is caused by failure of the retinal tamponade provided by the silicone oil bubble in the inferior quadrants and/or by residual, not completely relieved vitreoretinal tractions, which may or may not have created new rhegmatogenous lesions in the inferior retinal sectors. These new lesions, not being adequately tamponaded—potentially due to underfilling of the eye with silicone oil—can lead to a recurrence of inferior retinal detachment. Therefore, placing a segmental buckle in the lower 180 degrees of the retina would create an indentation in the inferior quadrants, bringing the retina closer to the silicone oil bubble and thereby enhancing the tamponade effect of the silicone oil itself. Additionally, this approach helps relieve any residual vitreoretinal tractions or address inferior retinal breaks, further contributing to the stabilization and reattachment of the retina.

The advantages of this technique over a 360-degree scleral buckle and additional vitrectomy are numerous, including minimal alterations in refractive error, reduced surgical time—typically requiring no more than 60 min for completion—lower invasiveness compared to performing a revitrectomy, decreased overall cost of the procedure, a significantly reduced risk of postoperative diplopia as the surgery involves only the inferior rectus muscle, and a relatively low risk of both anterior and posterior segment ischemia, making it a safer and more efficient option for managing early recurrent inferior retinal detachments.

As the study is retrospective in nature, includes a case series of only four eyes, and has a relatively short follow up of six months, further standardized, randomized, and multicentric clinical trials are needed to validate our findings. Nevertheless, we found the use of segmental scleral buckle in the early recurrence inferior RD encouraging, not only due to its positive anatomic and refractive outcomes but also in most efficiently managing precious theatre time with minimal postoperative patient recovery time.

5. Conclusions

In conclusion, this case series highlights the efficacy of segmental scleral buckle as a novel and promising strategy for addressing early recurrent inferior retinal detachment in silicone oil-filled eyes. The technique demonstrated favorable outcomes, including retinal reattachment and stability in visual acuity, without significant complications during the follow-up period. The advantages of segmental scleral buckle over traditional 360-degree scleral buckling and repeated pars plana vitrectomy include reduced surgical time, lower risk of refractive errors and postoperative complications, and overall cost-effectiveness. However, further large-scale studies are necessary to validate these findings and establish standardized protocols for wider clinical application.

Author Contributions: Conceptualization, L.V.; methodology, L.V., A.V. and E.M.; validation, L.V., A.V. and E.M.; formal analysis, G.D.S.; investigation, L.V.; resources, L.V. and A.V.; data curation, A.V., E.M., F.M. and G.P.; writing—original draft preparation, A.V. and E.M.; writing—review and editing, L.V. and G.D.S.; supervision, L.V. and G.D.S.; project administration, L.V. All authors have read and agreed to the published version of the manuscript.

Funding: Azienda USL della valle d'Aosta, Corso Saint-Martin-de-Corléans, 248, 11100 Aosta AO, Italy.

Informed Consent Statement: Informed consent was obtained from all subjects involved in the study.

Data Availability Statement: The data presented in this study are available on request from the corresponding author. The data are not publicly available due to privacy concerns.

Conflicts of Interest: The authors declare no conflicts of interest.

References

1. Ge, J.Y.; Teo, Z.L.; Chee, M.L.; Tham, Y.C.; Rim, T.H.; Cheng, C.Y.; Wong, T.Y.; SNEC Surgical Retina Research Group; Wong, E.Y.M.; Lee, S.Y.; et al. International incidence and temporal trends for rhegmatogenous retinal detachment: A systematic review and meta-analysis. *Surv. Ophthalmol.* **2024**, *69*, 330–336. [CrossRef] [PubMed]
2. Haimann, M.H.; Burton, T.C.; Brown, C.K. Epidemiology of retinal detachment. *Arch. Ophthalmol.* **1982**, *100*, 289–292. [CrossRef] [PubMed]
3. Mitry, D.; Fleck, B.W.; Wright, A.F.; Campbell, H.; Charteris, D.G. Pathogenesis of rhegmatogenous retinal detachment: Predisposing anatomy and cell biology. *Retina* **2010**, *30*, 1561–1572. [CrossRef] [PubMed]
4. Warren, A.; Wang, D.W.; Lim, J.I. Rhegmatogenous retinal detachment surgery: A review. *Clin. Exp. Ophthalmol.* **2023**, *51*, 271–279. [CrossRef] [PubMed]
5. Benson, W.E. *Retinal Detachment: Diagnosis and Management*, 2nd ed.; Lippincott: Philadelphia, PA, USA, 1988.
6. Wei, Y.; Wu, G.; Xu, K.; Wang, J.; Zu, Z.; Wang, R. The outcomes of scleral buckling versus re-vitrectomy for the treatment of recurrent inferior retinal detachment in silicone oil tamponade eyes. *Acta Ophthalmol.* **2016**, *94*, e624–e628. [CrossRef] [PubMed]
7. Solaiman, K.A.; Dabour, S.A. Supplemental scleral buckling for inferior retinal detachment in silicone oil-filled eyes. *Retina* **2014**, *34*, 1076–1082. [CrossRef] [PubMed]
8. Martínez-Mujica, M.T.; Retamal, J.; González, R. Scleral buckle versus pneumatic retinopexy for rhegmatogenous retinal detachments. *Medwave* **2018**, *18*, e7277. [CrossRef] [PubMed]
9. Papakostas, T.D.; Vavvas, D. Postoperative Complications of Scleral Buckling. *Semin. Ophthalmol.* **2018**, *33*, 70–74. [CrossRef] [PubMed]
10. Martins Melo, I.; Bansal, A.; Naidu, S.; Oquendo, P.L.; Hamli, H.; Lee, W.W.; Muni, R.H. Morphologic Stages of Rhegmatogenous Retinal Detachment Assessed Using Swept-Source OCT. *Ophthalmol. Retin.* **2023**, *7*, 398–405. [CrossRef] [PubMed]

11. Machemer, R.; Aaberg, T.M.; Freeman, H.M.; Irvine, A.R.; Lean, J.S.; Michels, R.M. An updated classification of retinal detachment with proliferative vitreoretinopathy. *Arch. Ophthalmol.* **1991**, *112*, 159–165. [CrossRef] [PubMed]
12. Adelman, R.A.; Parnes, A.J.; Ducournau, D.; European Vitreo-Retinal Society (EVRS) Retinal Detachment Study Group. Strategy for the management of uncomplicated retinal detachments: The European vitreo-retinal society retinal detachment study report 1. *Ophthalmology* **2013**, *120*, 1804–1808. [CrossRef] [PubMed]
13. Huang, D.; Starr, M.R.; Patel, L.G.; Ammar, M.J.; Kaiser, R.S.; Mehta, S.; Park, C.H.; Khan, M.A.; Gupta, O.P.; Kuriyan, A.E.; et al. Factors Affecting Retinal Redetachment After Silicone Oil Removal For Rhegmatogenous Retinal Detachments. *Retina* **2022**, *42*, 1248–1253. [CrossRef] [PubMed]
14. Wolf, S.; Schön, V.; Meier, P.; Wiedemann, P. Silicone oil-RMN3 mixture ("heavy silicone oil") as internal tamponade for complicated retinal detachment. *Retina* **2003**, *23*, 335–342. [CrossRef] [PubMed]
15. Wetterqvist, C.; Wong, D.; Williams, R.; Stappler, T.; Herbert, E.; Freeburn, S. Tamponade efficiency of perfluorohexyloctane and silicone oil solutions in a model eye chamber. *Br. J. Ophthalmol.* **2004**, *88*, 692–696. [CrossRef] [PubMed] [PubMed Central]
16. Acar, M.A.; Ünlü, N.; Hazirolan, D.; Demir, M.N.; Üney, G.Ö.; Örnek, F. Conventional surgery for complicated retinal detachment in silicone oil-filled eyes. *Eur. J. Ophthalmol.* **2011**, *21*, 290–295. [CrossRef] [PubMed]
17. Campochiaro, P.A. Pathogenic mechanisms in proliferative vitreoretinopathy. *Arch. Ophthalmol.* **1997**, *115*, 237–241. [CrossRef] [PubMed]
18. Fu, Y.; Xie, T.-H.; Gu, Z.-H.; Yang, N.; Geng, R.-F.; Zhang, Y.-L. Recurrent retinal detachment after pars plana vitrectomy with silicone oil tamponade for rhegmatogenous retinal detachment. *Int. Ophthalmol.* **2022**, *42*, 3813–3820. [CrossRef] [PubMed]
19. Yang, C.M.; Hsieh, Y.T.; Yang, C.H.; Liu, K.R. Irrigation-free vitreoretinal surgery for recurrent retinal detachment in silicone oil-filled eyes. *Eye* **2006**, *20*, 1379–1382. [CrossRef] [PubMed]
20. Sharma, T.; Gopal, L.; Shanmugam, M.P.; Bhende, P.S.; Agrawal, R.; Badrinath, S.S.; Samanta, T.K. Management of recurrent retinal detachment in silicone oil-filled eyes. *Retina* **2002**, *22*, 153–157. [CrossRef] [PubMed]
21. Kreissig, I.; Rose, D.; Jost, B. Minimized surgery for retinal detachments with segmental buckling and nondrainage. An 11-year follow-up. *Retina* **1992**, *12*, 224–231. [CrossRef] [PubMed]
22. Kreissig, I. View 1: Minimal segmental buckling without drainage. *Br. J. Ophthalmol.* **2003**, *87*, 782–784. [CrossRef] [PubMed] [PubMed Central]

life

MDPI

Hypothesis

Exploring a Novel Hypothesis: Could the Eye Function as a Radar or Ultrasound Device in Depth and Distance Perception? Neurophysiological Insights

Hüseyin Findik [1,*], Muhammet Kaim [1], Feyzahan Uzun [1], Ayhan Kanat [2], Osman Nuri Keleş [3] and Mehmet Dumlu Aydin [4]

[1] Department of Ophthalmology, School of Medicine, Recep Tayyip Erdogan University, 53100 Rize, Turkey; muhammet.kaim@erdogan.edu.tr (M.K.)
[2] Department of Neurosurgery, School of Medicine, Recep Tayyip Erdogan University, 53100 Rize, Turkey
[3] Department of Histology, School of Medicine, Ataturk University, 25030 Erzurum, Turkey
[4] Department of Neurosurgery, School of Medicine, Ataturk University, 25030 Erzurum, Turkey; nmda11@hotmail.com
* Correspondence: huseyin.findik@erdogan.edu.tr; Tel.: +90-05057501054

Abstract: Recent advancements in ocular physiology suggest that the eyes may function similarly to radar antennae or ultrasound probes, with the occipital cortex acting as a detector, challenging the traditional view of binocular vision as the primary mechanism for depth and distance perception. Methods: We conducted a comprehensive analysis of the neuroanatomical and histological architecture of the neuro-optico-cortical systems in a male wild rabbit model. The objective was to identify potential structural and functional similarities between the retino-optical system and radar/ultrasound effector-detector systems. Results: Histological examination revealed significant similarities between retinal morphology and radar/ultrasound systems. The outermost retinal layer resembled an acoustic lens, with underlying layers functioning as acoustic matching layers. The ganglion cell layer exhibited characteristics akin to the piezoelectric elements of transducers. Conclusions: Our findings support the hypothesis that the retinal apparatus functions similarly to radar antennae or ultrasound probes. Light-stimulated retinal-occipital cortex cells perceive objects and emit electromagnetic waves through the retina, which are reflected by objects and processed in the occipital cortex to provide information on their distance, shape, and depth. This mechanism may complement binocular vision and enhance depth and distance perception in the visual system. These results open new avenues for research in visual neuroscience and could have implications for understanding various visual phenomena and disorders.

Keywords: retina; radar; ultrasound; depth perception; distance perception; neurophysiology; visual system

1. Introduction

The evaluation of distance and depth perception is fundamental to human visual processing, playing a critical role in everyday activities. Traditionally, these abilities have been attributed to the integration of binocular vision with neuro-optical networks [1,2]. However, emerging evidence suggests the existence of alternative mechanisms, which may expand our understanding of how the visual system operates.

The study of visual physiology and perceptual mechanisms has a long and rich history, originating in antiquity [3,4]. Alcmaeon of ancient Greece hypothesized that vision arose from optic nerves channeling fire encased in water within the eyes [5]. Democritus suggested that objects emitted atom-like particles perceived as colors, while Hippocrates examined the anatomical structure of the eye to uncover its functional rationale [6]. During Galen's time, vision was believed to be mediated by the eyes as effector organs, relying on pneuma derived from brain ventricles [7,8]. Advances during the Renaissance unveiled the anatomical basis of vision, including the optic chiasm, optical radiation, and the laminar organization of the occipital lobes [9]. In modern times, the visual system has been demonstrated to function akin to a photomultiplier, with binocular vision identified as essential for depth and distance perception [10]. Moreover, studies have shown that the eyes generate electromagnetic waves similar to brain waves [11], and the light-stimulated retina produces resting potentials of 6–10 mV [12,13].

Despite these advances, alternative mechanisms for depth and distance perception have garnered growing interest. Beyond the conventional role of binocular vision, monocular cues such as motion parallax, size constancy, texture gradients, and occlusion significantly contribute to depth perception, particularly when binocular input is limited or absent [14]. The brain's remarkable adaptability in integrating these monocular cues underscores the complexity of the visual system [15].

Recent findings in visual neuroscience suggest that the retina and visual pathways may process information through mechanisms beyond classical optical theories. Specifically, electromagnetic wave interactions and bioelectric signaling within the retina raise the possibility that it may encode spatial and distance information in a manner analogous to radar or sonar systems [16,17].

Another fascinating avenue involves neural oscillations and synchrony within the occipital cortex [18]. Gamma-band activity and phase synchronization have been implicated in the brain's ability to integrate spatial and temporal information, potentially contributing to depth and distance encoding [19]. Additionally, proprioceptive and vestibular inputs may complement visual cues, creating an integrated sensory framework for spatial awareness [20,21]. This multimodal integration enables robust depth perception even in complex, dynamic environments.

Building on these principles, this study proposes a novel hypothesis that the retina may function similarly to radar antennas or ultrasound probes, with the occipital cortex processing reflected signals. In this model, light-stimulated retinal cells could emit electromagnetic waves toward surrounding objects, while the visual system analyzes the returning waves to aid in depth and distance perception. Through neurophysiological and histological approaches, this investigation examines structural and functional parallels between the retinal apparatus and radar or ultrasound systems.

The findings from this study may transform our understanding of the visual system, emphasizing its intricate network that integrates diverse physiological and neural processes to achieve depth and distance perception. This perspective could pave the way for new research directions in visual physiology, neuro-ophthalmology, and biomedical engineering, with significant implications for the understanding and treatment of visual disorders.

2. Materials and Methods

This study was conducted on a male wild rabbit model to analyze the anatomical and histological network architectures of the neuro-opticocortical system and investigate potential structural similarities between the retino-optical system and radar-ultrasound effector-detector systems.

Animal protocol was reviewed and approved by the Ethics Committee of Erzurum Atatürk University, Faculty of Medicine. The care of the animal model and the experimental procedures adhered to the guidelines established by the ethics committee to ensure humane treatment and ethical compliance. To minimize pain and mortality during the study, a balanced injectable anesthetic protocol was utilized. Anesthesia was initially induced with isoflurane administered via a face mask. Subsequently, a combination of ketamine hydrochloride (150 mg/1.5 mL), xylazine hydrochloride (30 mg/1.5 mL), and distilled water (1 mL) was prepared, and a dose of 0.2 mL/kg was administered subcutaneously prior to surgical procedures. During the experiment, an additional dose of 0.1 mL/kg of the same anesthetic combination was provided as required to maintain adequate anesthesia. Post-mortem analysis of the retinal and optical tissues was performed to obtain detailed histological and anatomical data.

Histopathological Procedures

To estimate neuronal density in the retina, bilateral retinal tissues were carefully excised. The specimens were horizontally embedded in paraffin blocks to ensure optimal visualization of all retinal layers during histopathological examination. Sections were stained using hematoxylin and eosin (H&E) (Merck GmbH, Darmstadt, Germany) and Masson's trichrome (MTC) (Sigma-Aldrich, St. Louis, MI, USA) stains to facilitate detailed morphological analysis.

Neuronal density was assessed using the physical dissector method, a reliable stereological technique. This method offers several advantages: it provides unbiased estimates of particle number, is straightforward to perform, does not rely on assumptions about particle shape, size, or orientation, and is unaffected by overprojection or truncation artifacts. Two consecutive sections (referred to as dissector pairs) were obtained from the tissue samples and mounted on each slide. The reference and look-up sections were alternated to effectively double the number of dissector pairs without the need for additional tissue sections.

Coronal sections of the ocular bulb, taken at the level of the ocular equator, were also prepared for analysis. These sections were stained with H&E to further investigate the structural and histological characteristics of the eye.

3. Results

3.1. Histological Analysis of the Retina

The histological structure of the retina, optic nerve, and retinal neurons was examined in detail, as shown in Figure 1. The retina consists of 10 distinct layers, as described before: (1) inner limiting membrane (ILM), (2) nerve fiber layer (NFL), (3) ganglion cell layer (GCL), (4) inner plexiform layer (IPL), (5) inner nuclear layer (INL), (6) outer plexiform layer (OPL), (7) outer nuclear layer (ONL), (8) outer limiting membrane (OLM), (9) photoreceptor layer (PL), and (10) the retinal pigmented epithelium (RPE) [22]. Notably, morphological similarities were identified between the retinal structure and the functional components of radar antennas and ultrasound probes. The outermost layer of the retina resembled the acoustic lens of these systems, while the underlying layer was analogous to the acoustic matching layer. Furthermore, the ganglion cell layer displayed structural characteristics akin to the piezoelectric elements of a transducer, which are essential for converting signals in radar and ultrasound systems.

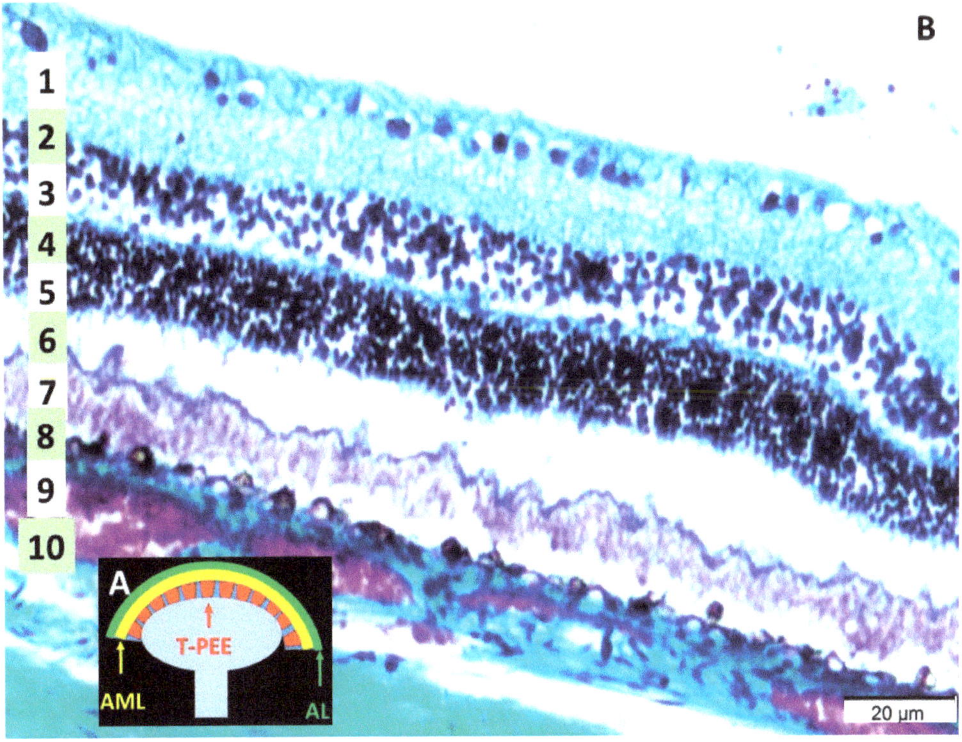

Figure 1. (**A**) Acoustic lens (AL) in the probe of an ultrasound device, transducer of piezoelectric transducer (T-PEE) and the acoustic matching layer (AML) (**B**) Histological appearance of choroid and retinal layers: (1) the inner limiting membrane, (2) the nerve fiber layer, (3) the ganglion cell layer, (4) the inner plexiform layer, (5) the inner nuclear layer, (6) the outer plexiform layer, (7) the outer nuclear layer, (8) the outer limiting membrane, (9) the photoreceptor layer, and (10) the retinal pigmented epithelium (LM, MTC, ×40).

3.2. Retinal Function and Radar Analogy

As illustrated in Figure 2, the functional analogy between the retina and radar systems was conceptualized using principles of reflected power. The reflected power (Pr) at the retina is influenced by factors such as the power density (Su), the antenna gain (G), and the variable retinal cross-section (σ). This relationship can be expressed as:

$$\mathrm{Su} \times \varsigma \times \mathrm{G}/\mathrm{R}^2{}_1$$

Pr = reflected power (WC = retinal cross-section (mm^2), R_1 = range, distance retina-to target (m).

In this analogy, the target can be regarded as a secondary radiator, reflecting power back to the retina. The reflected power serves as the emitted signal that the retina processes.

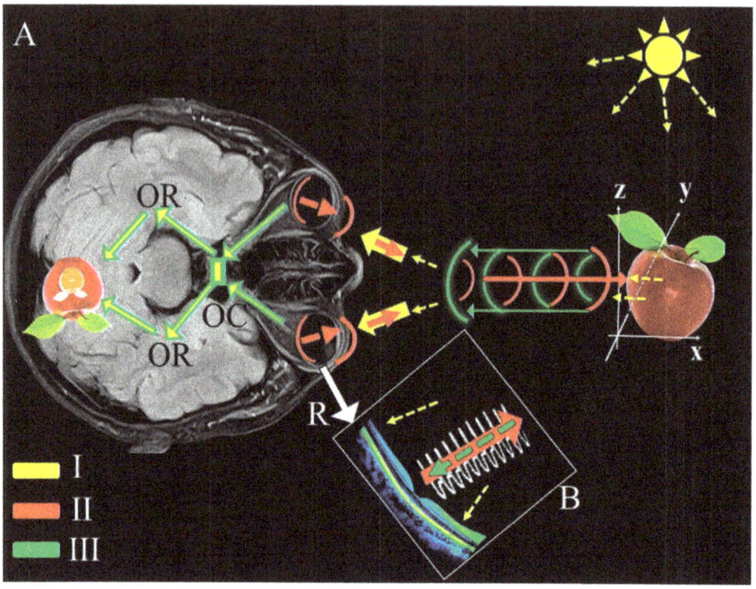

Figure 2. In the figure, a schematic summary explaining the formation of the sense of distance and depth according to our hypothesis is observed. In part (**A**); as a result of the rays emitted from the sun and hitting the apple and reaching the eye, passing through the retina (R), optic chiasm (OC), and optic radiation (OR) and reaching the occipital cortex, which is the visual field (yellow arrows), we first only notice the apple (yellow arrows). At this time, the electromagnetic waves (White wave beam (**B**)), formed at a value of 6–10 mV in the retina (R) stimulated by light, are spread from the retina, which is like a radar dish, to the external environment. In this way, the electromagnetic waves (Red arrows and bows (**A**,**B**)) leaving the retina and leaving the pupil hit the object and return (Green arrows and bows), while a certain amount of energy and time loss occurs depending on the characteristics of the external and internal environments. Neural networks, especially those located in the retina and occipital cortex and working like the signal processing chips and screens of radars, inform the consciousness about the distance, proximity, and depth of objects by taking advantage of the time and energy differences of the first and last signals that come to them. The order of emergence and flow of the rays involved in the formation of vision and depth is symbolized in the lower left corner of the picture.

3.3. Comparative Observations

Overall, the analysis revealed striking parallels between retinal morphology and the structural–functional elements of radar antennas and ultrasound probes. The outermost retinal layer functions analogously to an acoustic lens, focusing incoming signals, while the acoustic matching layer is mirrored in the subsequent layers. The ganglion cell layer exhibits functional similarities to piezoelectric elements, crucial for signal transduction. These findings highlight the potential for the retina to operate as an integrated biological system capable of complex signal processing, akin to engineered radar and ultrasound systems.

4. Discussion

This study investigated the hypothesis that the eyes might function analogously to radar or ultrasound devices, yielding compelling evidence in support of this concept. The findings highlight remarkable structural similarities between the retina and the components of radar antennas and ultrasound probes, reinforcing the premise that the eyes may possess the capacity to emit electromagnetic waves. Histological analysis of the retinas from a male rabbit model revealed morphological structures that closely parallel those found in these advanced technologies. Specifically, the outermost retinal layer exhibits similarities to an acoustic lens, the underlying layer resembles an acoustic coupling layer, and the ganglion cell layer shares structural features with piezoelectric transducer elements (Figure 1). These observations suggest that the retina's unique architecture may facilitate both the emission and detection of electromagnetic waves, providing a novel perspective on ocular function.

Wang et al. [23] presented groundbreaking research that offered a novel perspective on the electromagnetic properties of the visual system, demonstrating that the eye produces biophoton emissions. This discovery suggests that the retina is not merely a light-absorbing structure but also actively emits electromagnetic radiation. When considered alongside the intricate layered architecture of the retina and the potential electromagnetic properties of each layer, this phenomenon lends support to the hypothesis that the eye may possess radar- or ultrasound-like functional capabilities [24].

Uncertainties surrounding the coherence length and directional emission properties of biophotons raise questions about their suitability for spatial distance perception. However, recent findings indicate that biophotons contribute significantly to visual processing. Studies suggest that neuronal oscillations and phase correlations may enable biophotons to enhance contrast mechanisms in the retina and modulate optical feedback [23,25,26]. Moreover, the ordered alignment of Müller cells within the retina may serve as an intrinsic waveguide, facilitating the directional propagation of biophotons and enhancing their interactions with external light sources [27]. The ordered arrangement of photoreceptors could optimize the propagation of biophotons by concentrating their emission in specific directions [26]. Additionally, the retina's neural network supports visual processing by detecting and integrating weak biophoton signals [28]. To further investigate these mechanisms, experimental approaches utilizing ultra-sensitive photonic detection systems and artificial retina models are recommended [29–31]. The integration of biophotons into the brain's sensory processing system unveils a novel paradigm for depth perception, transcending traditional optical models.

The similarities between retinal morphology and radar and ultrasound systems provide a novel perspective on the functioning of the visual system. By examining the layers and functions of the retina, the hypothesis can be reassessed as follows: the RPE enhances image quality by preventing the back-reflection of light. Strauss [32] highlighted the high metabolic activity of this layer and its critical role in the phagocytosis of photoreceptor outer segments. This functionality is analogous to radar-absorbing materials (RAM) in radar systems, as both mechanisms effectively minimize unwanted reflections. Furthermore, the high metabolic activity and phagocytic processes of the RPE may contribute to the emission of biophotons [23,33]. Regarding the photoreceptor layer, photoreceptors undergo conformational changes in response to light stimuli [34,35] and play a critical role in converting light into electrical signals. This function is analogous to the role of antenna elements in radar systems, which detect electromagnetic waves and transform them into electrical signals. This analogy aligns with the well-established optical properties of the retina, as demonstrated in various studies [36–38]. The outer and inner nuclear and plexiform layers of the retina facilitate initial signal processing and transmission. Molnar et al. [39] demonstrated that the DNA structure within cell nuclei possesses the ability to absorb and emit electromagnetic waves. These retinal layers can be compared to signal processing circuits in radar systems, as both filter, amplify and prepare received signals for subsequent processing. This analogy is consistent with findings from studies on retinal signal processing mechanisms [40,41]. The ganglion cell layer comprises the primary neurons responsible for transmitting retinal signals to the brain. Kastner and Baccus [42] demonstrated that ganglion cells are sensitive to magnetic fields. The function of this layer can be compared to the output layer in radar systems. The ability of ganglion cells to process multiple streams of information is further supported by studies conducted by Escobar et al. [43] and Gollisch and Meister [37]. These findings support the hypothesis that ganglion cells may possess the capability to generate and/or sense electromagnetic waves. Additionally, the retinal nerve fiber layer can be likened to data transmission lines in radar systems, as both facilitate the transmission of processed signals to a central processing unit—be it the brain or a computer.

Electro-oculographic (EOG) measurements capture the electrical activity arising from the corneo-retinal potential difference. Due to the dipole properties of the eyeball (positive charge at the cornea and negative charge at the retina), changes in the electrical field during eye movements result in electromagnetic wave emissions, as predicted by Maxwell's equations. The observed linear correlation between eye movements and electromagnetic wave emissions in EOG measurements suggests that modulation of the corneo-retinal potential influences electromagnetic wave propagation [44–46]. This finding, combined with the biophoton emissions arising from the metabolic activity of the RPE and its electromagnetic properties, supports the hypothesis that the eye may function analogously to a radar system. These results align with the extensive research conducted by Arden and Constable on electroretinography, which demonstrated that light stimulation generates a potential of approximately 6–10 mV [12]. This electrical activity may underlie the electromagnetic wave emissions hypothesized in our study. Moreover, the electromagnetic waves generated and propagated by the electrical activity of retinal cells exhibit functional similarities to piezoelectric crystals in radar or ultrasound devices, as described by Bachofer et al. [47]. Bachofer's seminal study demonstrated that electromagnetic waves are produced in the retina when stimulated by X-rays, suggesting that the retina may respond to various forms of electromagnetic radiation, including, but not limited to, visible light, by generating electromagnetic waves. These findings provide further support for the hypothesis that the retina functions as a bidirectional electromagnetic transducer, contributing to a deeper understanding of its potential roles beyond light perception [47–49].

Building on these studies, our hypothesis can be summarized as follows: When light from an object stimulates the retina and the occipital cortex, the object is initially perceived. We propose that electromagnetic waves, generated by electrical activity in the retina stimulated by light, are emitted from the retina, which acts similarly to a dish antenna. These waves pass through the pupil, interact with objects in the external environment, and reflect back. The retina evaluates the phase difference and energy loss of these emitted and reflected waves, analogous to a radar mechanism, enabling the perception of the distance, shape, and depth of objects. The retina, in conjunction with the occipital cortex, functions similarly to the cache system in computers, facilitating the initial recognition of objects (Figure 2). This relationship suggests that the eyes are not merely passive receptors but may also actively transmit electromagnetic waves. Such a mechanism parallels the operation of an antenna in radar systems, enabling the eyes to discern the position and distance of surrounding objects. These findings lend further support to our hypothesis that the eyes might employ a radar- or ultrasound-like mechanism for depth and distance perception. Nevertheless, additional molecular and electrophysiological studies are required to elucidate the precise mechanisms underlying this process and its contribution to visual perception.

The findings of our study may complement existing theories on the functioning of the visual system. While the role of binocular vision in depth and distance perception is well established [50], the ability to perceive depth with a single eye highlights the presence of alternative mechanisms [51–53]. The radar- or ultrasound-like mechanism we propose may provide insights into how monocular depth cues are processed. Furthermore, our hypothesis raises intriguing questions about the role of the visual cortex. The suggestion that the occipital cortex might function as a radar or ultrasound detector necessitates a re-evaluation of how visual information is processed. In this context, Livingstone and Hubel's seminal work on parallel processing pathways in the visual cortex offers a framework that aligns with our hypothesis [54]. Additionally, our hypothesis aligns with the framework proposed by Marr [55], who suggested that visual perception can be analyzed at three levels: (1) the computational level, (2) the algorithmic level, and (3) the implementation level.

Our work presents several potential real-world applications. For instance, it may inspire novel strategies for the design of retinal prostheses. Current research on retinal implants seeks to stimulate retinal nerves through electrical impulses to evoke the perception of a point in space [56]. The radar- or ultrasound-like mechanism we propose could inform the development of new approaches and designs for such devices. Additionally, our findings may enhance the understanding of the pathophysiology of certain visual disorders. For example, the loss of retinal ganglion cells, as seen in glaucoma patients [57], can be understood not only in the context of visual field defects but also as a disruption of the proposed radar- or ultrasound-like mechanism. This loss not only impairs the transmission of visual signals but also affects the generation and modulation of electromagnetic signals, which may explain the observed deficits in depth perception. Similarly, retinal vascular diseases such as diabetic retinopathy offer new insights into how vascular damage impacts depth perception. The altered metabolism of the RPE due to vascular damage may disrupt biophoton emission and electromagnetic signal modulation, further impairing visual function.

Future research could include in vitro studies aimed at measuring electromagnetic wave emissions from retinal cells using more sensitive techniques. In this context, researchers employed advanced electrophysiological methods that could be adapted for this purpose [58,59]. Additionally, brain imaging techniques such as functional magnetic resonance imaging and magnetoencephalography could be utilized to investigate the cortical consequences of the proposed mechanism [60]. Psychophysical experiments could also be designed to examine the behavioral implications of the radar- or ultrasound-like mechanism. This approach could extend and refine the findings of Westheimer on depth perception [61,62]. Our hypothesis has the potential to inspire biomimetic applications [63], as studying the radar- or ultrasound-like functioning of the eye may lead to the development of advanced imaging systems and sensors.

To further validate our hypothesis and address the limitations identified, we propose a preliminary experimental model (Figure 3), detailed in the Section 4, which will investigate the propagation of electromagnetic waves (6–10 mV) from the human retina using a magnet–vacuum setup in a shielded environment. This model, involving an evacuated ellipsoid tube and a magnetic needle to detect directional changes (alpha angle) during eye movements by volunteers, will offer initial evidence for the radar-like function of the eye in depth and distance perception. Although this model is theoretical and will await ethical approval for human application, it will provide a robust framework for future hypothesis-driven research, enhancing our understanding of the electromagnetic properties of the visual system and guiding investigations into its role in spatial awareness.

However, our study has several limitations. The data are primarily derived from animal models, and direct applicability to the human eye requires further investigation. While our findings are promising, larger, controlled studies in humans are essential for validation. Furthermore, more detailed investigations into the neural mechanisms underlying the proposed radar- or ultrasound-like system are needed. Advanced techniques, such as electrophysiological and neuroanatomical studies, combined with computational models simulating eye function, could provide deeper insights into the nature and operation of this mechanism.

Experimental Model

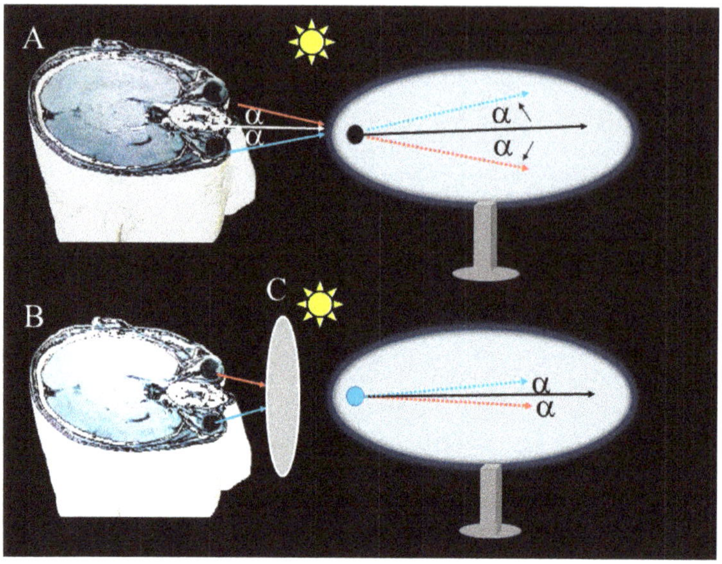

Figure 3. This model will investigate the propagation of electromagnetic waves (6–10 mV) from the human retina in a shielded, electronics-free room, using a magnet–vacuum setup with an evacuated ellipsoid tube (1 cm diameter, 4 cm long) and a magnetic needle (0.3 mm thick, 4 cm long) to detect directional changes (alpha angle) in these waves during eye movements by volunteers with normal vision. The eyes will be closed for 3 min, then opened in an illuminated environment, and horizontal/vertical eye movements will be recorded, showing that the magnetic needle will deflect with a varying alpha angle, suggesting wave propagation from the retina (**A**). A control condition, placing a wooden board between the eyes and the tube (**B**), will result in reduced or absent deflection, confirming the retinal origin of the waves (**C**). These preliminary findings, presented as a framework for future studies pending ethical approval, will offer initial evidence that electromagnetic waves emitted and absorbed by the retina could serve as a radar-like signal channel for spatial perception.

5. Conclusions

In conclusion, this study proposes a novel hypothesis for the functioning of the eyes, suggesting that the retina's complex, layered structure, with each layer potentially exhibiting distinct electromagnetic properties, may enable the eye to function as a radar- or ultrasound-like system. Combined with the observed electro-oculographic correlations, our findings indicate that the mechanisms underlying depth and distance perception may be more intricate than previously assumed. This perspective opens new avenues for research in visual physiology and neuroscience, offering deeper insights into the processes governing visual perception. If validated, this hypothesis could revolutionize vision science and neuro-ophthalmology, providing a foundation for new diagnostic and therapeutic advancements. Future studies should prioritize the validation of this hypothesis and undertake detailed investigations into the electromagnetic properties of the visual system.

Author Contributions: Methodology: M.D.A.; Software, M.K.; Validation, O.N.K.; Formal analysis, F.U.; Investigation, A.K.; Writing—original draft, H.F.; Writing—review and editing, H.F. All authors have read and agreed to the published version of the manuscript.

Funding: The authors thank the Recep Tayyip Erdogan University Development Foundation, which provided funding for the open-access publishing of this study (grant number: 02024012002188).

Institutional Review Board Statement: This study was conducted in accordance with the Declaration of Helsinki and was approved by the Institutional Ethics Committee of Atatürk University (protocol code E-42190979-050.01.04-2400431471; date: 2 January 2025).

Informed Consent Statement: Not applicable.

Data Availability Statement: The original contributions presented in this study are included in the article; further inquiries can be directed to the corresponding author.

Conflicts of Interest: The authors declare no conflicts of interest.

References

1. Sakano, Y.; Allison, R.S. Aftereffect of motion-in-depth based on binocular cues: Effects of adaptation duration, interocular correlation, and temporal correlation. *J. Vis.* **2014**, *14*, 21. [CrossRef]
2. Baburaj, V.P.; Gomez, G. Analysis of problems with distance determination using Night Vision Googles. *Indian J. Aerosp. Med.* **2009**, *53*, 1–9.
3. Gordon, B.L. Oculists and occultists: Demonology and the eye. *Arch. Ophthalmol.* **1939**, *22*, 25–65. [CrossRef]
4. Galst, J.M.; Van Alfen, P. *Ophthalmologia Optica & Visio in Nummis*; Wayenborgh Publishing: Piribebuy, Paraguay, 2018.
5. Panegyres, K.P.; Panegyres, P.K. The Ancient Greek discovery of the nervous system: Alcmaeon, Praxagoras and Herophilus. *J. Clin. Neurosci. Off. J. Neurosurg. Soc. Australas.* **2016**, *29*, 21–24. [CrossRef]
6. De Laey, J.J. The eye of Vesalius. *Acta Ophthalmol.* **2011**, *89*, 293–300. [CrossRef]
7. Siegel, R.E. Theories of vision and color perception of Empedocles and Democritus; some similarities to the modern approach. *Bull. Hist. Med.* **1959**, *33*, 145–159.
8. Werner, J.S.; Pinna, B.; Spillmann, L. Illusory color & the brain. Novel illusions suggest that the brain does not separate perception of color from perception of form and depth. *Sci. Am.* **2007**, *296*, 90–95.
9. Finger, S. *Origins of Neuroscience: A History of Explorations Into Brain Function*; Oxford University Press: Oxford, UK, 2001.
10. Pizzi, R.; Wang, R.; Rossetti, D. Human Visual System as a Double-Slit Single Photon Interference Sensor: A Comparison between Modellistic and Biophysical Tests. *PLoS ONE* **2016**, *11*, e0147464. [CrossRef]
11. Zheng, W.L.; Lu, B.L. A multimodal approach to estimating vigilance using EEG and forehead EOG. *J. Neural Eng.* **2017**, *14*, 026017. [CrossRef]
12. Arden, G.B.; Constable, P.A. The electro-oculogram. *Prog. Retin. Eye Res.* **2006**, *25*, 207–248. [CrossRef]
13. Kulyabin, M.; Zhdanov, A.; Dolganov, A.; Maier, A. Optimal Combination of Mother Wavelet and AI Model for Precise Classification of Pediatric Electroretinogram Signals. *Sensors* **2023**, *23*, 5813. [CrossRef]
14. Kim, H.R.; Angelaki, D.E.; DeAngelis, G.C. The neural basis of depth perception from motion parallax. *Philos. Trans. R. Soc. London. Ser. B Biol. Sci.* **2016**, *371*, 20150256. [CrossRef]
15. Rogers, B.; Graham, M. Motion parallax as an independent cue for depth perception. *Perception* **1979**, *8*, 125–134. [CrossRef]
16. Grimes, W.N.; Schwartz, G.W.; Rieke, F. The synaptic and circuit mechanisms underlying a change in spatial encoding in the retina. *Neuron* **2014**, *82*, 460–473. [CrossRef]
17. Purgert, R.J.; Lukasiewicz, P.D. Differential encoding of spatial information among retinal on cone bipolar cells. *J. Neurophysiol.* **2015**, *114*, 1757–1772. [CrossRef]
18. Fernandez-Ruiz, A.; Sirota, A.; Lopes-Dos-Santos, V.; Dupret, D. Over and above frequency: Gamma oscillations as units of neural circuit operations. *Neuron* **2023**, *111*, 936–953. [CrossRef]
19. Arab, F.; Rostami, S.; Dehghani-Habibabadi, M.; Mateos, D.M.; Braddell, R.; Scholkmann, F.; Ismail Zibaii, M.; Rodrigues, S.; Salari, V.; Safari, M.S. Effects of optogenetic and visual stimulation on gamma activity in the visual cortex. *Neurosci. Lett.* **2023**, *816*, 137474. [CrossRef]
20. Fetsch, C.R.; Deangelis, G.C.; Angelaki, D.E. Visual-vestibular cue integration for heading perception: Applications of optimal cue integration theory. *Eur. J. Neurosci.* **2010**, *31*, 1721–1729. [CrossRef]
21. Angelaki, D.E.; Klier, E.M.; Snyder, L.H. A vestibular sensation: Probabilistic approaches to spatial perception. *Neuron* **2009**, *64*, 448–461. [CrossRef]
22. Joyce, C.; Le, P.H.; Sadiq, N.M. Histology, Retina. In *StatPearls [Internet]*; StatPearls Publishing: Treasure Island, FL, USA, 2025; [Updated 8 August 2023]. Available online: https://www.ncbi.nlm.nih.gov/books/NBK546692/ (accessed on 4 January 2025).
23. Wang, C.; Bókkon, I.; Dai, J.; Antal, I. Spontaneous and visible light-induced ultraweak photon emission from rat eyes. *Brain Res.* **2011**, *1369*, 1–9. [CrossRef]
24. Cifra, M.; Pospíšil, P. Ultra-weak photon emission from biological samples: Definition, mechanisms, properties, detection and applications. *J. Photochem. Photobiol. B Biol.* **2014**, *139*, 2–10. [CrossRef]
25. Bókkon, I. Visual perception and imagery: A new molecular hypothesis. *Biosystems* **2009**, *96*, 178–184. [CrossRef]

26. Tang, R.; Dai, J. Biophoton signal transmission and processing in the brain. *J. Photochem. Photobiol. B Biol.* **2014**, *139*, 71–75. [CrossRef]
27. Rahnama, M.; Tuszynski, J.A.; Bókkon, I.; Cifra, M.; Sardar, P.; Salari, V. Emission of mitochondrial biophotons and their effect on electrical activity of membrane via microtubules. *J. Integr. Neurosci.* **2011**, *10*, 65–88. [CrossRef]
28. Sharkova, M.; Aparicio, G.; Mouzaaber, C.; Zolessi, F.R.; Hocking, J.C. Photoreceptor calyceal processes accompany the developing outer segment, adopting a stable length despite a dynamic core. *J. Cell Sci.* **2024**, *137*, jcs261721. [CrossRef]
29. Ahmadi, M.; Bolhasani, H. Photonic Neural Networks: A Compact Review. *arXiv* **2023**, arXiv:2302.08390.
30. Wang, M.; Chen, N. Three-dimensional cellular imaging in thick biological tissue with confocal detection of one-photon fluorescence in the near-infrared II window. *J. Biophotonics* **2019**, *12*, e201800459. [CrossRef]
31. Wu, Y.; Christensen, R.; Colón-Ramos, D.; Shroff, H. Advanced optical imaging techniques for neurodevelopment. *Curr. Opin. Neurobiol.* **2013**, *23*, 1090–1097. [CrossRef]
32. Strauss, O. The retinal pigment epithelium in visual function. *Physiol. Rev.* **2005**, *85*, 845–881. [CrossRef]
33. Pospíšil, P.; Prasad, A.; Rác, M. Role of reactive oxygen species in ultra-weak photon emission in biological systems. *J. Photochem. Photobiol. B Biol.* **2014**, *139*, 11–23. [CrossRef]
34. Tsai, C.J.; Marino, J.; Adaixo, R.; Pamula, F.; Muehle, J.; Maeda, S.; Flock, T.; Taylor, N.M.; Mohammed, I.; Matile, H.; et al. Cryo-EM structure of the rhodopsin-Gαi-βγ complex reveals binding of the rhodopsin C-terminal tail to the gβ subunit. *eLife* **2019**, *8*, e46041. [CrossRef]
35. Molday, R.S.; Moritz, O.L. Photoreceptors at a glance. *J. Cell Sci.* **2015**, *128*, 4039–4045. [CrossRef]
36. Baccus, S.A.; Olveczky, B.P.; Manu, M.; Meister, M. A retinal circuit that computes object motion. *J. Neurosci. Off. J. Soc. Neurosci.* **2008**, *28*, 6807–6817. [CrossRef]
37. Gollisch, T.; Meister, M. Eye smarter than scientists believed: Neural computations in circuits of the retina. *Neuron* **2010**, *65*, 150–164. [CrossRef]
38. Werblin, F.S. The retinal hypercircuit: A repeating synaptic interactive motif underlying visual function. *J. Physiol.* **2011**, *589*, 3691–3702. [CrossRef]
39. Molnar, A.; Hsueh, H.A.; Roska, B.; Werblin, F.S. Crossover inhibition in the retina: Circuitry that compensates for nonlinear rectifying synaptic transmission. *J. Comput. Neurosci.* **2009**, *27*, 569–590. [CrossRef]
40. Azeredo da Silveira, R.; Rieke, F. The Geometry of Information Coding in Correlated Neural Populations. *Annu. Rev. Neurosci.* **2021**, *44*, 403–424. [CrossRef]
41. Field, G.D.; Chichilnisky, E.J. Information processing in the primate retina: Circuitry and coding. *Annu. Rev. Neurosci.* **2007**, *30*, 1–30. [CrossRef]
42. Kastner, D.B.; Baccus, S.A. Insights from the retina into the diverse and general computations of adaptation, detection, and prediction. *Curr. Opin. Neurobiol.* **2014**, *25*, 63–69. [CrossRef]
43. Escobar, M.J.; Pezo, D.; Orio, P. Mathematical analysis and modeling of motion direction selectivity in the retina. *J. Physiol.* **2013**, *107*, 349–359. [CrossRef]
44. Noor, N.M.M.; Mustafa, M.A.M. Eye movement activity that affected the eye signals using electrooculography (EOG) technique. In Proceedings of the 2016 6th IEEE International Conference on Control System, Computing and Engineering (ICCSCE), Penang, Malaysia, 25–27 November 2016; pp. 91–95.
45. Polishchuk, O.V.; Tykhanova, O.F. Biophysical aspects of electromagnetic theory of human vision perception of light information in the visible range. *Ukr. Neurosurg. J.* **2022**, *28*, 17–24. [CrossRef]
46. Sun, Z. Neurons Can Generate Electromagnetic Waves. *Nat. Sci.* **2022**, *14*, 463–471. [CrossRef]
47. Bachofer, C.S.; Wittry, S.E. Electroretinogram in response to x-ray stimulation. *Science* **1961**, *133*, 642–644. [CrossRef]
48. Doly, M.; Isabelle, D.B.; Vincent, P.; Gaillard, G.; Meyniel, G. Mechanism of the formation of X-ray-induced phosphenes. I. Electrophysiological investigations. *Radiat. Res.* **1980**, *82*, 93–105. [CrossRef]
49. Feller, M.B. Retinal waves are likely to instruct the formation of eye-specific retinogeniculate projections. *Neural Dev.* **2009**, *4*, 24. [CrossRef]
50. Howard, I.P.; Rogers, B.J. *Binocular Vision and Stereopsis*; Oxford University Press: Oxford, UK, 1995.
51. Hibbard, P.B.; Goutcher, R.; Hornsey, R.L.; Hunter, D.W.; Scarfe, P. Luminance contrast provides metric depth information. *R. Soc. Open Sci.* **2023**, *10*, 220567. [CrossRef]
52. Linton, P. Minimal theory of 3D vision: New approach to visual scale and visual shape. *Philos. Trans. R. Soc. B Biol. Sci.* **2023**, *378*, 20210455. [CrossRef]
53. Vishwanath, D. Toward a new theory of stereopsis. *Psychol. Rev.* **2014**, *121*, 151–178. [CrossRef]
54. Livingstone, M.; Hubel, D. Segregation of form, color, movement, and depth: Anatomy, physiology, and perception. *Science* **1988**, *240*, 740–749. [CrossRef]
55. Marr, D. *Vision: A Computational Investigation into the Human Representation and Processing of Visual Information*; The MIT Press: Cambridge, MA, USA, 2010.

56. Shim, S.; Eom, K.; Jeong, J.; Kim, S.J. Retinal Prosthetic Approaches to Enhance Visual Perception for Blind Patients. *Micromachines* **2020**, *11*, 535. [CrossRef]
57. Qu, J.; Wang, D.; Grosskreutz, C.L. Mechanisms of retinal ganglion cell injury and defense in glaucoma. *Exp Eye Res* **2010**, *91*, 48–53. [CrossRef]
58. Guo, J.J.; Zhou, R.; Zhao, L.M.; Lu, B.L. Multimodal Emotion Recognition from Eye Image, Eye Movement and EEG Using Deep Neural Networks. In Proceedings of the 2019 41st Annual International Conference of the IEEE Engineering in Medicine and Biology Society (EMBC), Berlin, Germany, 23–27 July 2019; Volume 2019, pp. 3071–3074. [CrossRef]
59. Zheng, W.L.; Dong, B.N.; Lu, B.L. Multimodal emotion recognition using EEG and eye tracking data. In Proceedings of the 2014 36th Annual International Conference of the IEEE Engineering in Medicine and Biology Society, Chicago, IL, USA, 26–30 August 2014; pp. 5040–5043.
60. Singh, K.D. Which "neural activity" do you mean? fMRI, MEG, oscillations and neurotransmitters. *NeuroImage* **2012**, *62*, 1121–1130. [CrossRef]
61. Westheimer, G. Path dissociation of visual signals entering the cortex: Disparity, contour orientation and position. *Vis. Res.* **2011**, *51*, 1058–1063. [CrossRef]
62. Westheimer, G. Three-dimensional displays and stereo vision. *Proc. R. Soc. B Biol. Sci.* **2011**, *278*, 2241–2248. [CrossRef]
63. Bar-Cohen, Y. Biomimetics—Using nature to inspire human innovation. *Bioinspiration Biomim.* **2006**, *1*, P1. [CrossRef]

life

MDPI

Article

Pilot Study Evaluating the Early Clinical Outcomes Obtained with a Novel, Customized, Multifocal Corneo-Scleral Contact Lens for Presbyopia Correction

Laura Barberán-Bernardos [1], Daniel Soriano Salcedo [2], Sergio Díaz-Gómez [2] and David P. Piñero [1,3,*]

[1] Department of Optics, Pharmacology and Anatomy, University of Alicante, 03690 Alicante, Spain; laura.barberan@ua.es

[2] Centro Oftalmológico Integral Bilbao Berri SL, Miranza COI Bilbao, 48008 Bilbao, Spain; danielsoriano1989@gmail.com (D.S.S.); sergio.diaz@miranza.es (S.D.-G.)

[3] Department of Ophthalmology (IMQO-Oftalmar), Vithas Medimar International Hospital, 03016 Alicante, Spain

* Correspondence: david.pinyero@ua.es; Tel.: +34-965903400

Abstract: Background: The objective was to preliminarily evaluate the short-term clinical outcomes obtained in presbyopic patients with a novel, multifocal, customized corneo-scleral contact lens (CSCL). Methods: A total of 11 presbyopic subjects (age 45–80 years, corrected-distance visual acuity $\leq$ 0.1 LogMAR, near addition $\geq$ +1.00 D) were recruited and fitted with a multifocal corneo-scleral contact lens in this pilot study. Pre-fitting evaluations included stereopsis, contrast sensitivity (CS), and ocular aberrometry, with follow-up assessments conducted at 20 min and 1-month post-fitting. The defocus curve was also measured to assess visual performance across varying distances. Results: Twenty-two eyes from 11 participants (53.9 $\pm$ 4.7 years, 10 female) were included in this study. Significant changes were observed post-fitting for primary and secondary spherical aberration, coma, and stereopsis ($p \leq 0.033$). No significant changes in Strehl ratio and total root mean square were detected ($p \geq 0.182$). Binocular contrast sensitivity was better with spectacles than with the fitted CSCL at all frequencies ($p \leq 0.048$), but the change in monocular did not reach statistical significance for 18 cycles per degree ($p = 0.109$). All patients and 90.9% of patients achieved a visual acuity of 0.0 LogMAR or better at distance and at intermediate, respectively, and 91.8% achieved 0.3 LogMAR or better for near vision. Conclusions: The customized CSCL evaluated provided functional recovery of visual quality across distances, with acceptable reductions of CS and stereopsis that are comparable to those reported for other multifocal contact lenses.

Keywords: corneo-scleral contact lens; multifocal contact lens; defocus curve; contrast sensitivity; ocular high-order aberrations

1. Introduction

Presbyopia is an age-related condition characterized by a gradual reduction in the lens' accommodative capacity, leading to a progressive decline in near vision [1]. Symptoms typically become noticeable and worsen from the fourth decade of life, affecting approximately 1.8 billion people worldwide [1]. Given the global trend of population aging, the demand for effective presbyopia solutions is expected to rise significantly in the coming years.

The correction of presbyopia with contact lenses was first documented in the 1960s using bifocal designs [2]. However, it was not until the 1980s that the first generation

 https://doi.org/10.3390/life15050700

of multifocal contact lenses emerged, demonstrating clinically satisfactory outcomes [3]. Today, numerous optical designs are commercially available in both soft hydrogel and rigid gas-permeable (RGP) materials, employing various optical principles [4]. While extensive research has evaluated the performance of soft multifocal contact lenses, published data on the clinical efficacy of RGP multifocal designs remains limited [5]. It is important to note that multifocal rigid gas permeable (RGP) contact lenses are available in three distinct fitting designs: fully corneal, corneo-scleral, and fully scleral. While these designs may demonstrate comparable optical performance, previous experience suggests that lenses with scleral bearing typically provide superior comfort due to their reduced interaction with the sensitive corneal nerve endings [6].

Proper centration of multifocal contact lenses (CLs) is critical to prevent ghost images and maintain optimal optical quality. Lens movement during blinking or slight decentration can induce aberrations that compromise visual performance [7]. In this context, scleral contact lenses (SCLs) offer advantages by ensuring stable centration while preserving the superior optical quality of rigid gas-permeable (RGP) materials. However, evidence supporting their efficacy remains limited. Available studies have primarily evaluated miniscleral designs, with no published data on multifocal corneo-scleral contact lenses (CSCLs). Privado-Aroco et al. [8] demonstrated that multifocal miniscleral CLs provide enhanced intermediate and near vision while maintaining good distance acuity compared to monofocal designs. Additionally, SCLs with a customized, decentered optical zone have shown superior visual quality over conventional designs [9].

The tear film meniscus can significantly modulate visual quality and depth of focus in multifocal contact lens (CL) wear, with effects ranging from beneficial to detrimental depending on its optical properties [10]. Furthermore, the eye's inherent higher-order aberrations (HOAs)—particularly primary spherical aberration—critically influence multifocal CL performance since these lenses fundamentally work by inducing controlled amounts of HOAs [11,12]. This interaction between natural ocular aberrations and designed optical profiles underscores the importance of personalized fitting approaches. Thus, optimizing lens design to account for fitting dynamics and ocular optical properties is essential. A fully customized approach is recommended to maximize outcomes. Recently, the Presbycustom lens (Lenticon, Madrid, Spain) became the first commercially available multifocal CSCL for the compensation of presbyopia to incorporate customization based on primary and secondary spherical aberration profiles, compensating also for tear film meniscus effects. This innovation represents a significant advancement in personalized presbyopia correction.

This pilot study aimed to conduct a preliminary evaluation of the short-term clinical performance of a novel, customized, multifocal corneo-scleral contact lens (CSCL) in presbyopic patients, assessing both its clinical viability and potential efficacy. A one-month follow-up period was selected based on established neuroadaptation timelines, as demonstrated by functional magnetic resonance imaging studies showing that primary neural adaptations to new optical corrections typically stabilize within this timeframe [13,14].

2. Materials and Methods

2.1. Participants

This pilot study was conducted at Centro Oftalmológico Integral Bilbao Berri in Bilbao. All subjects signed an informed consent after they were informed of the details of the study. Ethical approval was obtained from the Ethics Committee of the Health Department of Alicante General Hospital (PI2020-084, ISABIAL 200071), and this study was conducted following the tenets of the Declaration of Helsinki.

Inclusion criteria were patients between the ages of 45 and 80 years with corrected-distance visual acuity of 0.1 LogMAR or better and a near addition value equal to or greater than 1 D. Additionally, subjects who presented any systemic pathology affecting the ocular surface, active ocular pathologies, or amblyopia with a difference in visual acuity between both eyes in two or more lines were excluded.

2.2. Pre-Fitting Examination

All participants underwent a complete visual examination by the same experienced optometrist (D.S.S.) before the fitting of the corneo-scleral contact lenses. This examination included objective refraction with retinoscopy, subjective refraction, a cover test, pupillometry, slit lamp biomicroscopy, corneal topography, ocular aberrometry, pachymetry, measurement of stereopsis, and measurement of monocular and binocular CS. The OPD-Scan III platform (Nidek Technologies, Gamagori, Japan) was used to evaluate corneal topography, ocular aberrometry, and pachymetry. Photopic binocular and monocular (dominant eye) contrast sensitivity for frequencies of 1.5, 6, 12, and 18 cycles/degree was assessed using the validated application ClinicCSF [14]. OptoTab (Smarthin4vision, Zaragoza, Spain) was used to evaluate stereopsis. With this data, the parameters of the first trial multifocal CSCL were calculated following the manufacturer's guidelines.

2.3. Contact Lens Design and Fitting

The Presbycustom contact lens (Roflufocon D, Dk 125 Fatt units, Contamac, Saffron Wilden, UK) is the result of a proof-of-concept research project developed by the Group of Optics and Visual Perception of the University of Alicante and licensed to Laboratorios Lenticon SA (Madrid, Spain) [15]. It is a corneo-scleral contact lens made of highly gas-permeable material and comprises three different areas: corneal, limbal, and scleral (Figure 1). This allows for optimal fitting of the CSCL to the different areas of the ocular surface, with alignment in the transition zone between the corneal and limbal zones, as shown in Figure 1.

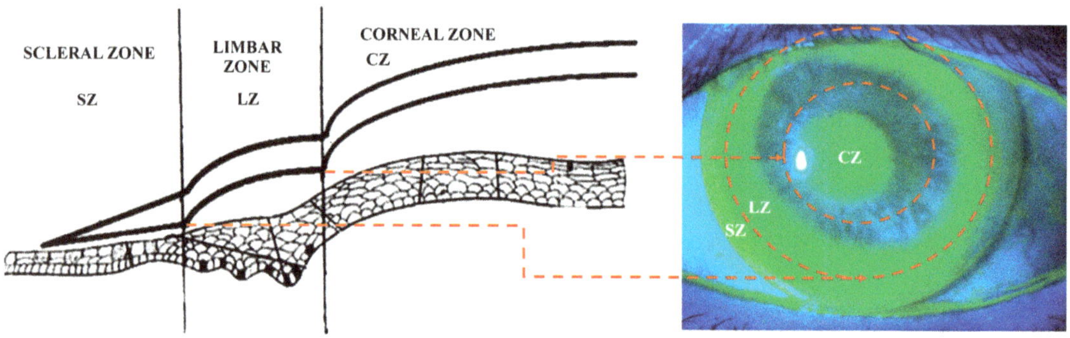

Figure 1. Ideal fluorogram of the corneo-scleral contact lens evaluated (**right**) and diagram of the different parts of the corneo-scleral contact lens (CSCL) (**left**): scleral (SZ), limbal (LZ), and corneal zone (CZ). The orange arrows and circles delimit the transition areas between zones.

The optics of the lens consist of a 4 mm optical zone modifiable to 3.5 mm, including two additional modalities (low or high) to provide less or greater depth of focus, respectively, and a customizable positive or negative spherical aberration induction depending on the patient's ocular spherical aberration. The back surface asphericity of the CSCL is fixed, whereas the central anterior surface asphericity is modified according to the aberrometric induction required. Specifically, the depth of focus achieved with the contact lens is set by customizing the induction of primary and secondary spherical aberration. It has been demonstrated that combining primary and secondary spherical aberrations of opposite signs is significantly more effective for expanding the depth of focus than other aberrometric options [16,17]. The scleral area of the contact lens allows for a smooth bearing over the sclero-conjunctival surface, facilitating comfortable wearing.

The optics were customized based on the level of ocular primary spherical aberration (measured for a 6 mm pupil aperture) in each eye. The target spherical aberration with the contact lens fitted was set close to −0.15 μm (combined with half the value of the secondary spherical aberration and with the opposite sign), as this has been shown to maximize the eye's depth of focus [17,18]. Using the OpTaLix-Pro® 10.1 software (Optenso™, Optical Engineering Software, Igling, Germany) and following a method previously described by our research group [12], specific designs (AB+ low addition, AB− low addition, AB+ high addition, and AB− high addition) were created for clinical use. The following fitting criteria were applied:

- Eyes with negative spherical aberration: Fitting with the AB+ low addition design, switching to AB+ high addition if near visual performance was unsatisfactory.
- Eyes with positive spherical aberration < 0.5 μm (6-mm pupil): Fitting with the AB− low addition design, switching to AB+ high addition if near visual performance was unsatisfactory.
- Eyes with positive spherical aberration > 0.5 μm (6-mm pupil): Case-specific simulation and creation of a fully customized design with the appropriate central anterior surface asphericity.

Multifocal CSCL fitting was performed using biomicroscopy, fluorogram with fluorescein, and optical coherence tomography (OCT) with a Cirrus HD 500 (Carl Zeiss Meditec, Dublin, CA, USA). The distribution of the tear film below the different areas of the CSCL generated a characteristic fluorogram consisting of central tear pooling with paracentral alignment and significant edge clearing (Figure 1).

2.4. Post-Fitting Examination

Two follow-up visits were scheduled by the same examiner who performed the pre-fitting examinations (D.S.): 20 min and a month after lens fitting. In these check-ups, stereopsis, contrast sensitivity, defocus curve, and aberrometry were measured.

2.5. Data Analysis

The SPSS statistical package version 28.0.0 (IBM SPSS Inc., Chicago, IL, USA) was used to perform the statistical analysis. Non-parametric statistics were used due to the limited sample size. The Wilcoxon and Friedman tests were used for the assessment of the statistical significance of differences between the measurements of two and three consecutive visits, respectively. A p-value < 0.05 was considered statistically significant for the analysis.

3. Results

A total of 22 eyes from 11 subjects (10 female) aged between 46 and 64 years were enrolled (mean age: 53.9 ± 4.7 years). All subjects were successfully fitted with the CSCL after one or more trials and no adverse effects were reported during the 1-month follow-up. Mean flattest and steepest keratometric readings were 7.83 ± 0.33 mm and 7.72 ± 0.26 mm, respectively, with a mean keratometry value of 7.77 ± 0.29 mm. Regarding the refractive error, the mean spherical equivalent was +1.14 ± 1.75 D (range: −1.00 to +3.25 D), while the mean presbyopic addition was +2.27 ± 0.32 D (range: +1.75 to +2.75 D). The mean value of the CSCL power that was fitted was −1.20 ± 2.17 D, with an average corneal base radius of 7.26 ± 0.51 mm. All eyes were fitted with contact lenses with a diameter of 14 mm.

Table 1 shows the results of the ocular aberrometric (5 mm pupil) and stereopsis analysis before and after the contact lens fitting. Significant changes were observed in primary spherical aberration (SA), secondary spherical aberration (SA2), primary coma root mean square (RMS), and stereopsis. In contrast, no significant changes were observed in Strehl ratio and total RMS between pre- and post-fitting visits. Specifically, there was a change towards negative primary spherical aberration, whereas the secondary spherical aberration experienced a change towards a positive value. Likewise, the level of primary coma increased. Regarding stereopsis, there was an increase in the threshold that represented a trend towards a lower level of stereopsis with the CSCL fitted.

Table 1. Aberrometry (5 mm pupil) and stereopsis measurements pre-fitting and 20 min post-fitting. Abbreviations: SD, standard deviation; RMS, root mean square; SA, primary spherical aberration; SA2, secondary spherical aberration.

	Pre-Fitting		**Post-Fitting**		
	Mean	**SD**	**Mean**	**SD**	***p*-Value**
Total RMS (µm)	1.90	1.77	3.16	2.13	0.182
Strehl ratio	0.020	0.027	0.018	0.018	0.965
SA (µm)	0.0127	0.103	−0.296	0.297	0.033
SA2 (µm)	−0.008	0.21	0.081	0.78	0.009
Coma RMS (µm)	0.173	0.130	0.882	0.557	0.008
Stereopsis (arc sec)	61.1	64.1	134.7	139.7	0.005

Contrast sensitivity was measured binocularly and monocularly (only in the dominant eye), as shown in Figure 2. Binocularly, contrast sensitivity was significantly better with spectacle correction than with the CSCL for all spatial frequencies: 1.5 (p = 0.027), 6 (p = 0.014), 12 (p = 0.011), and 18 cycles/degree (p = 0.048). Monocularly, significant changes were found for the spatial frequencies of 1.5 (p = 0.027), 6 (p = 0.049), and 12 (p = 0.009) cycles/degree, but changes in monocular CS for 18 cycles/degree did not reach statistical significance (p = 0.109). This is shown in Figure 2.

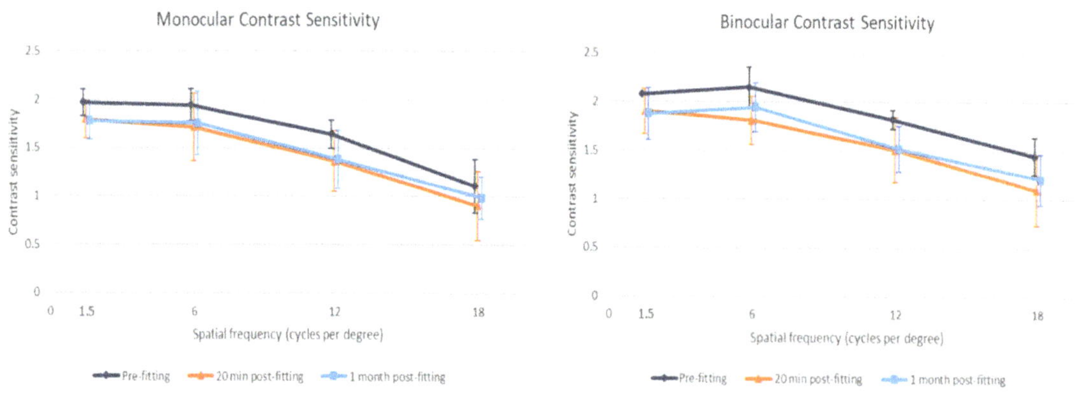

Figure 2. Monocular (dominant eye) and binocular contrast sensitivity before fitting, 20 min post-fitting, and 1-month post-fitting of the multifocal corneo-scleral contact lens evaluated.

Figure 3 shows the defocus curve of the CSCL measured under binocular and monocular conditions (both dominant and non-dominant eye). As shown, the mean corrected-distance visual acuity was 0.20 logMAR or better for defocus levels between 0.50 and −1.50 D under monocular conditions. When the visual acuity was measured binocularly, this range became wider, from +1.00 to −2.00 D.

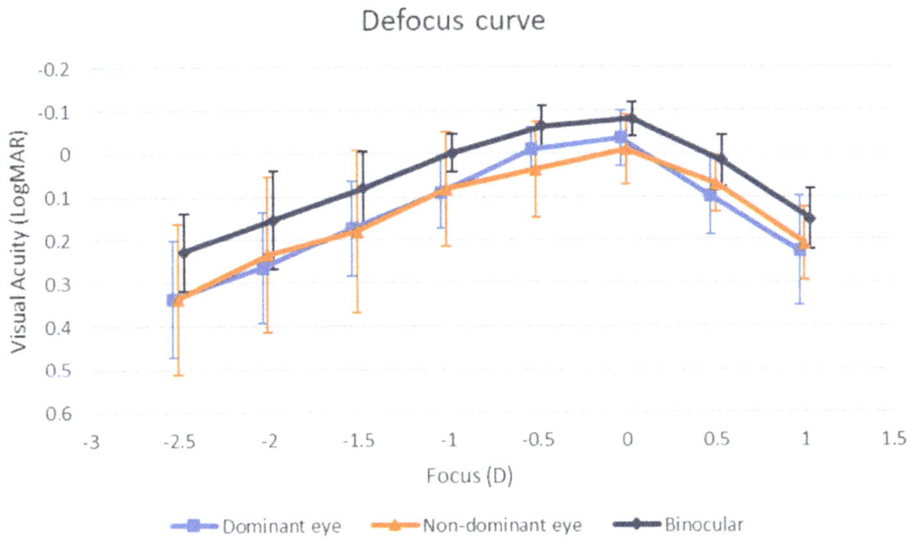

Figure 3. Defocus curve obtained with the multifocal corneo-scleral contact lens evaluated monocularly and binocularly.

Finally, Figure 4 shows the distribution of corrected-distance, intermediate, and near visual acuity achieved with the CSCL fitted. As shown, all patients presented a binocular corrected-distance visual acuity equal to or better than 0 LogMAR (defocus 0.00 D), and 90.9% of patients achieved this visual acuity level at intermediate vision (defocus −1.00 D). Concerning near vision (defocus −2.00 D), 91.8% of patients presented a binocular visual acuity equal to or better than 0.3 LogMAR.

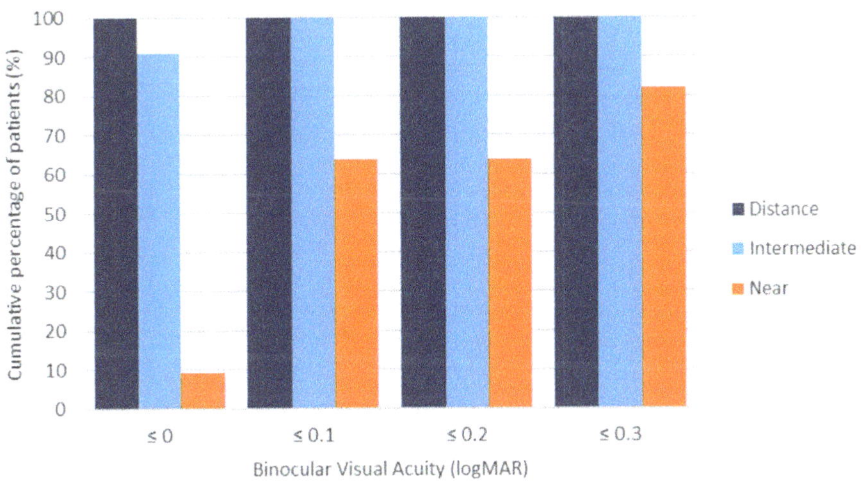

Figure 4. Cumulative percentage of patients with a binocular distance-corrected visual acuity equal to or better than 0.0, 0.1, 0.2, and 0.3 LogMAR for distance, intermediate, and near vision.

4. Discussion

Corneo-scleral contact lenses (CSCLs) offer several advantages for presbyopia correction. Their design creates a stable tear reservoir that simultaneously (1) reduces optical aberrations by smoothing irregular corneal surfaces and (2) maintains ocular surface hydration, particularly benefiting patients with corneal irregularities (e.g., keratoconus) or dry eye disease [19–21]. The mechanical stability of CSCLs provides additional optical benefits: minimal lens movement during blinking (<0.2 mm displacement) [22], reduced deformation, and the consistent induction of controlled aberrations for depth-of-focus enhancement [10]. These advantages have driven a growing interest in CSCLs for presbyopia management, though evidence remains limited. Recently, a breakthrough, customizable, multifocal CSCL (Presbycustom, Lenticon) has been introduced, featuring tear film meniscus compensation and ocular aberration customization. This study represents the first clinical evaluation of this innovative presbyopia correction approach, addressing a critical gap in the contact lens literature.

This study confirmed that the evaluated CSCL provides sufficient depth of focus to ensure functional visual acuity across various distances. Specifically, the mean binocular corrected-distance visual acuity was 0.20 logMAR or better for defocus levels between +1.00 and −2.00 D. These results are consistent with—and, in some cases, superior to—those previously reported for other soft and hybrid multifocal contact lenses [5,23–29]. In 2017, our research group [28] conducted a comparative study of one hybrid multifocal CL (Duette Multifocal, SynergEyes, Carlsbad, CA, USA) and two soft multifocal CLs (AirOptix from Alcon, Fort Worth, TX, USA and Biofinity from CooperVision, Pleasanton, CA, USA). The study found that the mean binocular corrected-distance visual acuity was 0.20 logMAR or better across a defocus range of +0.50 to −2.00 D for all three lenses, with no significant differences in visual acuity at any defocus level evaluated in the defocus curve. García-Lázaro et al. [29] compared the PureVision multifocal CL (Bausch & Lomb, Rochester, NY, USA) with a pinhole CL and observed no significant difference in presbyopia correction for intermediate distances (lens powers from −1.00 to −2.00 D). However, the PureVision Multifocal lens provided significantly better visual acuity at the −2.50 D vergence. In the current study, all patients achieved a binocular corrected-distance visual acuity of 0.00 logMAR or better at 0.00 D defocus, and 90.9% maintained this level at intermediate vision (−1.00 D defocus). These findings confirm the efficacy of the evaluated multifocal CL for far and intermediate distance correction. At near vision (−2.00 D defocus), 91.8% of patients exhibited a binocular visual acuity of $\leq$0.30 logMAR, suggesting functional near vision for most patients [30]. Future studies should explore whether near vision can be further improved with micromonovision, as demonstrated with other multifocal CL modalities [31].

This study provides the first preliminary evaluation of visual performance with a novel, multifocal CSCL. Our findings revealed a measurable reduction in stereopsis (134.7 $\pm$ 139.7 arcsec) after 20 min of lens wear, which contrasts with the better stereopsis outcomes reported by Privado-Aroco et al. for conventional (68.3 $\pm$ 33.3 arcsec) and decentered-optics multifocal scleral lenses (81.2 $\pm$ 60.9 arcsec) [9]. The literature presents conflicting evidence regarding stereopsis with multifocal corrections: while some studies of soft multifocal lenses report superior stereopsis [19–21], others demonstrate impairment comparable to our findings [22,32]. Notably, Privado-Aroco et al.'s pilot work also showed worse stereopsis with multifocal versus monofocal scleral lenses [8]. Several factors may explain this variability, including methodological differences, such as heterogeneity in stereopsis assessment protocols, lack of standardized testing conditions across studies, or variations in control group selection. In addition, the substantial standard deviation in our results ($\pm$139.7 arcsec) suggests considerable inter-subject variability, and the small sample size may have amplified the impact of individual outliers. For this reason, comparison between studies of multifocal CLs in terms of stereopsis should be conducted with care.

This highlights the need for larger, controlled studies with standardized protocols, with direct comparisons between different multifocal designs under matched conditions.

Although some high-order aberrations (coma, SA, SA2) increased after the fitting of the CSCL evaluated, the Strehl ratio and total ocular RMS did not experience significant changes. These changes in SA and SA2 were mainly induced by the lens design, which combines SA and SA2 with opposite signs, leading to an increase in the depth of focus [16,17]. Additionally, as the CSCL evaluated does not have peripheral toricity, some levels of decentration that were mainly due to the naso-temporal scleral asymmetry of the human eye may have been present, contributing potentially to the observed increase in coma [10,33]. In any case, the levels of SA, SA2, and primary coma found with the multifocal CSCL fitted were within the range of normality [34], with no abnormal inductions of high-order aberrations. It should also be noted here that the adjustment of the toricity of the landing zone of an SCL could be beneficial in reducing lens flexure and rotation [35], leading to an improvement in the level of neutralization of high-order aberrations.

As in most previous studies evaluating the impact of multifocal CLs in CS [8,9,36–38], a trend towards a reduction in contrast sensitivity was found when assessed with the multifocal CSCL compared to spectacle correction. However, compared to the range of normality defined for most of the CS tests that are available, the level of CS obtained with the CSCL evaluated was within the range of normality across all spatial frequencies, despite its reduction [39]. Therefore, the expansion of the depth of focus with the CSCL evaluated was generated by inducing a controlled increase of high-order aberrations, maintaining the levels of visual quality within an acceptable level. Indeed, as previously mentioned, the defocus curve showed that the CSCL evaluated enabled good visual performance at far and intermediate vision, with functional results in near vision [30]. The defocus curve presented a smooth profile, characterized by a gradual decrease in near vision and a peak in distance vision, indicating an effective distribution of focal power across distances.

This was a pilot study and, therefore, has several limitations. First, the small sample size may limit the generalizability of the results to a broader population, but the aim of the current study was to confirm the clinical viability of this novel CSCL. Further studies with larger sample sizes—including a more balanced sex distribution—are needed to analyze clinical outcomes across subgroups (e.g., refractive error, pupillometry, age). Moreover, the lack of a control group using multifocal soft CL or CSCL limits the ability to directly compare the performance of the CSCL against current options. However, it should be considered that this is a pilot study to confirm the viability of this type of CL, and a new, randomized, controlled clinical trial has been designed (including a control group) to confirm exactly the real benefit of the new CSCL over a commercially available multifocal soft CL. Another limitation is the potential decentration due to the lack of toricity in the peripheral area of the lens, which may have significantly impacted the visual quality. This limitation should be overcome in future modifications of the design of the CL.

5. Conclusions

The CSCL Presbycustom effectively restores visual acuity across distances in presbyopic patients while maintaining functional visual quality and stereopsis. Further research with larger sample sizes is needed to validate these preliminary findings and assess its comparative efficacy relative to existing multifocal contact lenses for presbyopia.

Author Contributions: Conceptualization, L.B.-B., D.S.S. and D.P.P.; methodology, D.S.S. and D.P.P.; software, L.B.-B.; validation, L.B.-B., D.S.S., S.D.-G. and D.P.P.; formal analysis, L.B.-B. and D.S.S.; investigation, L.B.-B., D.S.S. and D.P.P.; resources, D.S.S., S.D.-G. and D.P.P.; data curation, L.B.-B.; writing—original draft preparation, D.S.S. and L.B.-B.; writing—review and editing, L.B.-B., D.S.S., S.D.-G. and D.P.P.; visualization, D.S.S.; supervision, L.B.-B. and D.P.P.; project administration,

D.P.P.; funding acquisition, D.P.P. All authors have read and agreed to the published version of the manuscript.

Funding: The author Laura Barberán-Bernardos was supported by the Conselleria de Innovación, Universidades, Ciencia y Sociedad Digital de la Generalitat Valenciana, within the Program ACIF (Subvenciones para la contratación de personal investigador predoctoral), reference number CIACIF/2022/073, cofinanced by the European Social Fund. The rest of the authors did not receive funding for conducting this research.

Institutional Review Board Statement: This study was conducted in accordance with the Declaration of Helsinki and approved by the Ethics Committee of the Health Department of Alicante General Hospital (PI2020-084, ISABIAL 200071) on 27 May 2020.

Informed Consent Statement: Informed consent was obtained from all subjects involved in this study.

Data Availability Statement: Data are available upon reasonable request to the authors.

Conflicts of Interest: David P. Piñero is the author of the patent of the Presbycustom contact lens, whose commercialization has been licensed to Laboratorios Lenticon SA (Madrid, Spain). The rest of the authors have no proprietary or commercial interest in the medical devices that are involved in this manuscript.

Abbreviations

The following abbreviations are used in this manuscript:

CSCL	Corneo-scleral contact lens
CS	Contrast sensitivity
IOL	Intraocular lens
SCL	Scleral contact lens
CL	Contact lens
SA	Primary spherical aberration
SA2	Secondary spherical aberration
RMS	Root mean square

References

1. Fricke, T.R.; Tahhan, N.; Resnikoff, S.; Papas, E.; Burnett, A.; Ho, S.M.; Naduvilath, T.; Naidoo, K.S. Global prevalence of presbyopia and vision impairment from uncorrected presbyopia: Systematic review, meta-analysis, and modelling. *Ophthalmology* **2018**, *125*, 1492–1499. [CrossRef]
2. Fonda, G. Presbyopia corrected with single vision spectacles or corneal lenses in preference to bifocal corneal lenses. *Trans. Ophthalmol. Soc. Aus.* **1966**, *25*, 78–80.
3. Gussler, C.H.; Solomon, K.D.; Gussler, J.R.; Litteral, G.; Van Meter, W.S. A clinical evaluation of two multifocal soft contact lenses. *CLAO J.* **1992**, *18*, 237–239.
4. Kim, E.; Bakaraju, R.C.; Ehrmann, K. Power profiles of commercial multifocal soft contact lenses. *Optom. Vis. Sci.* **2017**, *94*, 183–196. [CrossRef]
5. Molina-Martín, A.; Piñero, D.P.; Martínez-Plaza, E.; Rodríguez-Vallejo, M.; Fernández, J. Efficacy of presbyopia-correcting contact lenses: A systematic review. *Eye Contact Lens* **2023**, *49*, 319–328. [CrossRef] [PubMed]
6. Shorter, E.; Schornack, M.; Harthan, J.; Nau, A.; Fogt, J.; Cao, D.; Nau, C. Keratoconus patient satisfaction and care burden with corneal gas-permeable and scleral lenses. *Optom. Vis. Sci.* **2020**, *97*, 790–796. [CrossRef] [PubMed]
7. Fedtke, C.; Ehrmann, K.; Thomas, V.; Bakaraju, R.C. Association between multifocal soft contact lens decentration and visual performance. *Clin. Optom.* **2016**, *8*, 57–69.
8. Privado-Aroco, A.; Valdes-Soria, G.; Romaguera, M.; Serramito, M.; Carracedo, G. Visual quality assessment and comparison of monofocal and multifocal scleral lens designs: A pilot study. *Eye Contact Lens* **2024**, *50*, 35–40. [CrossRef]
9. Privado-Aroco, A.; Romaguera, M.; Valdes-Soria, G.; Serramito, M.; Carracedo, G. Visual quality assessment and comparison of two multifocal scleral lens designs. *Contact Lens Anterior Eye* **2024**, *47*, 102098. [CrossRef]
10. Piñero, D.P.; Tolosa, Á.; Ariza-Gracia, M.A. Optical simulations of the impact of vault increase in scleral contact lenses in healthy eyes. *Contact Lens Anterior Eye* **2023**, *46*, 101847. [CrossRef]

11. Plainis, S.; Ntzilepis, G.; Atchison, D.A.; Charman, W.N. Through-focus performance with multifocal contact lenses: Effect of binocularity, pupil diameter and inherent ocular aberrations. *Ophthalmic Physiol. Opt.* **2013**, *33*, 42–50. [CrossRef] [PubMed]
12. Rosa, A.M.; Miranda, A.C.; Patricio, M.; McAlinden, C.; Silva, F.L.; Murta, J.N.; Castelo-Branco, M. Functional magnetic resonance imaging to assess the neurobehavioral impact of dysphotopsia with multifocal intraocular lenses. *Ophthalmology* **2017**, *124*, 1280–1289. [CrossRef]
13. Rosa, A.M.; Miranda, A.C.; Patricio, M.M.; McAlinden, C.; Silva, F.L.; Castelo-Branco, M.; Murta, J.N. Functional magnetic resonance imaging to assess neuroadaptation to multifocal intraocular lenses. *J. Cataract Refract. Surg.* **2017**, *43*, 1287–1296. [CrossRef]
14. Rodríguez-Vallejo, M.; Remón, L.; Monsoriu, J.A.; Furlan, W.D. Designing a new test for contrast sensitivity function measurement with iPad. *J. Optom.* **2015**, *8*, 101–108. [CrossRef]
15. Piñero, D.P.; Tolosa, A.; de Fez, D.; Camps, V.J.; Caballero, M.T. Lente de Contacto Multifocal Scleral. P201631236, 21 September 2016.
16. Yi, F.; Iskander, R.; Collins, M. Depth of focus and visual acuity with primary and secondary spherical aberration. *Vis. Res.* **2011**, *51*, 1648–1658. [CrossRef] [PubMed]
17. Benard, Y.; López-Gil, N.; Legras, R. Optimizing the subjective depth-of-focus with combinations of fourth- and sixth order spherical aberration. *Vis. Res.* **2011**, *51*, 2471–2477. [CrossRef]
18. Bakaraju, R.C.; Ehrmann, K.; Papas, E.B.; Ho, A. Depth-of-focus and its association with the spherical aberration sign. A ray-tracing analysis. *J. Optom.* **2010**, *3*, 51–59. [CrossRef]
19. Rathi, V.M.; Mandathara, P.S.; Taneja, M.; Dumpati, S.; Sangwan, V.S. Scleral lens for keratoconus: Technology update. *Clin. Ophthalmol.* **2015**, *9*, 2013–2018. [CrossRef] [PubMed]
20. Ruiz-Lozano, R.E.; Gomez-Elizondo, D.E.; Colorado-Zavala, M.F.; Loya-Garcia, D.; Rodriguez-Garcia, A. Update on indications, complications, and outcomes of scleral contact lenses. *Med. Hypothesis Discov. Innov. Ophthalmol.* **2022**, *10*, 165–178. [CrossRef]
21. Qiu, S.X.; Fadel, D.; Hui, A. Scleral lenses for managing dry eye disease in the absence of corneal irregularities: What is the current evidence? *J. Clin. Med.* **2024**, *13*, 3838. [CrossRef]
22. Ticak, A.; Marsack, J.D.; Koenig, D.E.; Ravikumar, A.; Shi, Y.; Nguyen, L.C.; Applegate, R.A. A comparison of three methods to increase scleral contact lens on-eye stability. *Eye Contact Lens* **2015**, *41*, 386–390. [CrossRef] [PubMed]
23. Kang, P.; Wildsoet, C.F. Acute and short-term changes in visual function with multifocal soft contact lens wear in young adults. *Contact Lens Anterior Eye* **2016**, *39*, 133–140. [CrossRef]
24. Ferrer-Blasco, T.; Madrid-Costa, D. Stereoacuity with balanced presbyopic contact lenses. *Clin. Exp. Optom.* **2011**, *94*, 76–81. [CrossRef] [PubMed]
25. Sha, J.; Bakaraju, R.C.; Tilia, D.; Chung, J.; Delaney, S.; Munro, A.; Ehrmann, K.; Thomas, V.; Holden, B.A. Short-term visual performance of soft multifocal contact lenses for presbyopia. *Arq. Bras. Oftalmol.* **2016**, *79*, 73–77. [CrossRef]
26. Tilia, D.; Munro, A.; Chung, J.; Sha, J.; Delaney, S.; Kho, D.; Thomas, V.; Ehrmann, K.; Bakaraju, R.C. Short-term comparison between extended depth-of-focus prototype contact lenses and a commercially-available center-near multifocal. *J. Optom.* **2017**, *10*, 14–25. [CrossRef]
27. Sivardeen, A.; Laughton, D.; Wolffsohn, J.S. Randomized crossover trial of silicone hydrogel presbyopic contact lenses. *Optom. Vis. Sci.* **2016**, *93*, 141–149. [CrossRef] [PubMed]
28. Piñero, D.P.; Carracedo, G.; Ruiz-Fortes, P.; Pérez-Cambrodí, R.J. Comparative analysis of the visual performance and aberrometric outcomes with a new hybrid and two silicone hydrogel multifocal contact lenses: A pilot study. *Clin. Exp. Optom.* **2015**, *98*, 451–458. [CrossRef]
29. García-Lázaro, S.; Albarrán-Diego, C.; Ferrer-Blasco, T.; Radhakrishnan, H.; Montés-Micó, R. Visual performance comparison between contact lens-based pinhole and simultaneous vision contact lenses. *Clin. Exp. Optom.* **2013**, *96*, 46–52. [CrossRef]
30. Ribeiro, F.; Cochener, B.; Kohnen, T.; Mencucci, R.; Katz, G.; Lundstrom, M.; Casanovas, A.S.; Hewlett, D. Definition and clinical relevance of the concept of functional vision in cataract surgery ESCRS Position Statement on Intermediate Vision: ESCRS Functional Vision Working Group. *J. Cataract Refract. Surg.* **2020**, *46* (Suppl. 1), S1–S3. [CrossRef]
31. Parekh, D.; Asokan, R.; Purkait, S.; Iqbal, A. Multifocal versus modified monovision corrections: A non-dispensing comparison of visual assessment in presbyopic neophytes. *Indian J. Ophthalmol.* **2023**, *71*, 1837–1842. [CrossRef]
32. Sha, J.; Tilia, D.; Kho, D.; Amrizal, H.; Diec, J.; Yeotikar, N.; Jong, M.; Thomas, V.; Bakaraju, R.C. Visual performance of daily-disposable multifocal soft contact lenses: A randomized, double-blind clinical trial. *Optom. Vis. Sci.* **2018**, *95*, 1096–1104. [CrossRef]
33. Kowalski, L.P.; Collins, M.J.; Vincent, S.J. Scleral lens centration: The influence of centre thickness, scleral topography, and apical clearance. *Contact Lens Anterior Eye* **2020**, *43*, 562–567. [CrossRef] [PubMed]
34. Wang, L.; Koch, D.D. Ocular higher-order aberrations in individuals screened for refractive surgery. *J. Cataract Refract. Surg.* **2003**, *29*, 1896–1903. [CrossRef] [PubMed]

35. Alexander, J.; Belaineh Aweke, Y.; Bhebhe, Z.; Cho, D.; Lay, S.; Ryan, I.; Collins, M.J.; Vincent, S.J. The effect of landing zone toricity on scleral lens fitting characteristics and optics. *Ophthalmic Physiol. Opt.* **2024**, *44*, 867–875. [CrossRef]
36. Kaymak, H.; Neller, K.; Schütz, S.; Graff, B.; Sickenberger, W.; Langenbucher, A.; Seitz, B.; Schwahn, H. Vision tests on spectacle lenses and contact lenses for optical myopia correction: A pilot study. *BMJ Open Ophthalmol.* **2022**, *7*, e000971. [CrossRef] [PubMed]
37. Nti, A.N.; Gregory, H.R.; Ritchey, E.R.; Wolffsohn, J.S.; Berntsen, D.A. Contrast sensitivity with center-distance multifocal soft contact lenses. *Optom. Vis. Sci.* **2022**, *99*, 342–349. [CrossRef]
38. Bickle, K.M.; Mitchell, G.L.; Walline, J.J. Visual performance with spherical and multifocal contact lenses in a pediatric population. *Optom. Vis. Sci.* **2021**, *98*, 483–489. [CrossRef]
39. Chung, S.T.L.; Legge, G.E. Comparing the Shape of Contrast Sensitivity Functions for Normal and Low Vision. *Investig. Opthalmology Vis. Sci.* **2016**, *57*, 198–207. [CrossRef]

life

MDPI

Article

Fixation Stability of the Right and Left Eyes Under Binocular and Monocular Viewing Conditions

Jae-Hyeon Noh, Sang-Yeob Kim, Byeong-Yeon Moon, Hyun Gug Cho and Dong-Sik Yu *

Department of Optometry, Kangwon National University, Samcheok 25949, Republic of Korea; nys3678@kangwon.ac.kr (J.-H.N.); syk@kangwon.ac.kr (S.-Y.K.); bymoon@kangwon.ac.kr (B.-Y.M.); hyung@kangwon.ac.kr (H.G.C.)

* Correspondence: yds@kangwon.ac.kr; Tel.: +82-33-540-3415; Fax: +82-33-540-3419

Abstract: Herein, we investigated changes in fixation stability between the right and left eyes during binocular and monocular viewing in young adults without strabismic binocular vision disorders. Fixation stability was assessed using the bivariate contour ellipse area (BCEA) in 34 healthy participants (15 males, 19 females) in their 20s. Eye-tracking was performed under three conditions: binocular viewing, monocular viewing, and monocular occlusion. Under these conditions, the median BCEA (deg^2) values for the right and left eyes were 0.95 and 0.75, 1.07 and 0.86, and 1.62 and 1.32, respectively. Fixation stability did not differ significantly between the right and left eyes under the same viewing conditions. However, the left eye demonstrated greater fixation stability under binocular viewing (closed loop/both eyes open) than the right eye under monocular viewing (open loop/one eye closed). Participants with a dominant left eye in binocular viewing had higher fixation stability than those with a dominant right eye. During monocular occlusion, the nondominant eye showed better fixation stability than the dominant eye. A significant quantitative correlation was observed between phoria and fixation stability in the left eye during binocular viewing. These findings show that fixation stability changes with different viewing conditions and is affected by which eye is covered. Therefore, when conducting tests such as ocular alignment, which involve covering one eye, it may be helpful to assess both right and left eye occlusion for ensuring a more comprehensive analysis.

Keywords: fixation stability; binocular viewing; monocular viewing; phoria; bivariate contour ellipse area (BCEA); dominant eye

1. Introduction

Fixation stability, along with saccadic and pursuit functions, is a key factor in evaluating ocular movements [1–3]. Clinically, fixation stability refers to the ability of the eye to maintain a steady gaze on a target. Disorders such as macular disease [4], amblyopia [5,6], strabismus [7,8], anisometropia [9], and neurological dysfunction [10] can compromise fixation stability, leading to impaired visual function. Advanced devices such as microperimeters [11,12] and eye trackers [13,14] have allowed for more precise evaluation of fixation stability, revealing impairments in both binocular coordination and monocular-independent eye movements [15–17] in individuals with these disorders. As a result, fixation stability assessment has become an essential tool in ophthalmological and neurological examinations [18]. Fixation stability is not only fundamental to ocular health but also contributes to a better understanding of eye movement dynamics, binocular coordination, and interactions within the oculomotor system. Furthermore, it can provide crucial insights into the detection of abnormalities associated with motor and neurological disorders such as Parkinson's disease [19]. Therefore, the objective assessment of fixation stability using eye tracking offers valuable implications for both clinical and research settings.

Eye trackers, which are precise and non-invasive, enable detailed analysis of fixation stability, including micro-eye movements. They can assess fixation stability in each eye separately or evaluate binocular coordination [20,21], making them particularly valuable for detecting subtle fixation disturbances. In previous studies [22–25], we utilized an eye tracker to conduct a more detailed analysis of micro-eye movements in individuals with non-strabismic binocular vision disorders such as phoria, which may be less apparent during binocular fixation. However, those studies analyzed the mean gaze positions of the right and left eyes collectively rather than examining each eye's individual gaze position during binocular viewing. Additionally, fixation stability could not be assessed during monocular viewing under covered conditions.

Because eye trackers detect fixation using infrared cameras, incorporating an infrared filter could allow for the assessment of fixation stability in both exposed and covered eyes. This approach may make it possible to measure fixation stability under both closed-loop binocular (both eyes open) and open-loop monocular viewing (one eye closed) conditions [26,27].

Fixation stability evaluation can improve patient care or diagnosis of eye fixation disorders related to ocular health. We aimed to evaluate fixation stability in the right and left eyes under three conditions: binocular viewing, gazing (fixating) during monocular viewing, and covered non-fixation during monocular occlusion. We also examined whether fixation stability is related to eye dominance and phoria. These findings provide insight into how fixation stability is influenced by binocular coordination, eye dominance, and phoria, offering valuable implications for both clinical and research settings.

2. Materials and Methods

2.1. Participants and Clinical Measures

The required minimum sample size was determined using G*Power 3.1 software (version 3.1.9.4; Heinrich-Heine-Universität Düsseldorf, Düsseldorf, Germany). The sample size needed for the Wilcoxon signed-rank test was calculated for the control group based on an effect size of 0.54. This effect size was derived by converting the mean $\pm$ standard deviation of log-transformed bivariate contour ellipse area ($\log_{10}$BCEA) for binocular and monocular viewing from the reference data [27] (-0.88 ± 0.28 and -0.59 ± 0.26, respectively) into exponent values (0.13 ± 0.18 and 0.26 ± 0.32, respectively). The calculation also incorporated the strongest correlation coefficient (0.663) between binocular and monocular viewing from the control group reference data [28], which were converted into exponent values. With a significance level (α) of 0.05 and statistical power (1-β) of 0.80, the minimum sample size was calculated as 31. In this study, 34 participants were recruited, exceeding the minimum required sample size by 10%.

This study included 34 healthy university students (15 males and 19 females) aged 20–27 years. The inclusion criteria required participants to have non-strabismic binocular vision, no history of refractive surgery, no current or past diagnosis of strabismus, and no use of medications that could affect visual function. This study was approved by the Kangwon National University Institutional Review Board (KWNUIRB-2023-02-007-001) and conducted in accordance with the tenets of the Declaration of Helsinki. Written informed consent was obtained from all participants before their inclusion.

All participants underwent clinical optometric examinations to assess habitual visual correction, with or without spectacles or contact lenses [29]. Distance visual acuity at 5 m ranged from 0.70 logMAR (logarithm of the minimum angle of resolution) (0.2 decimal) to

−0.08 logMAR (1.2 decimal). Near visual acuity at 40 cm was within normal limits, with no reported difficulty in performing daily activities such as reading and writing. Distance visual acuity was measured using a projection chart (ACP-8; Topcon, Tokyo, Japan), and the refractive power of corrective ophthalmic and contact lenses was measured using a lens meter (LM-15; Topcon, Tokyo, Japan). Ocular dominance was determined using the hole-in-the-card method. Phoria was assessed using the modified Thorington method with a Bernell muscle imbalance measure (MIM) card (BC/1209; Bernell, Mishawaka, IN, USA) by placing a Maddox rod in front of the right eye. Distance phoria was measured at 5 m, and near phoria was measured at a viewing distance of 55 cm using an MIM card calibrated to 40 cm and then converted. The measured prism diopters were recorded as negative for exophoria and positive for esophoria.

2.2. Apparatus and Procedure

Fixation stability was assessed using the Clinical Eye Tracker (version 18.04; Thomson Software Solutions, Hatfield, UK) [22–24]. This device is equipped with a 70 Hz remote Tobii Eye Tracker (Tobii EyeX; Tobii Technology, Stockholm, Sweden) and features a display that visually presents gaze positions. A 27-inch LCD monitor (1920 × 1080 pixels; LG, Seoul, Republic of Korea) was used to display gaze targets. Tobii eye trackers use near-infrared spectral light to illuminate the eyes and produce light reflection patterns for each eye. These patterns, combined with advanced image-processing algorithms, enable precise tracking of gaze positions. All participants underwent fixation stability testing during habitual visual correction, with or without spectacles, to minimize the influence of new spectacles. The participants were instructed to fixate on the center of the monitor, positioned 55 cm away, using a chin and forehead rest to minimize head movements.

The eye tracker was calibrated for each participant's eyes using built-in fixation targets (center, top center, bottom left, and bottom right). Gaze targets consisted of red circular stimuli (3.7 mm diameter, corresponding to approximately 0.66 logMAR) displayed against a black background at the center of the monitor. Participants were asked to fixate on the target for 15 s while measurements were recorded. Gaze data from the monitoring display were recorded as horizontal (x-axis) and vertical (y-axis) positions, while vergence states were classified as divergence (exo) and convergence (eso). Fixation stability was primarily analyzed based on horizontal and vertical gaze positions. Viewing conditions included binocular, monocular, and monocular non-fixation, as shown in Figure 1. For monocular viewing conditions, one eye was occluded using an infrared filter (Hoya R72 infrared filter; Hoya Corporation, Tokyo, Japan) that blocked light with wavelengths shorter than 720 nm, enabling simultaneous measurement of the viewing and occluded eyes.

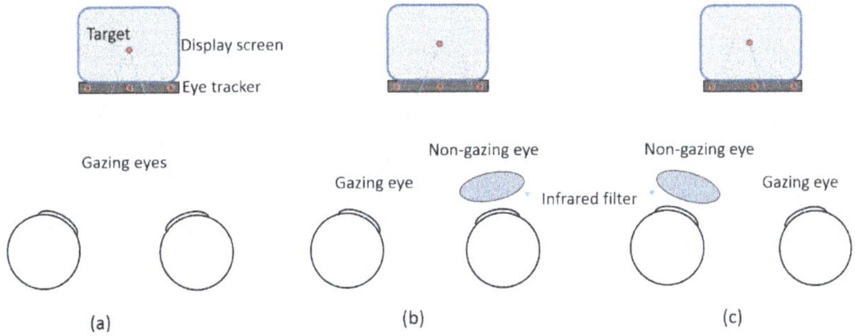

Figure 1. Schematic presentation of viewing conditions. (**a**) Binocular viewing; (**b**) monocular non-fixation for the right eye and monocular viewing for the left eye; (**c**) monocular viewing for the right eye and monocular non-fixation for the left eye.

Fixation stability data were exported to Excel files for analysis. Data extraction was performed over a 10-s interval, with the start point ranging from 0.5 to 3 s and the end point from 10.5 to 13 s, excluding spark-affected regions within the 15-s measurement period and disregarding eye blinks.

Gaze stability was assessed using the bivariate contour ellipse area (BCEA) [22–24,30], which integrates the horizontal and vertical gaze positions according to the following equation:

$$BCEA = 2k\pi\sigma_h\sigma_v(1-\rho^2) \quad (1)$$

where σ_h and σ_v represent the standard deviations (SD) of the horizontal and vertical gaze positions, respectively, and ρ denotes the Pearson product-moment correlation coefficient between the horizontal and vertical gaze positions. The constant k corresponds to the probability area, where k = 1.146 represents a 68.2% probability area (±1 SD). BCEA was expressed in the pixel area (pixel^2). To convert the units to degrees (deg^2), a conversion factor of 0.032°/pixel was applied, based on a reference distance of 55 cm. A smaller BCEA value indicates better gaze stability. If necessary, BCEA plots were generated using the RStudio software (version 1.3.1093; RStudio, Boston, MA, USA).

2.3. Statistical Analysis

All statistical analyses were performed using MedCalc (version 12.7.7.0; MedCalc Software, Ostend, Belgium). The D'Agostino-Pearson test was used to determine whether the sample data followed a normal distribution. To compare fixation stability between the eyes under different viewing conditions, the choice of statistical test was based on the normality test result. If the data did not follow a normal distribution, the Wilcoxon signed-rank test or Mann–Whitney U test was applied instead of the paired *t*-test or independent *t*-test. The high and low fixation stability ratios between viewing conditions were analyzed using a chi-square test. The correlation between fixation stability and phoria was assessed using Spearman's rank correlation coefficient (r_s). A *p*-value of less than 0.05 was considered statistically significant.

3. Results

3.1. Participants' Demographic and Refractive Characteristics

The demographic and refractive characteristics of the 68 eyes of the 34 participants included in the study are presented in Table 1. These characteristics provide insights into the participants' demographic composition, including age and sex distribution, refractive errors in non-strabismic binocular vision disorders (rather than strabismus), and the degree of ocular deviation, facilitating the interpretation of the study results.

All participants were in their 20s, with a mean age of 22.4 ± 2.1 years. The male-to-female ratio was 15:19, and the number of participants wearing spectacles was twice that of those who did not. Visual acuity below the amblyopia threshold of 0.20 logMAR [7,27] was identified in seven eyes. However, after excluding three eyes with uncorrected refractive errors and one eye with an interocular difference of fewer than two lines, only three eyes (3/68 eyes; 4.4%) were classified as amblyopic, indicating a very low prevalence of amblyopia. Refractive errors were predominantly myopic (67.6%), with no cases of hyperopia. The right eye was dominant in 60.3% of cases (61.8% for distance vision, 58.8% for near vision). Most participants exhibited non-strabismic binocular vision characterized by exophoria at near distances.

Table 1. Demographic and refractive characteristics of the study participants.

	Mean ± SD	Range
Male/female (*n*)	15/19	
Age (years)	22.4 ± 2.1	20—27
Refractive correction/no correction (*n*)	23/11	
Decimal visual acuity (logMAR)	0.07 ± 0.16	−0.08—0.70
Better than 0.15/worse than 0.20 (eyes)	61/7	no correction: 3
Refractive errors (*n*)		
Myopia/emmetropia/not confirmed (*n*)	23/6/5	
Corrected refractive power (D, diopters)		
Spherical power	−2.88 ± 1.42	0.25—−5.75
Cylindrical power	−1.24 ± 0.93	−0.25—−3.50
Spherical equivalent	−3.32 ± 1.53	−0.25—−6.50
Phoria (△, prism diopters)		
Distance	−2.24 ± 2.35	1.50—−9.50
Near	−5.91 ± 5.42	1.00—−24.00
Dominant eyes: right/left eyes (*n*)		
Distance	21/13	Distance ≠ near: 3
Near	20/14	

3.2. *Fixation Stability in Binocular and Monocualr Viewing*

Fixation stability under three viewing conditions—binocular viewing (closed loop/both eyes open), gazing eye during monocular viewing (open loop), and covered non-gazing eye during monocular viewing (open loop/one eye closed)—was evaluated using BCEA (deg^2), where lower BCEA values indicate better fixation stability. The median (25th to 75th percentile) and the mean ± standard deviation were as follows: for the right eye in binocular viewing (RE/BV), 0.95 (0.67–1.62) and 1.20 ± 0.87; for the left eye in binocular viewing (LE/BV), 0.75 (0.53–1.22) and 1.02 ± 0.84; for the right eye in monocular viewing (RE/MV), 1.07 (0.72–1.58) and 1.32 ± 0.92; for the left eye in monocular viewing (LE/MV), 0.86 (0.68–1.18) and 1.02 ± 0.58; for the right eye covered in monocular viewing (cRE/MV), 1.62 (1.09–2.30) and 1.87 ± 1.03; and for the left eye covered in monocular viewing (cLE/MV), 1.32 (0.91–2.31) and 1.61 ± 0.96. Across all viewing conditions, the left eye tended to show better fixation stability than the right eye. However, when data from both right and left eyes were combined to increase the sample size, the right eye had a significantly larger BCEA, indicating lower fixation stability (RE vs. LE, Wilcoxon signed-rank test, Z-score = 2.959, $p = 0.003$).

When fixation stability was visualized using box-and-whisker and violin plots, as shown in Figure 2, fixation stability was the highest under binocular viewing conditions (RE/BV and LE/BV), with smaller BCEA values and narrower data distributions. Under monocular viewing conditions (RE/MV and LE/MV), BCEA values increased, indicating slightly reduced fixation stability. For the covered eye conditions (cRE/MV and cLE/MV), the BCEA values increased significantly, showing the lowest fixation stability.

A significant difference in the proportion of high vs. low BCEA values between the right and left eyes observed across viewing conditions ($\chi^2(5) = 13.412$, $p = 0.020$). In 22 of the 34 cases (64.7%), LE/BV was smaller than RE/BV. Similarly, in 21 of the 34 cases (61.8%), both LE/MV and cLE/MV were smaller than RE/MV and cRE/MV, respectively. However, the difference in fixation stability between right and left eyes was not statistically significant.

As shown in Table 2, a comparison of fixation stability between binocular and monocular viewing showed that the difference in BCEA was statistically significant between the left eye in binocular viewing and the right eye in monocular viewing (LE/BV vs. RE/MV; Wilcoxon signed-rank test, $p = 0.029$), with the left eye demonstrating better fixation stability in binocular viewing. Moderate positive correlations were observed between the right eye during binocular viewing and the right eye during monocular viewing (r_s = 0.484, p = 0.005), while a weak positive correlation was observed between the left eye during binocular viewing and the left eye during monocular viewing (r_s = 0.345, p = 0.047).

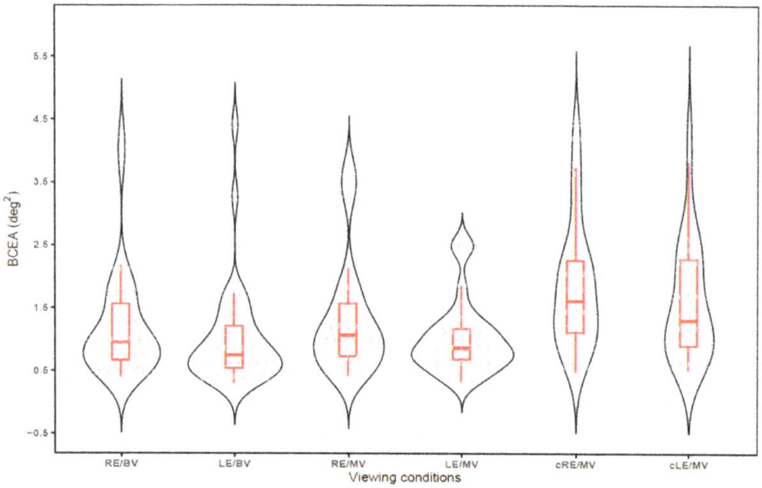

Figure 2. Fixation stability under different viewing conditions. BCEA = bivariate contour ellipse area, RE/BV = right eye in binocular viewing, LE/BV = left eye in binocular viewing, RE/MV = right eye in monocular viewing, LE/MV = left eye in monocular viewing, cRE/MV = right eye covered in monocular viewing, cLE/MV = left eye covered in monocular viewing.

Table 2. Comparison of BCEA during binocular and monocular viewing.

	n	Wilcoxon Signed-Rank Test		Correlation Coefficient	
		Z-Score	***p*-Value**	**r_s [1]**	***p*-Value**
RE/BV vs. RE/MV	34	−0.563	0.573	0.484	0.005 *
RE/BV vs. LE/MV	34	0.427	0.669	0.007	0.966
LE/BV vs. RE/MV	34	−2.188	0.029 *	0.308	0.077
LE/BV vs. LE/MV	34	−0.241	0.809	0.345	0.047 *

The abbreviations refer to the notes in Figure 2. [1] Spearman's rank correlation coefficient. * $p < 0.05$, significant difference.

3.3. BCEA in Gazing and Non-Gazing Eyes in Monocualr Viewing

The BCEA values of the gazing and non-gazing eyes during monocular viewing are presented in Table 3. The difference in BCEA between gazing and non-gazing eyes was statistically significant in all comparisons except between the right gazing eye and the left non-gazing eye (RE/MV vs. cLE/MV). All cases showed moderate to strong correlations (r_s = 0.401–0.646). However, no significant BCEA differences were found between the right and left eyes for either the gazing or non-gazing conditions. Nonetheless, fixation stability was consistently better in the gazing eye than in the non-gazing eye during monocular viewing.

Table 3. Comparison of BCEA between gazing and non-gazing eyes during monocular viewing.

	n	Wilcoxon Signed-Rank Test		Correlation Coefficient	
		Z-Score	p-Value	r_s [1]	p-Value
RE/MV vs. cRE/MV	34	−3.274	0.001 *	0.646	<0.001 *
RE/MV vs. cLE/MV	34	−1.903	0.057	0.580	0.001 *
LE/MV vs. cRE/MV	34	−4.197	<0.001 *	0.401	0.021 *
LE/MV vs. cLE/MV	34	−3.830	0.001 *	0.444	0.011 *

The abbreviations refer to the notes in Figure 2. [1] Spearman's rank correlation coefficient. * $p < 0.05$, significant difference.

3.4. Comparison of BCEA in Dominant and Non-Dominant Eyes

A comparison of the BCEA between the dominant and non-dominant eyes, which relates ocular dominance to visual functions, such as eye movement [31], is presented in Table 4. Under binocular viewing, monocular viewing with gazing, and monocular viewing without gazing conditions, the non-dominant eye exhibited better fixation stability than the dominant eye in the monocular viewing without gazing condition (Wilcoxon signed-rank test, $p = 0.008$). However, no significant differences were observed under the other conditions.

Table 4. Comparison of BCEA between dominant and non-dominant eyes.

	Dominant Eye (n = 34)		Non-Dominant Eye (n = 34)		Wilcoxon Signed-Rank Test	
	Median	Range	Median	Range	Z-Score	p-Value
BV	0.97	0.56–1.62	0.73	0.57–0.99	1.864	0.062
MV	1.01	0.69–1.85	1.06	0.77–1.35	0.060	0.952
cMV	1.65	0.96–2.38	1.11	0.71–2.14	2.653	0.008 *

BV, binocular viewing; MV, monocular viewing; cMV, covered monocular viewing. Range = 25th to 75th percentile. * $p < 0.05$, significant difference.

3.5. Comparison of BCEA Between Doinmant Eyes

A comparison of fixation stability according to viewing conditions for the dominant eye (right eye for 20 participants, left eye for 14 participants), is shown in Table 5. Under binocular viewing conditions, BCEA of the right eye differed significantly between right-eye and left-eye dominance (Mann–Whitney test, $p = 0.046$). However, no significant differences were observed under other conditions.

Table 5. Comparison of BCEA between dominant eyes.

	RE Dominant (n = 20)		LE Dominant (n = 14)		Mann–Whitney U Test	
	Median	Range	Median	Range	Z-Score	p-Value
RE/BV	1.12	0.84–1.73	0.73	0.58–0.96	1.995	0.046 *
LE/BV	0.71	0.57–1.26	0.83	0.50–1.22	0.157	0.875
RE/MV	1.17	0.76–1.63	0.97	0.63–1.28	0.980	0.327
LE/MV	0.77	0.65–1.22	0.94	0.77–1.18	−0.490	0.624
cRE/MV	2.03	1.21–2.70	1.41	0.94–1.95	1.505	0.132
cLE/MV	1.26	0.80–2.42	1.44	0.91–1.80	0.192	0.847

The abbreviations refer to the notes in Figure 2. Range = 25th to 75th percentile. * $p < 0.05$, significant difference.

3.6. Correction Between BCEA and Phoria

A correlation analysis to investigate the relationship between the degree of phoria, a latent form of eye misalignment [32], and BCEA is presented in Table 6. Under binocular viewing conditions, a significant correlation was observed between the left eye and phoria ($r_s = 0.413$, $p = 0.018$). No significant correlations were found under other conditions.

Table 6. Correlation between phoria and BCEA.

	r_s [1]	*p*-Value
RE/BV	0.091	0.600
LE/BV	0.413	0.018 *
RE/MV	−0.020	0.908
LE/MV	−0.075	0.665
cRE/MV	−0.179	0.305
cLE/MV	−0.314	0.072

The abbreviations refer to the notes in Figure 2. [1] Spearman's rank correlation coefficient. * $p < 0.05$, significant difference.

4. Discussion

Fixation stability has primarily been observed with the naked eye in clinical practice. However, an objective and detailed assessment can be conducted using an eye tracker, enabling the detection of subtle eye movements and allowing for the development of a more precise evaluation method. In this study, we investigated fixation stability under three conditions: binocular viewing, monocular viewing with gaze, and monocular viewing without gaze in participants with non-strabismic binocular vision, a key focus in optometry. Fixation stability was generally better during binocular and monocular viewing with gaze than during monocular viewing without gaze. Although no statistically significant differences in fixation stability were observed between the right and left eyes, the left eye tended to exhibit greater stability. When comparing the dominant and non-dominant eyes, fixation stability in the left eye during binocular viewing was higher when the left eye was dominant. In monocular viewing without gaze, the non-dominant eye demonstrated better fixation stability than the dominant eye. Additionally, a significant quantitative correlation was found between fixation stability and the degree of phoria, particularly in the left eye during binocular viewing.

Previous studies on fixation stability assessment [27] suggested using multiple methods due to differences in BCEA, kernel density estimation, and scanpath methods. However, to facilitate comparisons with other studies, this study evaluated the fixation stability using BCEA, a widely applied method.

The results of fixation stability evaluations under the three conditions showed an average BCEA ranging from 1.01 to 1.87 deg^2, which was higher than the values reported in other studies, such as 0.56 deg^2 [33] and 0.57 deg^2 [34]. In contrast, a previous study on subjects with normal phoria reported lower values, ranging from 0.24 to 0.52 deg^2 [24]. A recent study evaluating monocular non-viewing in patients with amblyopia reported BCEA values in the control group ranging from 0.63 to 1.23 deg^2 [35]. These differences may be attributed to variations in the study populations [27,34,36], experimental conditions such as fixation targets [37], and measurement devices [13,38]. Most notably, differences were likely influenced by degree of refractive error, binocular vision disorders, and whether the non-gazing eye was assessed.

When comparing fixation stability between binocular and monocular viewing, both eyes generally exhibited better stability in binocular viewing than in monocular viewing [28]. However, in contrast to previous studies, which reported better fixation stability in binocular viewing for both eyes, this study found that only the left eye demonstrated better fixation stability in binocular viewing compared to the right eye in monocular viewing. No other statistically significant differences were observed, although BCEA values for binocular viewing tended to be lower than those for monocular viewing. Contrary to previous findings that reported differences in fixation stability between the amblyopic and fellow eye [7], this study found no statistically significant difference between the right and left eyes. This may be due to the low prevalence of amblyopia (4.4%) among the participants, which likely had minimal impact on fixation stability. Applying these results to closed- and open-loop systems offers an alternative perspective. In both binocular and monocular views (with and without gaze), the eyes maintain retinal image stability through accommodative vergence eye movements [39]. This study confirmed that binocular viewing occurred in a closed-loop condition, while gazing and non-gazing eyes in monocular viewing occurred in an open-loop condition. Under both conditions, both eyes moved simultaneously and the vergence movements of both eyes continued even in the open-loop state. Additionally, in the open-loop condition, the covered eye exhibited larger movements [26].

Fixation stability of the gazing and non-gazing eyes in monocular viewing is consistent with previous research [28], which found that gazing eyes exhibit better fixation stability than non-gazing eyes in monocular viewing. The results correspond to previous findings [40] showing that the BCEA is larger in the covered eye than in the gazing eye under monocular conditions and that the gazing eye exhibits a larger BCEA than either eye under binocular conditions. While the gazing eye continuously followed the target, the covered eye deviated from it, as suggested by prior studies [41]. This supports the conclusion that the fixation stability of the covered eye is lower. However, these results contradict Hering's law, which states that eye movements are governed by a single neural command. These findings suggest the presence of asymmetric eye movements deviating from Hering's law [42,43]. A rare vertical movement pattern can occur during a cover test, where one eye remains stationary while the other moves during the transition from covering to uncovering. This temporary disobedience of Hering's law is followed by realignment once fixation is regained [44].

The frequency of right-eye dominance was 60.3%, which is lower than the reported range of 61.3–71.5% [31,45]. In contrast to previous studies [3], which found no difference in fixation stability between the dominant and non-dominant eyes, this study observed that the non-dominant eye exhibited better fixation stability than the dominant eye in the gazing state. Earlier research [46] found that in 7- and 8-year-olds, fixation in the dominant eye was more stable than that in the non-dominant eye, with no differences observed in older age groups. In this study, monocular fixation stability, as measured by the BCEA, ranged from 1.02 to 1.87 deg^2, which was greater than the binocular fixation stability values reported in previous studies [24,33], which ranged from 0.24 to 0.52 deg^2 and 0.8 deg^2. These findings indicate that fixation stability varies depending on measurement equipment, experimental conditions, and participant characteristics.

When comparing fixation stability in the dominant eye, fixation stability was better when the left eye was dominant. This result is probably due to the possibility that the monocular deviation with changes in fixation distance was larger in the rightward direction than the leftward direction, regardless of the dominant eye's direction [47]. Moreover, research using the von Graefe method for phoria testing revealed that the right eye showed more exotropic deviations than the left eye [48]. This suggests that the fixation stability of the left eye may be better than that of the right eye. While fixation stability is generally better in the dominant eye than in the non-dominant eye [7,12,35], there is no clear evidence that the right eye is more stable than the left. In this study, the non-dominant and left eyes exhibited better fixation stability than the right dominant eye in individuals with a dominant right eye. According to previous studies [46], fixation is more stable in the dominant eye at a younger age and improves with age, with no significant differences between the two eyes in adulthood. Furthermore, when dominance was not considered, no differences were observed between the right and left eyes. Another study involving adults reported that the non-dominant eye was less stable than the dominant eye [49], while another report found no difference [50].

Phoria showed a distinct quantitative correlation with BCEA of the left eye during binocular viewing. The correlation with the left eye in binocular viewing was measured by positioning the Maddox rod in front of the right eye and measuring phoria, while the left eye remained open during the modified Thorington phoria test. This suggests a relationship between maintaining the gaze in the left eye. This relationship is believed to be associated with horizontal phoria when one eye is occluded, as the apparent position of the subject correlates with phoria [32,51]. In a previous study [22], no correlation was found between fixation stability and phoria when using binocular gaze position, which averaged the gaze positions of the right and left eyes. However, a correlation was observed between the amount of deviation in the gazing plane, both in the front and behind, and abnormal phoria. In this study, a correlation between fixation stability and phoria was observed when the left eye was gazing at the binocular view. This suggests that evaluating the gazing position of each eye separately, rather than using the average binocular gaze, reflects the gazing state more accurately. Therefore, considering the previous findings that fixation stability differences exist between monocular gazing and non-gazing eyes and that there is a correlation between the position of the occluded eye and phoria, it is necessary to reflect both right and left eye occlusion when assessing eye movements or ocular alignment abnormalities during monocular occlusion tests.

This study had some limitations. It focused only on individuals with phoria, excluding those with strabismus, and did not analyze factors that may influence fixation stability, such as visual acuity, refractive power, and binocular vision abnormalities. Additionally, the small sample size and use of non-parametric methods for analysis may limit generalizability. The need for future expansion in terms of clinical application and consideration of diagnostic accuracy should be addressed. However, a previous study [24] showed no significant difference in fixation stability between normal and abnormal groups in binocular vision when comparing the averages before and after blinking. Moreover, of the 68 eyes included in the study, only 4 showed the possibility of amblyopia, suggesting that amblyopia did not significantly impact the results. Despite these limitations, the evaluation and comparison of fixation stability between the right and left eyes in both binocular and monocular views are still feasible.

Fixation stability holds fundamental scientific importance and contributes to a deeper understanding of oculomotor dynamics, binocular coordination, and interactions within the visual system. Furthermore, it offers critical insights for detecting abnormalities associated with motor and neurological disorders, such as Parkinson's disease [19]. Therefore, objective assessment of fixation stability using eye-tracking technology presents valuable implications for both clinical and research settings. The findings of the present study will enhance clinicians' comprehension of gaze stability under varying viewing conditions, potentially improving diagnostic accuracy and treatment strategies for patients with gaze-related disorders. For optometrists, this knowledge aids in conducting more precise evaluations, thereby elevating the quality of patient care during eye examinations. As a result, patients benefit from more accurate diagnoses and personalized treatment plans, leading to better management of conditions affecting gaze stability, such as binocular vision disorders or visual instability. In addition, the precision offered by eye tracking could facilitate earlier detection of visual dysfunctions and support the development of tailored therapeutic interventions. This study is currently in an experimental stage; however, it lays the groundwork for future clinical integration, highlighting the potential of fixation stability analysis in routine eye examinations to monitor treatment progress and assess the effectiveness of visual therapies.

5. Conclusions

In a study of healthy individuals in their 20s, the fixation stability in non-strabismic eyes, including those with phoria, was measured using eye tracking. The results showed that fixation stability in the left eye during binocular viewing was better than that in the right eye during monocular viewing. During monocular viewing, the gazing eye demonstrated better fixation stability than the non-gazing eye, indicating a trend in fixation stability as follows: binocular viewing, monocular viewing, and non-fixating monocular conditions. However, no significant differences in fixation stability were observed between the right and left eyes across the three conditions.

When comparing the dominant and non-dominant eyes, fixation stability in the left eye during binocular viewing was better when the left eye was dominant than when the right eye was. Similarly, in the non-gazing monocular condition, the non-dominant eye showed better fixation stability than the dominant eye. Furthermore, the link between phoria and fixation stability—depending on which eye is covered—highlights the need to test both eyes separately when checking for issues such as eye movement and ocular alignment in tests that involve occlusion.

Author Contributions: Conceptualization, J.-H.N. and D.-S.Y.; methodology, J.-H.N. and D.-S.Y.; software, J.-H.N.; validation, S.-Y.K., B.-Y.M., and H.G.C.; formal analysis, J.-H.N. and S.-Y.K.; investigation, J.-H.N.; resources, J.-H.N. and D.-S.Y.; data curation, J.-H.N. and D.-S.Y.; writing—original draft preparation, J.-H.N. and D.-S.Y.; writing—review and editing, B.-Y.M., H.G.C. and D.-S.Y.; visualization, S.-Y.K.; supervision, D.-S.Y. All authors have read and agreed to the published version of the manuscript.

Funding: The authors have received no specific funding for this study.

Institutional Review Board Statement: This study was approved by the Kangwon National University Institutional Review Board (KWNUIRB-2023-02-007-001) and adhered to the tenets of the Declaration of Helsinki.

Informed Consent Statement: Informed consent was obtained from all the participants involved in the study.

Data Availability Statement: The data presented in this study are available upon request from the corresponding author.

Conflicts of Interest: The authors declare no conflicts of interest.

References

1. Krauzlis, R.J.; Goffart, L.; Hafed, Z.M. Neuronal control of fixation and fixational eye movements. *Phil. Trans. R. Soc. B* **2017**, *372*, 20160205. [CrossRef]
2. Rucci, M.; Poletti, M. Control and functions of fixational eye movements. *Annu. Rev. Vis. Sci.* **2015**, *1*, 499–518. [CrossRef] [PubMed]
3. Raveendran, R.N.; Bobier, W.R.; Thompson, B. Binocular vision and fixational eye movements. *J. Vis.* **2019**, *19*, 9. [CrossRef]
4. Kumar, G.; Chung, S.T. Characteristics of fixational eye movements in people with macular disease. *Investig. Ophthalmol. Vis. Sci.* **2014**, *55*, 5125–5133. [CrossRef] [PubMed]
5. Schor, C.; Hallmark, W. Slow control of eye position in strabismic amblyopia. *Investig. Ophthalmol. Vis. Sci.* **1978**, *17*, 577–581.

6. Scaramuzzi, M.; Murray, J.; Otero-Millan, J.; Nucci, P.; Shaikh, A.G.; Ghasia, F.F. Fixation instability in amblyopia: Oculomotor disease biomarkers predictive of treatment effectiveness. *Prog. Brain Res.* **2019**, *249*, 235–248.
7. Mompart-Martínez, R.; Argilés, M.; Cardona, G.; Cavero-Roig, L.; González-Sanchís, L.; Pighin, M.S. The relationship between fixation stability and retinal structural parameters in children with anisometropic, strabismic and mixed amblyopia. *Life* **2023**, *13*, 1517. [CrossRef]
8. Kelly, K.R.; Cheng-Patel, C.S.; Jost, R.M.; Wang, Y.Z.; Birch, E.E. Fixation instability during binocular viewing in anisometropic and strabismic children. *Exp. Eye Res.* **2019**, *183*, 29–37. [CrossRef]
9. Birch, E.E.; Subramanian, V.; Weakley, D.R. Fixation instability in anisometropic children with reduced stereopsis. *J. AAPOS* **2013**, *17*, 287–290. [CrossRef]
10. Subramanian, P.S. Fixation Instability: A new measure of neurologic dysfunction in multiple sclerosis. *Investig. Ophthalmol. Vis. Sci.* **2018**, *59*, 202. [CrossRef]
11. Tarita-Nistor, L.; Brent, M.H.; Steinbach, M.J.; González, E.G. Fixation stability during binocular viewing in patients with age-related macular degeneration. *Investig. Ophthalmol. Vis. Sci.* **2011**, *52*, 1887–1893. [CrossRef]
12. Subramanian, V.; Jost, R.M.; Birch, E.E. A quantitative study of fixation stability in amblyopia. *Investig. Ophthalmol. Vis. Sci.* **2013**, *54*, 1998–2003. [CrossRef] [PubMed]
13. Crossland, M.D.; Rubin, G.S. The use of an infrared eyetracker to measure fixation stability. *Optom. Vis. Sci.* **2002**, *79*, 735–739. [CrossRef]
14. Zhao, X.; Zhao, C.; Liu, N.; Li, S. Investigating the eye movement characteristics of basketball players executing 3-point shot at varied intensities and their correlation with shot accuracy. *PeerJ* **2024**, *12*, e17634. [CrossRef]
15. Krauskopf, J.; Cornsweet, T.N.; Riggs, L.A. Analysis of eye movements during monocular and binocular fixation. *J. Opt. Soc. Am.* **1960**, *50*, 572–578. [CrossRef] [PubMed]
16. Liversedge, S.P.; White, S.J.; Findlay, J.M.; Rayner, K. Binocular coordination of eye movements during reading. *Vision Res.* **2006**, *46*, 2363–2374. [CrossRef]
17. Jakobsen, N.S.; Larsen, D.A.; Bek, T. Binocular fixation reduces fixational eye movements in the worst eye of patients with center-involving diabetic macular edema. *Ophthalmic Res.* **2017**, *58*, 142–149. [CrossRef]
18. Corbett, J.J. The bedside and office neuro-ophthalmology examination. *Semin. Neurol.* **2003**, *23*, 63–76.
19. Wu, C.; Cao, B.; Dali, V.; Gagliardi, C.; Barthelemy, O.J.; Salazar, R.D.; Pomplun, M.; Cronin-Golomb, A.; Yazdanbakhsh, A. Eye movement control during visual pursuit in Parkinson's disease. *PeerJ* **2018**, *6*, e5442. [CrossRef]
20. Otero-Millan, J.; Macknik, S.L.; Martinez-Conde, S. Fixational eye movements and binocular vision. *Front. Integr. Neurosci.* **2014**, *8*, 52. [CrossRef]
21. González-Vides, L.; Hernández-Verdejo, J.L.; Cañadas-Suárez, P. Eye tracking in optometry: A systematic review. *J. Eye Mov. Res.* **2023**, *16*, 1–55. [CrossRef] [PubMed]
22. Kim, S.Y.; Moon, B.Y.; Cho, H.G.; Yu, D.S. Quantitative evaluation of the association between fixation stability and phoria during short-term binocular viewing. *Front. Neurosci.* **2022**, *16*, 721665. [CrossRef] [PubMed]
23. Kim, S.Y.; Moon, B.Y.; Cho, H.G.; Yu, D.S. Comparison of image-based quantification methods in evaluating fixation stability using a remote eye tracker in abnormal phoria. *J. Int. Med. Res.* **2022**, *50*, 3000605221098183. [CrossRef] [PubMed]
24. Kim, S.Y.; Moon, B.Y.; Cho, H.G.; Yu, D.S. Comparative analysis of fixation stability before and after blinking during binocular viewing. *J. Korean Ophthalmic Opt. Soc.* **2023**, *28*, 9–17. [CrossRef]
25. Blignaut, P.; van Rensburg, E.J.; Oberholzer, M. Visualization and quantification of eye tracking data for the evaluation of oculomotor function. *Heliyon* **2019**, *5*, e01127. [CrossRef]
26. Saida, S.; Ono, H.; Mapp, A.P. Closed-loop and open-loop accommodative vergence eye movements. *Vision Res.* **2001**, *41*, 77–86. [CrossRef]
27. González, E.G.; Wong, A.M.; Niechwiej-Szwedo, E.; Tarita-Nistor, L.; Steinbach, M.J. Eye position stability in amblyopia and in normal binocular vision. *Investig. Ophthalmol. Vis. Sci.* **2012**, *53*, 5386–5394. [CrossRef]
28. Samet, S.; González, E.G.; Mandelcorn, M.S.; Brent, M.H.; Tarita-Nistor, L. Changes in fixation stability with time during binocular and monocular viewing in maculopathy. *Vision* **2018**, *2*, 40. [CrossRef]
29. Reilly, J.; Gaiser, H.; Young, B. *Clinical Procedures for Ocular Examination*, 5th ed.; McGraw Hill: New York, NY, USA, 2023; pp. 61–147.
30. Castet, E.; Crossland, M. Quantifying eye stability during a fixation task: A review of definitions and methods. *Seeing Perceiving* **2012**, *25*, 449–469. [CrossRef]
31. Linke, S.J.; Baviera, J.; Munzer, G.; Steinberg, J.; Richard, G.; Katz, T. Association between ocular dominance and spherical/astigmatic anisometropia, age, and sex: Analysis of 10,264 myopic individuals. *Investig. Ophthalmol. Vis. Sci.* **2011**, *52*, 9166–9173. [CrossRef]
32. Ono, H.; Gonda, G. Apparent movement, eye movements and phoria when two eyes alternate in viewing a stimulus. *Perception* **1978**, *7*, 75–83. [CrossRef] [PubMed]

33. Morales, M.U.; Saker, S.; Wilde, C.; Pellizzari, C.; Pallikaris, A.; Notaroberto, N.; Rubinstein, M.; Rui, C.; Limoli, P.; Smolek, M.K.; et al. Reference clinical database for fixation stability metrics in normal subjects measured with the MAIA microperimeter. *Transl. Vis. Sci. Technol.* **2016**, *5*, 6. [CrossRef]
34. Altemir, I.; Alejandre, A.; Fanlo-Zarazaga, A.; Ortín, M.; Pérez, T.; Masiá, B.; Pueyo, V. Evaluation of fixational behavior throughout life. *Brain Sci.* **2021**, *12*, 19. [CrossRef]
35. Ghasia, F.; Tychsen, L. Inter-ocular fixation instability of amblyopia: Relationship to visual acuity, strabismus, nystagmus, stereopsis, vergence, and age. *Am. J. Ophthalmol.* **2024**, *267*, 230–248. [CrossRef]
36. Vikesdal, G.H.; Langaas, T. Optically induced refractive errors reduces fixation stability but saccade latency remains stable. *J. Eye Mov. Res.* **2016**, *9*, 1–8. [CrossRef]
37. Hirasawa, K.; Oka, K.; Koshiji, R.; Funaki, W.; Shoji, N. Smaller fixation target size is associated with more stable fixation and less variance in threshold sensitivity. *PLoS ONE* **2016**, *11*, e0165046. [CrossRef]
38. Liu, H.; Bittencourt, M.G.; Sophie, R.; Sepah, Y.J.; Hanout, M.; Rentiya, Z.; Annam, R.; Scholl, H.P.; Nguyen, Q.D. Fixation stability measurement using two types of microperimetry devices. *Transl. Vis. Sci. Technol.* **2015**, *4*, 3. [CrossRef] [PubMed]
39. Argilés, M.; Cardona, G. The interaction between vergence and accommodation cues in the assessment of fusional vergence range. *Life* **2024**, *14*, 1185. [CrossRef]
40. Watamaniuk, S.N.J.; Heinen, S.J.; Singh, D.; Chandna, A. Occluding one eye during fixation increases wandering of both eyes. *J. Vision* **2023**, *23*, 5670. [CrossRef]
41. Chandna, A.; Badler, J.; Singh, D.; Watamaniuk, S.; Heinen, S. A covered eye fails to follow an object moving in depth. *Sci. Rep.* **2021**, *11*, 10983. [CrossRef]
42. Sharma, P.; Prakash, P.; Menon, V. Saccadic underaction in concomitant strabismus and Hering's law: A new neurophysiologic model for binocular motor correspondence. *Indian J. Ophthalmol.* **1993**, *41*, 117–120.
43. King, W.M. Binocular coordination of eye movements-Hering's Law of equal innervation or uniocular control? *Eur. J. Neurosci.* **2011**, *33*, 2139–2146. [CrossRef]
44. Peli, E.; McCormack, G. Dynamics of cover test eye movements. *Am. J. Optom. Physiol. Opt.* **1983**, *60*, 712–724. [CrossRef]
45. Lopes-Ferreira, D.; Neves, H.; Queiros, A.; Faria-Ribeiro, M.; Peixoto-de-Matos, S.C.; González-Méijome, J.M. Ocular dominance and visual function testing. *Biomed. Res. Int.* **2013**, *2013*, 238943. [CrossRef] [PubMed]
46. Serpa, E.; Alecka, M.; Ceple, I.; Krumina, G.; Svede, A.; Kassaliete, E.; Goliskina, V.; Volberga, L.; Berzina, A.; Mikelsone, R.; et al. The impact of eye dominance on fixation stability in school-aged children. *J. Eye Mov. Res.* **2023**, *16*, 1–8. [CrossRef] [PubMed]
47. Shim, J.B.; Shim, H.S. Direction changes in the dominant eye and comparison of single-eye inset amounts depending on the view distance. *J. Korean Ophthalmic Opt. Soc.* **2020**, *25*, 19–24. [CrossRef]
48. Kim, J.S.; Shim, J.B. Comparison of amount of at distance and near phoria in dominant eye and non-dominant eye by von Graefe method. *J. Korean Ophthalmic Opt. Soc.* **2018**, *23*, 111–116. [CrossRef]
49. Vikesdal, G.H.; Langaas, T. Saccade latency and fixation stability: Repeatability and reliability. *J. Eye Mov. Res.* **2016**, *9*, 1–13. [CrossRef]
50. Mestre, C.; Otero, C.; Díaz-Doutón, F.; Gautier, J.; Pujol, J. An automated and objective cover test to measure heterophoria. *PLoS ONE* **2018**, *13*, e0206674. [CrossRef]
51. Park, K.; Shebilske, W.L. Phoria, Hering's laws, and monocular perception of direction. *J. Exp. Psychol. Hum. Percept. Perform.* **1991**, *17*, 219–231. [CrossRef]

life

MDPI

Article

Comparative Effects of Red and Blue LED Light on Melatonin Levels During Three-Hour Exposure in Healthy Adults

Ana Sanchez-Cano [1,2,*], María José Luesma-Bartolomé [3], Estela Solanas [3] and Elvira Orduna-Hospital [1,2,*]

1 Department of Applied Physics, University of Zaragoza, 50009 Zaragoza, Spain
2 Aragon Institute for Health Research (IIS Aragon), 50009 Zaragoza, Spain
3 Department of Human Anatomy and Histology, University of Zaragoza, 50009 Zaragoza, Spain; mjluesma@unizar.es (M.J.L.-B.); esolanas@unizar.es (E.S.)
* Correspondence: anaisa@unizar.es (A.S.-C.); eordunahospital@unizar.es (E.O.-H.)

Abstract: Circadian rhythms, essential for regulating human physiology and behavior, are influenced by light exposure, particularly at night. This study examined the impact of red (631 nm) and blue (464 nm) LED light on melatonin secretion, a key circadian marker. Twelve participants aged 19–55 years were exposed to red and blue light for three hours (9:00 p.m.–midnight), with hourly saliva samples analyzed via ELISA to track melatonin levels. Initially, melatonin levels were comparable under both light conditions. After one hour, both lights suppressed melatonin, but differences emerged after two hours: blue light-maintained suppression, with levels at 7.5 pg/mL, while red light allowed recovery to 26.0 pg/mL ($p = 0.019$). This pattern persisted at the third hour. Blue light had stronger suppression effects, particularly in younger participants and men. These results underscore blue light's disruptive effects on circadian health and highlight red light as a less disruptive alternative for nighttime environments.

Keywords: circadian rhythms; melatonin; integrative lighting; LED light; blue light; red light; non-visual effects; salivary biomarkers

1. Introduction

Human physiology and behavior are governed by circadian rhythms, which are synchronized to the 24-h solar day by the circadian clock located in the suprachiasmatic nucleus (SCN) of the hypothalamus. The SCN receives environmental light information via the retinohypothalamic tract (RHT), aligning internal biological time with the external light-dark cycle. This synchronization underlies various physiological processes, such as hormone secretion, body temperature regulation, and cognitive performance, even in the absence of external cues, melatonin production, alertness, and cognitive functions, collectively referred to as non-visual effects of light [1–3]. These effects are mediated by a photoreceptive system that includes rods, cones, and the recently known intrinsically photosensitive retinal ganglion cells (ipRGCs), which express the photopigment melanopsin [4,5]. Advancements in physiology have transformed our understanding of retinal structure and its neural connections. While the classical visual photoreceptors, rods and cones, have been well-studied, the ipRGCs have been uncovered [4,6]. Their photosensitivity is driven by the photopigment melanopsin, which exhibits peak sensitivity in the short-wavelength region of the visible spectrum and encodes ambient light intensity independent of rods and cones [7,8]. The characteristics and responses of all five photoreceptor types have been extensively documented [9]. The ipRGCs established their role in light-induced melatonin suppression during the biological night, emphasizing their importance in non-image-forming (NIF) processes such as circadian rhythm regulation, the pupillary light reflex (PLR), and the modulation of sleep, mood, and alertness [10–12]. Emerging evidence suggests interconnected roles among photoreceptors, rather than strictly independent functions [13]. Disruptions in light exposure, particularly at night, can desynchronize circadian rhythms, as seen in shift work, jet lag, and prolonged evening light exposure, delaying sleep onset and suppressing sleepiness. Optimizing light exposure is essential to enhance health benefits while mitigating adverse effects on circadian health [14].

These effects vary significantly between individuals, influenced by factors such as timing, intensity, wavelength, and prior light exposure history [15–19]. These individual differences in the NIF effects of light via ipRGCs are shaped by age, health, sensitivity, and light characteristics. Younger adults respond to dim, colored light with heart rate changes, whereas older adults require higher intensities, indicating age-related sensitivity decline [20]. This also has clinical implications; desynchronized circadian rhythms in the elderly often reduce light therapy efficacy, highlighting the need to study ipRGC function [11]. This research is crucial for developing targeted light therapies to improve cognitive function, mood, and quality of life, especially as conditions such as diabetic retinopathy impair ipRGC function, disrupting circadian rhythms and sleep [11,21].

The CIE S 026/E:2018 international standard by the International Commission on Illumination (CIE) marked a key advancement, defining spectral weighting functions for cones, rods, and melanopsin to standardize light measurement for NIF effects [22,23]. This milestone supports mechanistic models of circadian and neuroendocrine phototransduction and has enabled the development of consensus guidelines for optimizing light exposure to enhance sleep, alertness, and overall health [14]. These recommendations are derived from a meta-analysis of data from healthy young adults [24]. The guidelines propose a minimum melanopic Equivalent Daylight Illuminance (mEDI) of 250 melanopic lux at the eye during daytime hours, with a maximum of 10 mEDI during the three hours preceding bedtime. During sleep, it should not exceed 1 mEDI; however, if visual tasks are required during nighttime hours, the melanopic mEDI can be increased to a maximum of 10 lux [14,23].

Meanwhile, recommendation by the WELL building standard [25] ensures occupants receive adequate light exposure, in Equivalent Melanopic Light (EML), to support circadian health by aligning rhythms with the natural day-night cycle, addressing deficiencies caused by indoor environments with insufficient lighting. For places during the daytime, electric lighting should be designed to achieve thresholds of at least 150 EML (136 mEDI) or 120 EML (109 mEDI) for the minimum standard for compliance, and at least 275 EML (250 mEDI) or 180 EML (163 mEDI) for a more advanced level of performance, measured on the vertical plane at eye level for at least four hours by noon, ensuring effective stimulation of the circadian system while avoiding overstimulation at night.

On the other hand, the revised model proposed by Rea et al. [26,27] has been widely used in research papers since it optimizes the CL_A (Circadian Light) spectral sensitivity framework while preserving key features: the relationship between (Circadian Stimuli) CS and predicted nocturnal melatonin suppression, such that a CS of 0.5 corresponds to 50% melatonin suppression after a 1-h reference light exposure [28].

This preliminary study aims to compare the effects of two LED light exposures on nighttime melatonin levels in human saliva, utilizing antibody-based assays such as ELISA, which are considered the gold standard for measuring salivary biomarkers [2]. These two selected LEDs were fully characterized using the three models previously described, providing a robust basis for evaluating their impact on circadian regulation. By measuring melatonin concentration changes under each light condition, we seek to clarify how different spectra could influence melatonin regulation and circadian rhythms, with implications for optimizing lighting environments for health and well-being.

2. Materials and Methods

2.1. Experimental Setup Configuration

To determine the spectral power distribution (SPD) and total irradiance (W·m^{-2}) of the two selected LEDs used in the experiments, a calibrated spectroradiometer (model StellarNet-Black Comet, StellarNet, Inc., Tampa, FL, USA) was used. A blue LED with a peak emission wavelength of 464 nm and a full width at half maximum (FWHM) of 24 nm, and a red LED with a peak emission wavelength of 631 nm and an FWHM of 18 nm were selected (see Figure 1). Other characteristics are specified in Table 1.

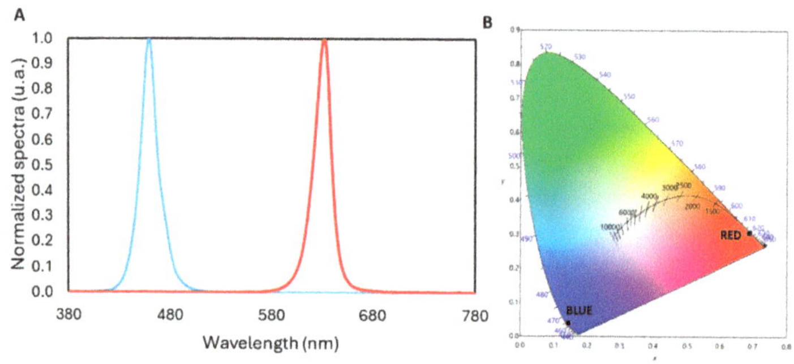

Figure 1. Spectral power distribution (**A**) and CIE 1931 chromaticity diagram (**B**) for the two LED light sources used in this study. (**A**) The blue LED shows a peak in the short-wavelength region (464 nm), while the red LED peaks in the long-wavelength region (631 nm). (**B**) Chromaticity coordinates plotted on the CIE diagram indicate the distinct color characteristics of each LED, corresponding to their spectral peaks.

Table 1. Properties of two LED light conditions (Blue and Red) at an illuminance level of 80 lx, including Irradiance, and chromaticity coordinates (x, y).

	Blue	**Red**
Irradiance (W·m^{-2})	1.628	0.407
Chromaticity Coordinates (x, y)	(0.1438, 0.0389)	(0.6898, 0.3068)

Two custom-made luminaires, Figure 2, were then built with these LEDs to be used during the experiments, with the objective of providing a photopic illuminance level of 80 lux on the corneal plane of the participants. This was controlled using a calibrated luxmeter (model Delta-Ohm, HD2102.1 and LP471PHOT Probe, Senseca Italy Srl, Padua, Italy), and it was determined that the red LED was located 40 cm from the corneal plane and the blue LED was positioned 55 cm from the corneal plane, oriented at a 45° angle, from the same vertical plane.

2.2. Theoretical Background

Both the CIE and WELL documents address lighting's impact on human health. The CIE Position Statement offers technical guidance on integrative lighting, while the WELL Building Standard v2 provides a framework for health-promoting environments. To quantify the biological effects of light, metrics such as mEDI from CIE S 026 and EML from WELL are used. Previous research shows that the equation EML = 1.104·mEDI links the two systems, derived from spectral data calculations [29].

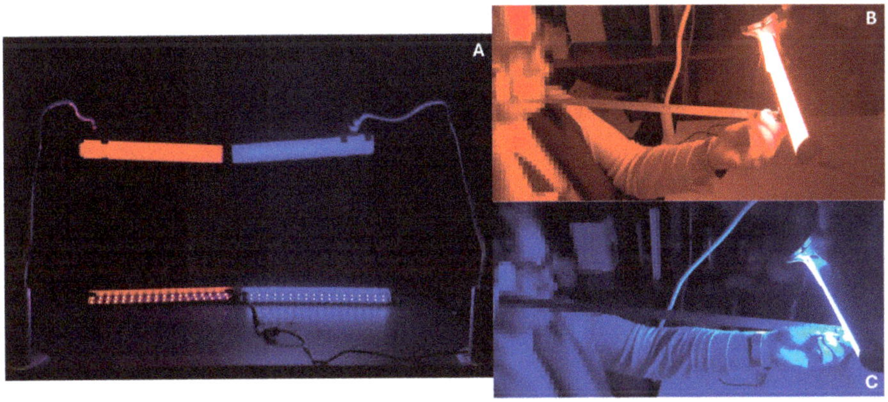

Figure 2. (**A**) Luminaires used in the experiments: at the top, the custom-built luminaires, and at the bottom, the luminaires without the diffuser, showing the LEDs. (**B**) Luminaire with red LEDs, calibrating the distance for the experiment. (**C**) Luminaire with blue LEDs, adjusted using a meter to ensure the correct distance.

Meanwhile, the CS metric outlined in the "Design Guideline for Promoting Circadian Entrainment with Light for Day-Active People" (DG 24480) guideline recommends a target CS value of 0.3 for at least 2 h in the morning to promote circadian entrainment [26,27]. The required circadian light dose (CSd) of 0.43 can be achieved by varying the CL_A intensity or exposure duration, with a reciprocal relationship between the two within limits of 0.5–3 h [30]. The updated version of the CS calculation incorporates these parameters, enabling the calculation of CL_A based on any SPD and photopic illuminance, thus determining the exposure duration needed to meet the CSd = 0.43 target. These recent model revisions have refined the CL_A spectral sensitivity curve, preserving the correlation between CS and nocturnal melatonin suppression, updating the description for CL_A (CL_A 2.0) allowing to align with reference illuminants, yielding a CL_A of 813 at 1000 lux from CIE Illuminant A and adjusting equivalencies for diverse lighting conditions for improving accuracy [28], such as CIE Illuminant D65 (daylight at 6500 K). It was designed to maintain the relationship between CS and predicted nocturnal melatonin suppression (e.g., CS of 0.5 results in 50% nocturnal melatonin suppression following a reference light exposure duration of 1 h), and to achieve these values, CL_A 2.0 approximates photopic illuminance for general "white" light, with conversion factors of 1.23 for CIE Illuminant A and 0.66 for CIE daylight Illuminant D65 (Figure 3 and Table 2).

Table 2. Spectral and photometric characteristics under blue and red light conditions at an illuminance level of 80 lx on the corneal plane, including α-opic efficacy ratios, melanopic equivalent daylight (D65) illuminance (mEDI), equivalent melanopic lux (EML), melanopic ratio (M/P), circadian stimulus (CS), and circadian light (CL_A 2.0).

	Illuminance 80 lx		**Blue**	**Red**
CIES026 [22,23,31]	Irradiance ($W \cdot m^{-2}$)	S-cone	1.256	6.71×10^{-4}
		M-cone	0.339	3.23×10^{-2}
		L-cone	0.196	1.59×10^{-1}
		Rhodopic	0.913	3.76×10^{-3}
		Melanopic	1.123	1.42×10^{-3}

Table 2. *Cont.*

Illuminance 80 lx			Blue	Red
CIES026 [22,23,31]	α-opic DER for (α-opic daylight (D65) efficacy ratio is 1.000)	S-cone-opic	19.2131	0.0103
		M-cone-opic	2.9101	0.2775
		L-cone-opic	1.5070	1.2199
		Rhodopic	7.8763	0.0324
		Melanopic	10.5823	0.0134
	$E^{D65}_{v,\alpha}$ Melanopic Equivalent Daylight (D65) Illuminance [lux]; mEDI		847	1
WELL [25]	Equivalent Melanopic Lux [m-lux]; EML		934	1
	Melanopic Ratio, R (M/P)		11.68	0.01
Rea et al. [26,27]	CS		0.588	0.003
	CL_A 2.0		1600	2

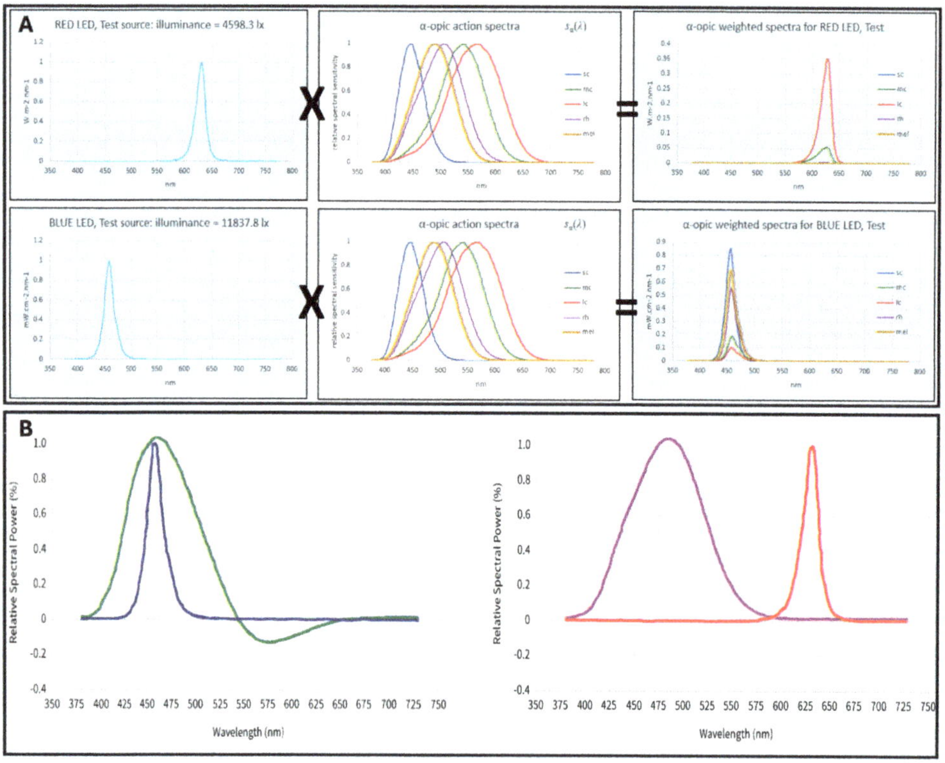

Figure 3. (**A**) Calculation of α-opic weighted spectra for red and blue LED test sources from CIE S 026 Toolbox (v1.49a—November 2020) [22]. The left figures show the spectral power distributions (SPDs) of the red LED top (illuminance = 4598.3 lx) and the blue LED bottom (illuminance = 11837.8 lx). The middle panels illustrate the α-opic action spectra for S-cones, M-cones, L-cones, rhodopic, and melanopic sensitivities. The right figures display the resulting α-opic weighted spectra for the red and blue LED test sources, obtained by multiplying the SPDs with the respective α-opic action spectra. (**B**) Calculation of the relative spectral contribution to the circadian response for cool (green) and warm (purple) lights, as well as blue and red LEDs, respectively, according to Rea et al. [26,27].

This revised circadian light model [26,27] optimized spectral sensitivity using photoreceptor fundamentals that differ slightly from CIE S 026 standards [22,23,31]. For melanopsin, the model uses the Wyszecki and Stiles [32] template, with a peak sensitivity at 485 nm and half-max sensitivity of 89 nm, rather than the CIE's 490 nm peak and 84 nm half-max from Govardovskii et al. [33]. While this choice had minimal impact on broadband predictions, it significantly improved accuracy for narrowband sources, suggesting it better characterizes melanopsin's in vivo action spectrum. This model indirectly tests the suitability of the CIE melanopic function for circadian sensitivity. The CL_A equation incorporates four unitless, normalized photoreceptor action spectra (M(λ), V(λ), V′(λ), and S-cone(λ)), each scaled to a maximum value of 1. These spectra represent in vivo photoreceptor sensitivities, accounting for preretinal filtering, such as lens absorption. The CIE photopic (V(λ)) and scotopic (V′(λ)) functions represent the L- and M-cone achromatic channel and the rod achromatic channel, respectively. Adjustments to the melanopsin (485 nm) response for lens transmission and the S-cone sensitivity for macular pigment removal required renormalizing each spectrum to a peak value of 1 [34,35]. This part is a different method from CIE, but it can also be computed from this standard when considering the transmittance of the crystalline lens depending on the age of the observer [36].

2.3. Sample Description

This study was conducted in accordance with the principles outlined in the Declaration of Helsinki and received approval from the Ethics Committee for Research of the Community of Aragón (CEICA), with registration code PI24/483. The participants provided informed consent prior to their inclusion in the study and were required to be healthy adults, aged 18 to 55, with no diagnosed ocular or systemic diseases and not undergoing pharmacological treatments that could affect melatonin secretion. Regarding clinical status, all participants self-reported good general health and were screened to exclude any history of neurological, psychiatric, sleep, or endocrine disorders. Besides, participants who were excluded from the experiment met one or more of the following exclusion criteria: presence of ophthalmological or systemic pathologies affecting vision; use of electronic devices one hour before the measurements, stimulating accommodation; consumption of coffee; smoking; and/or engaging in high-intensity sports activities.

2.4. Saliva Sample Collection

For saliva sample collection, participants did not eat, drink, chew gum, or brush their teeth for at least 30 min before sample collection. Samples were not taken if there were oral diseases, inflammations, or lesions to avoid blood contamination, as indicated by a reddish color in the saliva. Participants who had consumed multivitamins or supplements containing biotin within the previous 48 h were also excluded. During the study period, medications that affect melatonin secretion, such as benzodiazepines, fluvoxamine, caffeine, vitamin B12, and certain non-steroidal anti-inflammatory drugs, were avoided. Five minutes before collection, participants rinsed their mouths with cold water. A minimum of 0.5 mL of saliva was collected in an Eppendorf tube every hour. Samples were then stored at 2–8 °C for up to 5 days and delivered to the laboratory on ice, preferably dry ice, avoiding heat and direct sunlight. Once in the laboratory, samples were frozen at −20 °C for up to 2 weeks until analysis.

2.5. Experimental Protocol

The experiment was conducted on two separate days, each day with a different light source. Participants were exposed to the light (red or blue) in a random order to prevent any bias in the results. Regardless of which light was used first, once the setup was arranged with the appropriate distances for each illumination, participants remained under the light for 3 h without wearing glasses or contact lenses to avoid any wavelength interference. During this period, they were not allowed to use devices or screens of any kind, including mobile phones or tablets, nor watch television; only reading printed material was permitted. The experiment took place in March, from 9:00 p.m. to midnight, meaning that it was already dark at that time in the location of Zaragoza in Spain (41°38′31″ N, 0°53′60″ W; 243 m above sea level) to ensure participants were in the initial phase of melatonin secretion. After one hour under the designated light, at 10:00 p.m., participants collected a saliva sample in an Eppendorf tube, which was then stored in a refrigerator at the specified temperature. This process was repeated at the second (11:00 p.m.) and third hours (00:00 a.m.), resulting in a total of three saliva samples collected per light condition. For further information, four participants had saliva samples collected at 3:00 a.m. to evaluate the trend in melatonin secretion after sleeping, before being exposed to the lights.

2.6. Determination of Melatonin in Saliva Samples

Melatonin concentration in collected at predetermined time points saliva samples was determined using a direct high-sensitivity enzyme-linked immunosorbent assay (ELISA) kit for human saliva samples (Melatonin direct Saliva ELISA, Tecan, IBL International GmbH, Hamburg, Germany) according to the manufacturer's protocol. For this purpose, prior to analysis, samples were thawed, mixed, and centrifuged at $2500\times g$ for 10 min to remove particulate material. For each run, a melatonin standard curve (0–50 pg/mL) was used to calculate the melatonin concentration in the samples, expressed in pg/mL, and quality controls were included to validate the assay's accuracy. Standards, controls, and samples were analyzed in duplicate to ensure reliability. Absorbance readings on the plates were performed using a Synergy™ Multi-Detection Microplate Reader (BioTek Instruments, Winooski, VT, USA) controlled with Gen5™ Data Analysis Software (version 3.04), measuring at 450 nm wavelength with 600 nm wavelength as reference.

2.7. Data Processing and Statistical Analysis

The absorbance data obtained for the standards in the ELISA assays were fitted to a four-parameter logistic curve (4PL) using the free online program MyCurveFit® (MyAssays Ltd., Brighton, UK), from which the melatonin concentration of the samples was extrapolated. The data collected for the variables during the study were exported to Excel and processed using the Statistical Package for the Social Sciences (SPSS 24.0 Inc., Chicago, IL, USA) for analysis. Descriptive statistics, including the mean and standard error (SE), were calculated for the numerical variables. The Kolmogorov-Smirnov test indicated that the variables did not follow a normal distribution, prompting the use of non-parametric tests for related samples. The Wilcoxon signed-rank test was employed to assess differences in melatonin concentration between the two lighting conditions, with statistical significance set at a p-value < 0.05.

3. Results

The sample consisted of 12 participants, among whom seven (58.33%) were women and five (41.67%) were men, ranging from 19 to 55 years with a mean age of 30.08 ± 12.91 years, all of whom met the inclusion criteria.

3.1. Melatonin Concentration Across All Participants

The analysis included all 12 participants, comparing mean salivary melatonin concentrations under blue and red light conditions at baseline and after 1, 2, and 3 h of exposure (Figure 4A). At baseline, melatonin levels were similar on the day of exposure to blue light (19.5 pg/mL) and red light (19.7 pg/mL), with no significant difference (p = 1.00). After 1 h of exposure, both lighting conditions resulted in a notable decrease in melatonin concentration, with levels of 6.6 pg/mL under blue light and 6.8 pg/mL under red light, without any significant difference between them ($p = 0.754$). Significant differences between the two lighting conditions emerged after 2 h of exposure. Melatonin concentration under blue light was 7.5 pg/mL, whereas it increased to 26.0 pg/mL under red light, yielding a statistically significant difference ($p = 0.019$). This difference persisted after 3 h of exposure, with melatonin levels of 8.3 pg/mL under blue light and 16.6 pg/mL under red light ($p = 0.013$). These results indicate that blue light significantly suppresses melatonin secretion after 2 h of exposure, highlighting its impact on the circadian rhythm.

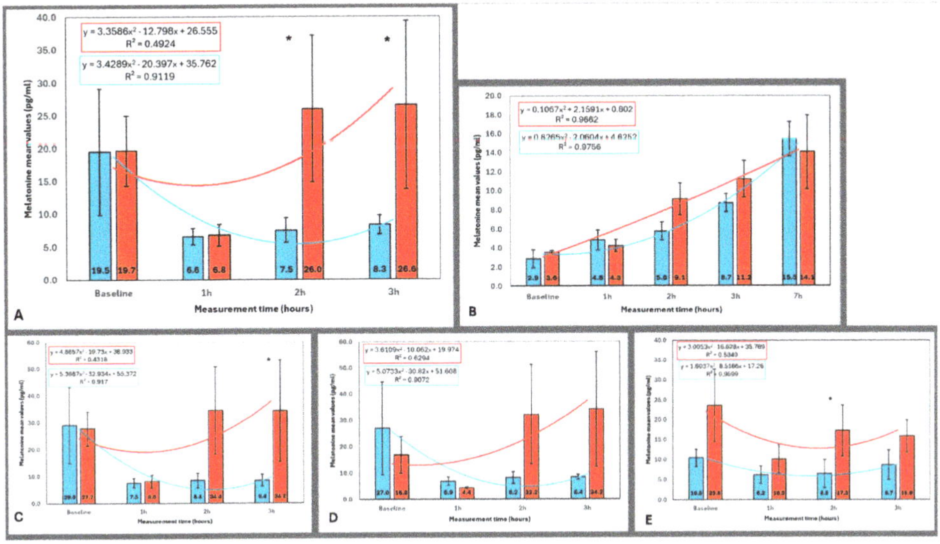

Figure 4. Mean (± standard deviation) melatonin concentration (pg/mL) across the four time points (baseline, 1 h, 2 h, and 3 h) under blue and red light conditions for different participant groups: (**A**) all participants (n = 12), (**B**) older female participants (n = 4, ages 32–55), including a 7-h measurement at 3 a.m., (**C**) young participants (n = 8), (**D**) all female participants (n = 7), and (**E**) all male participants (n = 5). The *X*-axis represents the time points of saliva sample collection, and the *Y*-axis shows the mean melatonin concentration for each lighting condition. Trend lines with equations illustrate melatonin secretion over time for both lighting conditions. Significant differences ($p < 0.05$) between blue and red light conditions at the same specific time points are marked with an asterisk (*). Statistical analysis was performed using the Wilcoxon signed-rank test for related samples.

3.2. Melatonin Concentration in Older and Younger Participants

The results for the 4 older female participants, aged between 32 and 55 years, with a mean age of 46 ± 9.83 years, were calculated separately (Figure 4B). In the baseline measurement, the melatonin concentrations were 2.9 pg/mL under blue light and 3.6 pg/mL under red light ($p = 0.465$). After 1 h of exposure, the concentrations were 4.8 pg/mL with blue light and 4.3 pg/mL with red light ($p = 0.465$). After 2 h, the melatonin levels were 5.8 pg/mL under blue light and 9.1 pg/mL under red light ($p = 0.068$), approaching statistical significance. At 3 h, the concentrations were 8.7 pg/mL with blue light and 11.2 pg/mL with red light ($p = 0.285$). Finally, at 7 h (coinciding with 3 a.m., when melatonin concentration typically peaks), the melatonin levels were 15.5 pg/mL with blue light and 14.1 pg/mL with red light ($p = 0.715$). No statistically significant differences were found between the lighting conditions at any time point, although at 2 h of exposure, the difference between blue and red light approached significance ($p = 0.068$), with higher melatonin concentrations observed under red light. By 7 h, the concentrations were similar between the two light conditions.

The group of young participants (Figure 4C) included 8 individuals (5 men and 3 women) with a mean age of 22.13 ± 1.81 years. Baseline melatonin concentrations were 29.0 pg/mL for the blue light condition and 27.7 pg/mL for the red light condition ($p = 1$). After 1 h of exposure, melatonin levels decreased to 7.5 pg/mL under blue light and 8.0 pg/mL under red light ($p = 0.889$). At 2 h, concentrations were 8.4 pg/mL for blue light and 34.4 pg/mL for red light, with the difference approaching statistical significance ($p = 0.069$). By the 3-h mark, melatonin levels were 8.4 pg/mL for blue light and 34.2 pg/mL for red light, showing a statistically significant difference in melatonin concentrations between the two lighting conditions ($p = 0.028$). These results indicate a clear suppression of melatonin secretion under blue light exposure at 2 and 3 h in young participants, as illustrated in Figure 4C.

3.3. Melatonin Concentration in Female and Male Participants

The sample of female participants was made up of 7 women who had a mean age of 36 ± 14.4 years, ranging from 19 to 55 years. Baseline melatonin concentrations in saliva were 27.0 pg/mL under blue light and 16.8 pg/mL under red light, with no significant difference between the two ($p = 0.463$). After 1 h of exposure, melatonin concentrations were 6.9 pg/mL with blue light and 4.4 pg/mL with red light ($p = 0.128$). After 2 h, the concentrations were 8.2 pg/mL with blue light and 32.2 pg/mL with red light ($p = 0.128$). At 3 h, concentrations were 8.4 pg/mL with blue light and 34.2 pg/mL with red light ($p = 0.116$). No significant differences in melatonin concentrations between the blue and red light conditions were observed. However, as shown in Figure 4D, after 2 h of exposure to blue light, melatonin concentration in saliva was notably lower, a trend that persisted after 3 h of exposure.

The male group consisted of 5 participants (Figure 4E) with a mean age of 21.8 ± 0.45 years, ranging between 21 and 22 years. At baseline, the melatonin concentration in saliva was 10.5 pg/mL under blue light and 23.6 pg/mL under red light, with no significant difference ($p = 0.225$). After 1 h of exposure, the concentrations were 6.2 pg/mL with blue light and 10.2 pg/mL with red light ($p = 0.225$). After 2 h, concentrations were 6.5 pg/mL with blue light and 17.3 pg/mL with red light, showing a statistically significant difference ($p = 0.043$), with higher melatonin levels under red light. At 3 h, the concentrations were 8.7 pg/mL with blue light and 15.9 pg/mL with red light, nearing statistical significance ($p = 0.068$). As shown in Figure 4E, melatonin concentrations increased significantly under red light exposure at the 2-h time point and approached significance at the 3-h time point, while blue light exposure showed consistently lower melatonin concentrations.

3.4. Comparison of Melatonin Levels Across Time Points for Each Lighting Condition

In Table 3, the p-values obtained from the Wilcoxon signed-rank test for paired samples are presented. These values compare the melatonin concentrations after 1 h of exposure to each lighting condition (blue and red) with the melatonin levels recorded at baseline, as well as the concentrations after 2 and 3 h of each exposure.

The choice of 1 h as the reference point for comparison was made because, across all participant groups, this is the time point where the most pronounced decrease in salivary melatonin concentration was observed, regardless of the lighting condition.

After 1 h of exposure to blue light, a substantial decrease in salivary melatonin concentration was observed when considering all participants together ($p = 0.182$), the group of young participants ($p = 0.063$), the group of women ($p = 0.917$), and the group of men ($p = 0.225$) compared to baseline levels. Melatonin levels increased slightly after 2 and 3 h of exposure in all cases, as shown in Figure 4A,C–E, respectively, without reaching statistical significance in any group (Table 3).

Table 3. p-values obtained using the Wilcoxon signed-rank test for paired samples, comparing melatonin concentrations at 1 h of exposure to blue and red light with baseline, 2 h, and 3 h melatonin levels for each lighting condition (blue and red). The analysis was conducted separately for each participant group. A p-value < 0.05 was considered statistically significant, and significant results are highlighted in bold with an asterisk (*).

Group	Blue Light 1 h vs.			Red Light 1 h vs.		
	Baseline	2 h	3 h	Baseline	2 h	3 h
All (n = 12) Figure 4A	0.182	0.583	0.386	**0.041** *	**0.028** *	**0.012** *
Younger (n = 8) Figure 4B	0.063	1.000	0.735	**0.025** *	0.093	0.093
Older (n = 4) Figure 4C	0.068	0.273	0.109	0.465	0.068	0.068
Female (n = 7) Figure 4D	0.917	0.398	0.249	0.237	**0.018** *	**0.028** *
Male (n = 5) Figure 4E	0.225	0.686	0.715	0.138	0.500	0.225

In contrast, after 1 h of exposure to red light, a significant decrease in salivary melatonin concentration compared to baseline was observed when considering all participants together (p = 0.041) and the group of young participants (p = 0.025). Although decreases were also noted in the group of women (p = 0.237) and the group of men (p = 0.138), these did not reach statistical significance. Furthermore, melatonin levels significantly increased in all participants and nearly all subgroups after 2 and 3 h of exposure (Table 3), as illustrated in Figure 4A,C–E.

4. Discussion

This study examined the effects of blue and red LED light on salivary melatonin concentrations, focusing on how their spectral characteristics influence circadian regulation. The findings highlight the significant role of the light spectrum in modulating melatonin secretion.

Blue light (peak 464 nm, overlapping with the melanopsin action spectrum) showed greater circadian stimulation and stronger, time-dependent melatonin suppression, particularly after 2 h. In contrast, red light (peak 631 nm, minimal overlap) preserved higher melatonin levels, indicating less circadian disruption. These differences may be influenced by prior light exposure, which modulates melatonin responses, with the greatest suppression occurring early and diminishing over time [16,18].

This study highlights age-specific differences in the effects of blue and red light on melatonin suppression. In older participants, no significant differences were observed between light conditions, though red light preserved slightly higher melatonin levels after 2 h. In younger participants, blue light significantly suppressed melatonin compared to red light, particularly after 2 and 3 h. Age-related declines in melatonin production have been attributed to factors such as reduced pupil size and lens yellowing, which limit retinal light exposure [16,19]. These changes lead to less light reaching the retina, which could theoretically impact circadian regulation, especially since retinal ganglion cells are more sensitive to blue light. However, in the context of our study, we consider the influence of these age-related ocular changes to be minimal. This is due to the substantial difference in the circadian effectiveness of light in the blue versus red spectrum selected to perform the experiments. Consequently, these pupillary changes, while important in a broader physiological context, seem to have limited influence on the circadian effects observed in our experiment, as reported by other authors [17].

The analysis by gender showed that in women, melatonin levels tended to be lower under blue light after 2 and 3 h, suggesting stronger circadian activation. However, the differences between light conditions were not significant, aligning with previous inconclusive findings [19]. For men, melatonin levels were significantly higher under red light after 2 h and approached significance at 3 h, while blue light consistently suppressed melatonin more, highlighting blue light's stronger impact and red light's circadian-friendly effects in both groups. These subgroup analyses were exploratory and based on a small sample, so the findings should be interpreted with caution. Larger and more balanced studies are needed to confirm these trends.

Globally, our results confirm red light's circadian-friendly properties, particularly for females and younger participants, while blue light consistently suppressed melatonin across groups. This variability may stem from factors such as age-related ocular changes, pupil size differences, health status, medications, hormonal levels, and genetic variations affecting melanopsin pathways, as well as long-term light exposure patterns, such as seasonal changes [18,19]. Achieving 250 mEDI outdoors during the day is feasible, but evening exposure should be limited to 10 mEDI, with near-darkness at night (very low mEDI) being crucial for maintaining a healthy circadian rhythm, improving sleep quality, and enhancing overall well-being [14,23]. While this may conflict with visibility needs, it is recommended in integrative lighting design. Existing guidelines, based on healthy young adults, need to be extended to other populations, with future research focusing on personal light dosimetry to better understand exposure patterns. Current lighting standards, based on averages, often overlook individual variability [15]; as sensitivity to light can differ by up to 50–60 times [37], with some people suppressing melatonin at minimal light levels while others require much higher intensities, the need for flexible controls and tailored recommendations could be necessary for individuals active at night, taking into consideration their distinct activities and light exposure outside of work.

NIF functions vary in response speed, with rapid pupil reactions and slower EEG Gamma responses, highlighting individual variability in how light affects cognitive alertness and brain activity [38]. Recent findings show that non-visual response systems, including those involving the brain, cardiovascular system, and thermoregulation, activate within 1 to 5 min of light exposure, suggesting a faster response than previously thought [38]. Blue light enhances NIF effects, such as brain activation, while blocking green light may amplify polychromatic white light's impact [39,40]. Psychological and behavioral responses to light also differ widely due to individual exposure and subjective alertness. Understanding these differences is crucial for tailoring light therapies to improve cognitive function, mood, and quality of life, especially in older populations. These variations arise because light impacts mood and behavior through ipRGCs, which mediate its effects on behavioral states [41]. However, the relationship between light exposure and daytime alertness varies significantly, with most dose-response analyses showing non-significant correlations [42].

Moreover, melanopic illuminance has become a key metric for predicting circadian effects, offering a valuable tool for assessing light's impact on human physiology [24]. Our findings show that blue light suppresses melatonin within 1 h of exposure, maintaining this suppression with minimal recovery over the next hours. In contrast, red light also suppresses melatonin initially but allows a significant rebound after 2 and 3 h, restoring secretion to higher levels. This suggests red light may be beneficial for preserving circadian regulation. Additionally, light color affects both physiological and psychological responses; blue light is associated with relaxation, while red light evokes alertness or even danger, which might initially inhibit melatonin. However, as the brain adapts, this effect diminishes, leading to melatonin rebound. It is also important to note that our results may be influenced by the S-cone response, which overlaps with the melatonin absorption spectrum, and their mutual influence is still under discussion [10,43]. These results also emphasize the need for refined methodologies to assess circadian light hygiene, beyond static or solely melanopic-based metrics. While recent tools such as CircaLight offer reliable spectral-spatial simulations of circadian metrics [44], and conceptual frameworks [45] emphasize the importance of spatial, spectral, and temporal components in light assessment over 24 h, our findings contribute complementary biological evidence by characterizing melatonin suppression and rebound in response to spectrally distinct light over time. This time-resolved physiological approach may support future developments in circadian light hygiene assessment by integrating not only spectral and spatial, but also temporal responsiveness of human physiology to light.

Existing lighting guidelines are primarily based on healthy young adults, indicating a need for further research to adapt these recommendations for diverse populations, particularly older adults or those with disrupted circadian rhythms. Future studies should focus on personal light dosimetry to better understand individual light exposure patterns. Additionally, current lighting standards often overlook individual variability, highlighting the need for adaptable lighting controls and tailored recommendations, especially for individuals active at night. While these findings offer valuable insights, more research is needed to fully understand the mechanisms involved and optimize lighting strategies.

5. Conclusions

In conclusion, our findings demonstrate that blue light causes a stronger and more sustained melatonin suppression than red light, highlighting its significant impact on the circadian system. In contrast, red light, while initially lowering melatonin, allowed for notable recovery, suggesting it is less disruptive to circadian rhythms. These results underline the importance of the light spectrum in circadian regulation and suggest red light as a potential option to reduce circadian disruption. This study represents a preliminary step toward understanding these effects, and future research should include a larger and more diverse sample to validate these findings, particularly with respect to age and gender differences.

Author Contributions: Conceptualization, A.S.-C., M.J.L.-B., E.S. and E.O.-H.; methodology, A.S.-C., M.J.L.-B., E.S. and E.O.-H.; validation, A.S.-C., M.J.L.-B., E.S. and E.O.-H.; formal analysis, A.S.-C., M.J.L.-B., E.S. and E.O.-H.; investigation, A.S.-C., M.J.L.-B., E.S. and E.O.-H.; resources, A.S.-C., M.J.L.-B., E.S. and E.O.-H.; data curation, A.S.-C., M.J.L.-B., E.S. and E.O.-H.; writing—original draft preparation, A.S.-C., M.J.L.-B., E.S. and E.O.-H.; writing—review and editing, A.S.-C., M.J.L.-B., E.S. and E.O.-H.; visualization, A.S.-C., M.J.L.-B., E.S. and E.O.-H.; supervision, A.S.-C., M.J.L.-B., E.S. and E.O.-H.; project administration, A.S.-C., M.J.L.-B., E.S. and E.O.-H.; funding acquisition, A.S.-C., M.J.L.-B., E.S. and E.O.-H. All authors have read and agreed to the published version of the manuscript.

Funding: This research was supported by the Gobierno de Aragón Departamento de Ciencia, Universidad y Sociedad del Conocimiento, under grant No. LMP39_21, Fundación Ibercaja, and the University of Zaragoza under project No. JIUZ-2021-CIE-03.

Institutional Review Board Statement: The study adhered to the Declaration of Helsinki and was approved by the Clinical Research Ethics Committee of Aragón (CEICA) (approval number PI24/483. 4 December 2024).

Informed Consent Statement: Written informed consent has been obtained from the patients to publish this paper.

Data Availability Statement: The data presented in this study are available within the article.

Conflicts of Interest: The authors declare no conflicts of interest.

Abbreviations

The following abbreviations are used in this manuscript:

SCN	Suprachiasmatic nucleus
RHT	Retinohypothalamic tract
ipRGCs	Intrinsically photosensitive retinal ganglion cells
NIF	Non-image-forming
PLR	Pupillary light reflex
CIE	Commission International de l'Eclairage
mEDI	Melanopic equivalent daylight (D65) illuminance
EML	Equivalent melanopic lux
CL_A	Circadian Light
CS	Circadian stimulus
SPD	Spectral power distribution
FWHM	Full width at half maximum
CSd	Circadian light dose
SE	Standard error

References

1. Wahl, S.; Engelhardt, M.; Schaupp, P.; Lappe, C.; Ivanov, I.V. The Inner Clock—Blue Light Sets the Human Rhythm. *J. Biophotonics* **2019**, *12*, e201900102. [CrossRef] [PubMed]
2. Pundir, M.; Papagerakis, S.; De Rosa, M.C.; Chronis, N.; Kurabayashi, K.; Abdulmawjood, S.; Prince, M.E.P.; Lobanova, L.; Chen, X.; Papagerakis, P. Emerging Biotechnologies for Evaluating Disruption of Stress, Sleep, and Circadian Rhythm Mechanism Using Aptamer-Based Detection of Salivary Biomarkers. *Biotechnol. Adv.* **2022**, *59*, 107961. [CrossRef]
3. Figueiro, M.G.; Nagare, R.; Price, L.L.A. Non-Visual Effects of Light: How to Use Light to Promote Circadian Entrainment and Elicit Alertness. *Light. Res. Technol.* **2018**, *50*, 38–62. [CrossRef] [PubMed]
4. Berson, D.M.; Dunn, F.A.; Takao, M. Phototransduction by Retinal Ganglion Cells That Set the Circadian Clock. *Science (1979)* **2002**, *295*, 1070–1073. [CrossRef]
5. Foster, R.G. Fundamentals of Circadian Entrainment by Light. *Light. Res. Technol.* **2021**, *53*, 377–393. [CrossRef]
6. Provencio, I.; Rodriguez, I.R.; Jiang, G.; Hayes, W.P.; Moreira, E.F.; Rollag, M.D. A Novel Human Opsin in the Inner Retina. *J. Neurosci.* **2000**, *20*, 600–605. [CrossRef]
7. Thapan, K.; Arendt, J.; Skene, D.J. An Action Spectrum for Melatonin Suppression: Evidence for a Novel Non-Rod, Non-Cone Photoreceptor System in Humans. *J. Physiol.* **2001**, *535*, 261–267. [CrossRef]
8. Brainard, G.C.; Hanifin, J.P.; Greeson, J.M.; Byrne, B.; Glickman, G.; Gerner, E.; Rollag, M.D. Action Spectrum for Melatonin Regulation in Humans: Evidence for a Novel Circadian Photoreceptor. *J. Neurosci.* **2001**, *21*, 6405–6412. [CrossRef]
9. Lucas, R.J.; Peirson, S.N.; Berson, D.M.; Brown, T.M.; Cooper, H.M.; Czeisler, C.A.; Figueiro, M.G.; Gamlin, P.D.; Lockley, S.W.; O'Hagan, J.B.; et al. Measuring and Using Light in the Melanopsin Age. *Trends Neurosci.* **2014**, *37*, 1–9. [CrossRef]
10. Brown, T.M.; Thapan, K.; Arendt, J.; Revell, V.L.; Skene, D.J. S-Cone Contribution to the Acute Melatonin Suppression Response in Humans. *J. Pineal. Res.* **2021**, *71*, e12719. [CrossRef]
11. Novotny, P.; Plischke, H. Pupillary Light Reflex and Circadian Synchronization in the Elderly. *Psych. J.* **2017**, *6*, 292–293. [CrossRef] [PubMed]
12. Mure, L.S. Intrinsically Photosensitive Retinal Ganglion Cells of the Human Retina. *Front. Neurol.* **2021**, *12*, 636330. [CrossRef]
13. Najjar, R.P.; Prayag, A.S.; Gronfier, C. Melatonin Suppression by Light Involves Different Retinal Photoreceptors in Young and Older Adults. *J. Pineal. Res.* **2024**, *76*, e12930. [CrossRef] [PubMed]
14. Brown, T.M.; Brainard, G.C.; Cajochen, C.; Czeisler, C.A.; Hanifin, J.P.; Lockley, S.W.; Lucas, R.J.; Münch, M.; OHagan, J.B.; Peirson, S.N.; et al. Recommendations for Daytime, Evening, and Nighttime Indoor Light Exposure to Best Support Physiology, Sleep, and Wakefulness in Healthy Adults. *PLoS Biol.* **2022**, *20*, e3001571. [CrossRef]
15. Chellappa, S.L. Individual Differences in Light Sensitivity Affect Sleep and Circadian Rhythms. *Sleep* **2021**, *44*, zsaa214. [CrossRef] [PubMed]
16. Nagare, R.; Plitnick, B.; Figueiro, M.G. Effect of Exposure Duration and Light Spectra on Nighttime Melatonin Suppression in Adolescents and Adults. *Light. Res. Technol.* **2019**, *51*, 530–543. [CrossRef] [PubMed]

17. Eto, T.; Higuchi, S. Review on Age-Related Differences in Non-Visual Effects of Light: Melatonin Suppression, Circadian Phase Shift and Pupillary Light Reflex in Children to Older Adults. *J. Physiol. Anthropol.* **2023**, *42*, 11. [CrossRef]
18. Lee, S.-I.; Kinoshita, S.; Noguchi, A.; Eto, T.; Ohashi, M.; Nishimura, Y.; Maeda, K.; Motomura, Y.; Awata, Y.; Higuchi, S. Melatonin Suppression during a Simulated Night Shift in Medium Intensity Light Is Increased by 10-Minute Breaks in Dim Light and Decreased by 10-Minute Breaks in Bright Light. *Chronobiol. Int.* **2020**, *37*, 897–909. [CrossRef]
19. Swope, C.B.; Rong, S.; Campanella, C.; Vaicekonyte, R.; Phillips, A.J.K.; Cain, S.W.; McGlashan, E.M. Factors Associated with Variability in the Melatonin Suppression Response to Light: A Narrative Review. *Chronobiol. Int.* **2023**, *40*, 542–556. [CrossRef]
20. Ju, J.; He, L.; Li, Z.; Wu, Z.; He, Z.; Liang, R. Biological Effects of Color Lighting for Different Ages. *Appl. Mech. Mater.* **2012**, *236–237*, 787–791. [CrossRef]
21. Reutrakul, S.; Crowley, S.J.; Park, J.C.; Chau, F.Y.; Priyadarshini, M.; Hanlon, E.C.; Danielson, K.K.; Gerber, B.S.; Baynard, T.; Yeh, J.J.; et al. Relationship between Intrinsically Photosensitive Ganglion Cell Function and Circadian Regulation in Diabetic Retinopathy. *Sci. Rep.* **2020**, *10*, 1560. [CrossRef] [PubMed]
22. *CIE S 026/E:2018*; CIE System for Metrology of Optical Radiation for IpRGC-Influenced Responses to Light. CIE Central Bureau: Vienna, Austria, 2018.
23. *Position Statement CIE Position Statement on Integrative Lighting Recommending Proper Light at the Proper Time*, 3rd ed.; CIE: Vienna, Austria, 2024. [CrossRef]
24. Brown, T.M. Melanopic Illuminance Defines the Magnitude of Human Circadian Light Responses under a Wide Range of Conditions. *J. Pineal. Res.* **2020**, *69*, e12655. [CrossRef] [PubMed]
25. IWBI International Well Building Institute. *WELL Building Standard v2 Pilot, Q3 2021 Version. Section L03: Circadian Lighting Design*; IWBI International Well Building Institute: New York, NY, USA, 2021.
26. Rea, M.S.; Nagare, R.; Figueiro, M.G. Modeling Circadian Phototransduction: Quantitative Predictions of Psychophysical Data. *Front. Neurosci.* **2021**, *15*, 615322. [CrossRef] [PubMed]
27. Rea, M.S.; Nagare, R.; Figueiro, M.G. Modeling Circadian Phototransduction: Retinal Neurophysiology and Neuroanatomy. *Front. Neurosci.* **2021**, *14*, 615305. [CrossRef]
28. Rea, M.S.; Figueiro, M.G.; Bullough, J.D.; Bierman, A. A Model of Phototransduction by the Human Circadian System. *Brain Res. Rev.* **2005**, *50*, 213–228. [CrossRef]
29. Sánchez-cano, A.; Aporta, J. Optimization of Lighting Projects Including Photopic and Circadian Criteria: A Simplified Action Protocol. *Appl. Sci.* **2020**, *10*, 8068. [CrossRef]
30. Schlangen, L.J.M.; Belgers, S.; Cuijpers, R.H.; Heynderickx, I.E.J. Invited Comment on "The Law of Reciprocity Holds (More or Less) for Circadian-Effective Lighting", by M Rea, Accepted for Publication in LRT 2022. *Light. Res. Technol.* **2022**, *54*, 756–757.
31. *CIE Position Statement on Non-Visual Effects of Light Recommending Proper Light at the Proper Time*, 2nd ed.; CIE: Vienna, Austria, 2019; Volume 1.
32. Wyszecki, G.; Stiles, W.S. *Color Science: Concepts and Methods, Quantitative Data and Formulae*; John Wiley & Sons: Hoboken, NJ, USA, 2000; Volume 40, ISBN 0471399183.
33. Govardovskii, V.I.; Fyhrquist, N.; Reuter, T.O.M.; Kuzmin, D.G.; Donner, K. In Search of the Visual Pigment Template. *Vis. Neurosci.* **2000**, *17*, 509–528. [CrossRef]
34. Smith, V.C.; Pokorny, J. Spectral Sensitivity of the Foveal Cone Photopigments between 400 and 500 Nm. *Vis. Res.* **1975**, *15*, 161–171. [CrossRef]
35. Commission International de l'Eclairage (CIE). *Light as a True Visual Quantity: Principles of Measurement*; CIE Central Bureau CIE: Vienna, Austria, 1978; Volume 41.
36. Sanchez-Cano, A.; Orduna-Hospital, E.; Fernández-Espinosa, G.; Aporta, J. Method to Calculate Melanopic Light Reaching the Retina Depending on the Optical Density of an Aging Crystalline Lens. *Appl. Sci.* **2023**, *13*, 2569. [CrossRef]
37. Phillips, A.J.K.; Vidafar, P.; Burns, A.C.; McGlashan, E.M.; Anderson, C.; Rajaratnam, S.M.W.; Lockley, S.W.; Cain, S.W. High Sensitivity and Interindividual Variability in the Response of the Human Circadian System to Evening Light. *Proc. Natl. Acad. Sci. USA* **2019**, *116*, 12019–12024. [CrossRef] [PubMed]
38. Prayag, A.S.; Jost, S.; Avouac, P.; Dumortier, D.; Gronfier, C. Dynamics of Non-Visual Responses in Humans: As Fast as Lightning? *Front. Neurosci.* **2019**, *13*, 126. [CrossRef]
39. Morioka, H.; Ozawa, H.; Kato, T. Physiological Study of Visual and Non-Visual Effects of Light Exposure. *Appl. Sci.* **2023**, *13*, 5785. [CrossRef]
40. Lee, S.; Kakitsuba, N.; Katsuura, T. Do Green-Blocking Glasses Enhance the Nonvisual Effects of White Polychromatic Light? *J. Physiol. Anthropol.* **2018**, *37*, 29. [CrossRef]
41. Milosavljevic, N. How Does Light Regulate Mood and Behavioral State? *Clocks Sleep* **2019**, *1*, 319–331. [CrossRef] [PubMed]
42. van Duijnhoven, J.; Aarts, M.P.J.; van den Heuvel, E.R.; Kort, H.S.M. Exploring the Relationship between Light and Subjective Alertness Using Personal Lighting Conditions. *J. Phys. Conf. Ser.* **2021**, *2042*, 012119. [CrossRef]

43. Fazlali, F.; Lazar, R.; Yahya, F.; Epple, C.; Spitschan, M.; Stefani, O.; Cajochen, C. Lack of Evidence for the Contribution of Cone Photoreceptors to Human Melatonin Suppression and Alerting Response to Light at Night. *bioRxiv* **2024**. [CrossRef]
44. Aguilar-Carrasco, M.T.; Acosta, I.; Domínguez-Amarillo, S. CircaLight, a New Circadian Light Assessment Tool for Grasshopper Environment: Development and Reliability Testing. *J. Build. Eng.* **2023**, *71*, 106527. [CrossRef]
45. Gubin, D.G.; Borisenkov, M.F.; Kolomeichuk, S.N.; Markov, A.A.; Weinert, D.; Cornelissen, G.; Stefani, O. Evaluating Circadian Light Hygiene: Methodology and Health Implications. *Russ. Open Med. J.* **2024**, *13*, e0415. [CrossRef]

life

MDPI

Article

The Effect of Pupil Size on Cone Contrast Sensitivity

Ali Almustanyir [1,*,†], Meznah S. Almutairi [1,†], Amal Aldrwish [1], Nabeela Hasrod [2], Bader A. Alqhtani [1], Tahani Alqahtani [1], Muteb Alanazi [1], Mansour Alghamdi [1], Essam Almutleb [1], Balsam Alabdulkader [1], Faisal Fakhouri [3] and Mosaad Alhassan [1]

[1] Optometry Department, College of Applied Medical Sciences, King Saud University, Riyadh 11362, Saudi Arabia; mzalmutairi@ksu.edu.sa (M.S.A.); aaldarweesh@ksu.edu.sa (A.A.); 441100921@student.ksu.edu.sa (B.A.A.); talqahtani@ksu.edu.sa (T.A.); mkalanazi@ksu.edu.sa (M.A.); algmansour@ksu.edu.sa (M.A.); esalsarhani@ksu.edu.sa (E.A.); alabdulkader@ksu.edu.sa (B.A.); malhassan@ksu.edu.sa (M.A.)

[2] Department of Optometry, Faculty of Health Sciences, University of Johannesburg, Johannesburg 2025, South Africa; nabeelah@uj.ac.za

[3] Department of Biomedical Technology, College of Applied Medical Sciences, King Saud University, Riyadh 11362, Saudi Arabia; ffakhouri@ksu.edu.sa

* Correspondence: aalmustanyir@ksu.edu.sa

† These authors contributed equally to this paper.

Abstract: Background: Measuring contrast sensitivity for each of the three cone types separately allows for a more precise and clinically valuable assessment of color vision. This study examined how pupil size affects cone contrast sensitivity (CCS). Methods: This study included 50 participants of equal gender. The mean age was 20.88 (±1.8) years. Using the ColorDx, a Landolt C stimulus of various sizes in an adaptive screening mode, we sequentially determined contrast sensitivity for long-, medium-, and short-wavelength stimuli. Two consecutive measurements were performed on participants, one with their natural pupil size (range 4–5 mm diameter) and, subsequently, with six artificial eye pupils (1 mm to 6 mm). Results: Generally, the 1 mm pupil size caused the greatest reduction in contrast sensitivity for two of the three cones. There was no significant main effect of sex ($F = 0.96$, $df = 1$, $p = 0.32$) on the log cone contrast sensitivity of the L-cone. However, pupil size had a significant main effect ($F = 116.1$, $df = 6$, $p < 0.001$). Within each sex, the log CCS was significantly reduced as the pupil size decreased compared with the normal pupil size. Conclusions: New technologies that assess individual cone pathway functions could potentially assist in identifying early or progressive conditions that may impact color vision pathways from the retina to the brain. Standardized protocols—such as controlled retinal illumination—are critical to avoid misinterpretation.

Keywords: pupil size; cone contrast sensitivity; wavelength cone systems; color vision

1. Introduction

Color vision testing evaluates an individual's capacity to perceive and differentiate various shades of color. These tests primarily diagnose color vision deficiencies, which affect approximately 8% of males [1]. Several types of color vision tests have been designed for specific purposes and varying levels of precision. For example, pseudoisochromatic plate tests are often employed to screen for inherited color vision disorders and exhibit high sensitivity [2]. However, these tests do have limitations. The determination of a specific type or severity of inherited color vision deficiencies is somewhat constrained, and tests rarely assess short-wavelength sensitivity. Furthermore, color plate tests are not commonly used in routine eye examinations, perhaps due to their limited ability to detect acquired color vision problems [3–5]. Notably, acquired color vision deficits may appear before the loss of high-contrast visual acuity or visual field defects [3,4,6].

Recent advancements in color perception testing technology have introduced methods for independently measuring color contrast thresholds for long (L), medium (M), and short (S) wavelength cone systems. This innovation enables the quantitative assessment of color perception without the need for specialized lighting conditions, which are required for color vision tests such as the Farnsworth D15 or 100-hue and pseudoisochromatic plate tests. It also removes the necessity for complex data interpretation generated by the gold-standard anomaloscope used in color-matching tests. Although pseudoisochromatic color plates, arrangement tests, matching tests, and contrast sensitivity tests evaluate different aspects of color perception, comparative studies involving individuals with normal vision and those with known inherited color vision deficiencies have demonstrated that these tests show comparable sensitivity and specificity in distinguishing between normal and anomalous trichromacy or dichromacy [6].

The cone contrast sensitivity (CCS) test, developed in the late 1990s, has been validated on military personnel [7]. In a 1996 study focusing on quantifying color perception using CCS, researchers employed a uniform stimulus size (6/95) for all three chromatic stimuli based on British Standard Institution letters [6]. This large stimulus size was specifically chosen to minimize the effect of defocus when viewing chromatic stimuli against an achromatic background [7]. It revealed that, for normal trichromatic vision, the CCS for the short-wavelength (S) stimulus was nearly one log unit lower than for the medium-wavelength cone (M) and long-wavelength cone (L) stimuli, respectively. This significant difference in sensitivity among the different cone types offers valuable insights into the varying sensitivities of the human visual system to different wavelengths [7,8].

In the 2011 test iteration, the S-wavelength stimulus was enlarged to 6/132 to align with the peak spatial frequency for the contrast detection of the S-wavelength neural mechanism [9]. This adjustment resulted in a higher CCS in individuals with normal trichromatic vision. Notably, using an S-wavelength stimulus larger than L- and M-wavelength stimuli is consistent with other studies investigating visual acuity and contrast sensitivity in cone-specific pathways utilizing letter charts and visually evoked potentials [10,11]. The enlarged S-wavelength stimulus also engaged a significant number of S-cones while remaining within the 3° macular region containing the macular pigment [12]. Additionally, in this version, each stimulus was displayed as a single letter on a monitor for 1.0–1.6 s.

As reported in 1996 and 2004, in comparing the CCS to other clinical color vision tests, including the gold-standard anomaloscope, the CCS test demonstrated comparable effectiveness in distinguishing between normal trichromacy and red–green anomalous trichromacy or dichromacy [7,8]. Moreover, the CCS test successfully identified defective color vision in patients with high-contrast acuity visual pathologies, sometimes detecting issues missed by other tests [9]. Konan Medical, Inc., in collaboration with the U.S. Air Force School of Aerospace Medicine, enhanced the original CCS clinical instrument by [13]:

- Expanding the evaluable contrast range;
- Substituting letter stimuli with Landolt C stimuli;
- Implementing a four-direction keypad for responses;
- Introducing an "adaptive screening mode" for efficiency.

Cisarik and Kampwerth evaluated the effects of pupil size on CCS using ColorDx technology (Konan Medical, Inc., Irvine, CA, USA) in young healthy adults [14]. They found that CCS decreased when retinal illumination was reduced in healthy individuals with normal color vision. This reduction was achieved by having the participants view through an artificial pupil smaller than their natural pupil size. Such effects are expected, as previous research has shown, that the thresholds for achromatic (black and white) contrast increase under conditions of reduced retinal illumination [15,16]. Notably, while a 2.5 mm pupil has been previously identified as optimal for enhancing contrast sensitivity and visual acuity, this study found that using an artificial pupil of this size negatively affected the CCS of participants. Their performance was better when using their larger natural pupils compared to the artificially created 2.5 mm pupils. Cisarik and Kampwerth suggested that the relationship between pupil size and color perception is complex and that what may be optimal for some aspects of vision (such as achromatic contrast sensitivity and visual acuity), such as cone contrast sensitivity, may not be ideal for others. Nevertheless, this study extended previous works to evaluate the effect of different retinal illumination sizes on CCS assessed using ColorDx technology (Konan Medical, Inc.) in normal adults.

Previous studies have also suggested that, in conditions such as early glaucoma, diabetic retinopathy, and optic neuropathies, contrast sensitivity deficits may precede measurable changes in high-contrast visual acuity or visual fields [17,18].

By having a better understanding of the effect of pupil size on cone contrast sensitivity, this study could potentially help clinicians with a better interpretation of contrast sensitivity tests specifically in non-standard lighting conditions, or in the presence of miosis or mydriasis, which could help reduce false positives/negative findings in early retinal or optic nerve dysfunction diagnosis.

Similarly, when assessing for early retinal or optic nerve dysfunction, as senile miosis may influence cone contrast responses, the findings could guide clinicians' expectations in older adults [19].

This study may also lead to developing best practices for clinicians for pupil control and ambient lighting during cone contrast sensitivity testing.

Knowing the impact of pupil size on contrast sensitivity could also help manage patients' expectations of visual quality under different lighting conditions when wearing multifocal contact lenses or post refractive surgery [20,21]. This study aims to evaluate the effect of different retinal illumination sizes on the CCS assessed with the ColorDx technology (Konan Medical, Inc.) in normal adults.

2. Materials and Methods

This study was approved by the Institutional Review Board (IRB) of the College of Medicine at King Saud University, Saudi Arabia. This study followed the Declaration of Helsinki's tenets and was approved by King Saud University through the Institution Review Board Office of Research Ethics (E-23-8128). After obtaining written informed consent as per the IRB-approved protocol, a group of 25 male and 25 female healthy young adults between the ages of 21 and 31 took part in the study. All participants had undergone different color vision tests. All subjects were found to have normal trichromatic vision. All participants had healthy visual systems. The use of tinted contact lenses or glasses was not permitted, and any history of eye disease was ruled out through a brief questionnaire. To further minimize the risk of including individuals with bilateral disorders linked to acquired color vision defects, only those with binocular distance visual acuity of 6/9 or better were selected. Presbyopic participants wore their usual near correction during testing.

2.1. Instrumentation

Pseudoisochromatic plate tests were used to test the normality of color vision. The pseudoisochromatic plate tests used were the 38-plate edition of the Ishihara test (Kanhara & Co., Ltd., 1996, Tokyo, Japan) and the Hardy, Rand, and Rittler tests (4th edition, Richmond Products, Albuquerque, NM, USA). The normality of individual color vision was classified according to Rayleigh color matching using an HMC Oculus anomaloscope

(Oculus Optikgeräte GmbH, Wetzlar, Germany). Tinted contact lenses or spectacles were not used in this study. The sequences of all tests were randomized using a random block design. The failure criterion for the Ishihara screening plates was ≥3 errors on plates 1–17, >2 errors on the red–green screening plate, and >0 errors on the blue–yellow plates of HRR. The illuminance for the tests was 800 lux (±5%) in the horizontal plane. The ColorDx test was performed to measure the CCS of all cones (L, M, and S). Tropicamide eye drops (1%) were used to control pupil size. The drop was instilled 30 min before the examination started.

The test was repeated for different pupil sizes (1–6 mm) using artificial pupils.

Six circular artificial pupils were 3D-printed with the same outer diameter of 37 mm and a thickness of 2 mm. Each artificial pupil had a hole in the center of the circle with a diameter ranging from 1 to 6 mm, as shown in Figure 1. Each artificial pupil was installed on the trial frame on the right eye, and the left eye was covered by the frame occluder. 3D printing was performed using a Prusa MK3S+ (Prusa Research Inc., Prague, Czech Republic) fused deposition modeling (FDM) 3D printer. The 3D-printed objects were printed using an opaque dark blue eSun PLA+ filament (Shenzhen Esun Industrial Co., Ltd., Shenzhen, China), a poly lactic acid-based (PLA) 3D printing material. The 3D printing parameters were as follows: layer height 0.1 mm, infill percentage 100%, printing nozzle temperature 210 °C, printing bed temperature 60 °C with a smooth finish, and a printing time of 2 h and 52 min.

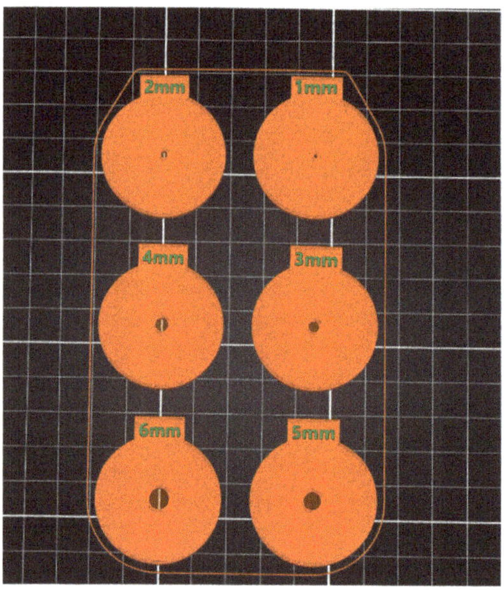

Figure 1. Illustration of the artificial pupil sizes used in this study. There were 6 sizes (1 to 6 mm) in 1 mm steps. The diameter of each of the artificial pupils was 37 mm. Each artificial pupil was marked with the pupil size at the top in mm.

The ColorDx test was used to evaluate CCS. This system comprises proprietary software (version 1.0.079), a Dell all-in-one computer with a 21.5-inch FHD LED-backlit IPS monitor, a 4-arrow response keypad, and a colorimeter for periodic screen calibration [22,23]. The software presents Landolt-C stimuli using the Bayesian [24] adaptive technique to determine the thresholds and standard errors. This technique adaptively targets nuisance parameters only when optimizing the estimation of the primary parameters of interest [24]. The monitor, with a maximum resolution of 1920 × 1080 pixels and a 60 Hz refresh rate, features an anti-glare color-calibrated screen with wide viewing angles. Before data collection, the monitor was calibrated using an OEM i1Pro USB colorimeter (Konan Medical). During testing, the luminance of the monitor was set to 65 candela/square meter, as measured by a Konica Minolta LS-150 luminance meter.

2.2. Procedure

The target was Landolt C, and participants needed to determine the direction of the letter 'C'. The viewing distance was 40 cm, which subtended 1.8° at the retina. The letter 'C' appears in the center of the screen, oriented in a specific direction. The options faced upward, downward, right, or left. The participants pressed the arrow key corresponding to the direction they perceived. The stimulus (letter) remained visible for 5 s before it disappeared. Whenever the participant answered correctly, the contrast decreased, and vice versa. Next, the tropicamide eye drops were administered to the right eye three times. Five minutes were spent waiting between the first and second drops, and the third drop after 15 min. The participants waited until the eye expanded completely (at least 45 min). The next step was to randomly place the artificial eye pupil on a trial frame (if the participant had a correction, we placed the prescription on the trial). There was a 1–2 min rest between each measurement. This was completed to ensure that the cones (L, M, and S) were fatigued. Figure 2 shows an example of a Landolt C presented. The Logarithm (Log) CCS was one of the outcomes from the test. Generally, the Log CCS is a logarithmic measure of the eye's ability to detect differences in contrast between an object and its background based on color, quantifying how well a person can see objects that do not stand out clearly from their surroundings.

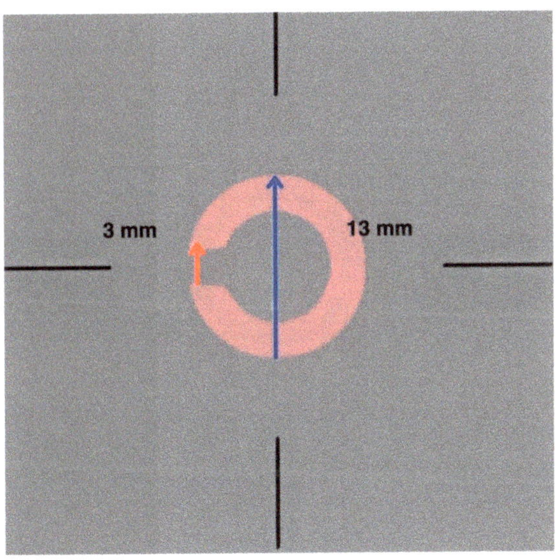

Figure 2. A screenshot of the Landolt C that was used in the CCS test for the L cone. Red arrow indicate the size of the opening gap of the Landolt C, and the blue arrow indicates the size of the Landolt C.

2.3. Statistical Analysis

Repeated measures analysis of variance (ANOVA) was employed to investigate the impact of sex and pupil size on log cone contrast sensitivity (log CCS). The mean, standard deviation of the mean, and the 95% confidence interval were calculated. The statistical significance level was set at 5% ($p < 0.05$). All statistical analyses were conducted using IBM SPSS Statistics version 29 (IBM, Armonk, NY, USA).

3. Results

The participants' mean age was 20.88 (±1.8) years. There were 50% male and 50% female participants. Natural pupil sizes ranged from 4 to 5 mm. All participants tested with their natural pupils demonstrated normal trichromacy, as indicated by their CCS measurements, pseudoisochromatic plate tests, and anomaloscope.

A two-way mixed-effects ANOVA was conducted to investigate the impact of sex and pupil size on log cone contrast sensitivity (log CCS). There was no significant main effect of sex (F = 0.96, df = 1, $p = 0.32$) on the log CS of the L-cone. However, pupil size had a significant main effect (F = 116.1, df = 6, $p < 0.001$). Within each sex, the log CCS was significantly reduced as the pupil size decreased compared with the normal pupil size (Table 1). The pairwise comparison test showed a significant difference between the genders with a 2 mm pupil size (mean difference = 0.086, $p = 0.043$).

Table 1. The mean Log contrast sensitivity (log CCS) of the L-cone.

Gender	Pupil Size (mm)	Mean ± SD	95% Confidence Interval	Mean Difference from Normal	*p*-Value
Males	Normal	2.183 ± 0.044	2.095–2.270	—	—
	1 mm	1.341 ± 0.025	1.292–1.390	0.842	<0.001
	2 mm	1.641 ± 0.028	1.585–1.697	0.542	<0.001
	3 mm	1.789 ± 0.032	1.724–1.853	0.394	<0.001
	4 mm	1.812 ± 0.033	1.746–1.878	0.371	<0.001
	5 mm	1.861 ± 0.028	1.805–1.917	0.322	<0.001
	6 mm	1.872 ± 0.035	1.801–1.943	0.311	<0.001
Females	Normal	2.092 ± 0.051	1.989–2.195	—	—
	1 mm	1.389 ± 0.029	1.331–1.447	0.703	<0.001
	2 mm	1.726 ± 0.033 *	1.660–1.792	0.366	<0.001
	3 mm	1.798 ± 0.037	1.722–1.873	0.294	<0.001
	4 mm	1.880 ± 0.039	1.803–1.958	0.211	0.026
	5 mm	1.905 ± 0.033	1.839–1.971	0.187	0.050
	6 mm	1.910 ± 0.042	1.827–1.994	0.181	0.089

The 95% confidence interval, mean difference from normal, and *p*-value are presented. * Significant mean difference in log CCS in the females compared to males ($p = 0.043$).

Similarly, there was no significant main effect of sex on the log CCS of M-cones (F = 1.35, df = 1, $p = 0.25$; Table 2) or S-cones (F = 0.198, df = 1, 0.66; Table 3). Pupil size had a significant effect on the M-cone (F = 131.2.1, df = 6, $p < 0.001$) and S-cones (F = 125.3, df = 6, $p < 0.001$). The pairwise comparison test showed a significant difference between the genders with a 1 mm pupil size in the M-cone (mean difference = 0.106, $p = 0.041$). No significant difference was found between males and females using a multiple comparison test for the S-cone.

Table 2. The mean Log contrast sensitivity (log CCS) of the M-cone.

Gender	Pupil Size (mm)	Mean ± SD	95% Confidence Interval	Mean Difference from Normal	*p*-Value
Males	Normal	1.917 ± 0.012	1.893–1.942	—	—
	1 mm	1.226 ± 0.033	1.160–1.292	0.691	<0.001
	2 mm	1.637 ± 0.037	1.563–1.710	0.280	<0.001
	3 mm	1.768 ± 0.031	1.705–1.831	0.149	<0.001
	4 mm	1.832 ± 0.037	1.756–1.907	0.086	0.037
	5 mm	1.853 ± 0.037	1.779–1.928	0.064	0.120
	6 mm	1.819 ± 0.036	1.746–1.891	0.099	0.013
Females	Normal	1.899 ± 0.014	1.870–1.928	—	—
	1 mm	1.332 ± 0.039 *	1.255–1.410	0.566	<0.001
	2 mm	1.638 ± 0.043	1.551–1.724	0.261	<0.001
	3 mm	1.779 ± 0.037	1.704–1.853	0.120	0.007
	4 mm	1.919 ± 0.044	1.831–2.007	−0.020	0.664
	5 mm	1.847 ± 0.043	1.759–1.934	0.052	0.279
	6 mm	1.930 ± 0.043	1.845–2.016	−0.032	0.481

The 95% confidence interval, mean difference from normal, and *p*-value are presented. * Significant mean difference in log CCS in the females compared to males ($p = 0.041$).

Table 3. The mean Log contrast sensitivity (log CCS) of the S-cone.

Gender	Pupil Size (mm)	Mean ± SD	95% Confidence Interval	Mean Difference from Normal	*p*-Value
Males	Normal	0.904 ± 0.029	0.845–0.963	—	—
	1 mm	0.907 ± 0.008	0.892–0.922	−0.003	1.0
	2 mm	0.280 ± 0.03	0.220–0.341	0.623	<0.001
	3 mm	0.612 ± 0.038	0.535–0.689	0.292	<0.001
	4 mm	0.713 ± 0.039	0.635–0.792	0.190	<0.001
	5 mm	0.810 ± 0.036	0.737–0.883	0.094	0.29
	6 mm	0.910 ± 0.031	0.853–0.979	−0.012	1.0
Females	Normal	0.851 ± 0.034	0.782–0.921	—	—
	1 mm	0.899 ± 0.009	0.881–0.916	−0.047	1.0
	2 mm	0.242 ± 0.035	0.171–0.314	0.609	<0.001
	3 mm	0.640 ± 0.045	0.549–0.731	0.211	<0.001
	4 mm	0.771 ± 0.046	0.679–0.864	0.080	1.0
	5 mm	0.798 ± 0.043	0.712–0.883	0.054	1.0
	6 mm	0.841 ± 0.037	0.768–0.915	0.010	1.0

The 95% confidence interval, mean difference from normal, and *p*-value are presented.

Figure 3 provides the descriptive statistics for the log CCS measurements for each cone stimulus for the six different pupil sizes. Boxplots present the CCS data for the six pupil sizes for the L-cone (Figure 3 top), M-cone (Figure 3 middle), and S-cone (Figure 3 bottom) stimuli. A reduction in log CCS occurred with the smallest pupil size (1 mm) for all three types of cones. The CCS increased as pupil size increased across the three types of cones.

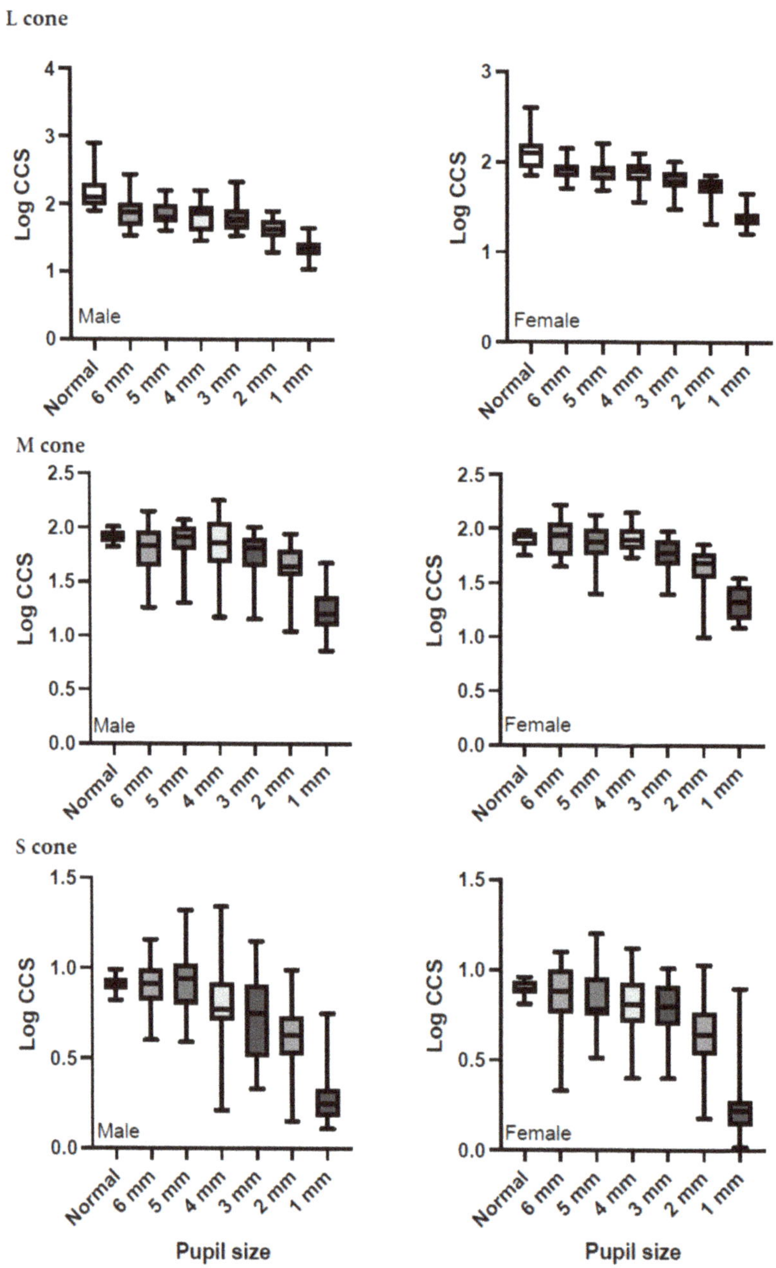

Figure 3. Boxplots showing the log cone contrast sensitivity (CCS) data (female: right figures and male: left figures) for each chromaticity stimulus (top: L-cone; middle: M-cone; last: S-cone) displayed at six pupil sizes. Results obtained with the natural pupil are presented as (Normal).

4. Discussion

In healthy participants with normal color vision, reducing retinal illumination using an artificial pupil smaller than their natural pupil size led to a significant decline in cone contrast sensitivity (CCS). This aligns with the known effects of lower illumination on the achromatic contrast thresholds, which also increase under dimmer conditions [15,16]. Specifically, this study showed that, generally, the 1 mm pupil size caused the greatest reduction in contrast sensitivity for two of the three cones (L-cone: [0.703: 0.84]; M-cone [0.566: 0.691]).

Data analysis employing two-way mixed-effect ANOVA and boxplots illustrated that, within each sex, the log CCS was significantly reduced as the pupil size was reduced compared to the normal pupil size for all three chromaticities. Pupil size had a significant main effect ($F = 116.1$, $df = 6$, $p < 0.001$) on the log CCS of L-cone, M-cone ($F = 131.2.1$, $df = 6$, $p < 0.001$), and S-cones ($F = 125.3$, $df = 6$, $p < 0.001$).

Generally, although there was no significant main effect of gender on the log CS of the L-cone ($F = 0.96$, $df = 1$, $p = 0.32$), M-cone ($F = 1.35$, $df = 1$, $p = 0.25$, Table 2), and S-cone ($F = 0.198$, $df = 1$, 0.66, Table 3), the pairwise comparison test did show a significant difference between the genders with 2 mm pupil size (mean difference = 0.086, $p = 0.043$) for the log CS of L-cone, and with 1 mm pupil size in the M-cone (mean difference = 0.106, $p = 0.041$).

Regarding the reduction in log CCS across all three chromaticities, it was found that the 1 mm pupil size produced the greatest mean differences between the normal for the L-cone (male: 0.84; female: 0.703) and M-cone (male: 0.691; female: 0.566). However, for the S-cone, the 2 mm pupil size produced the greatest mean difference from the normal (male: 0.623; female: 0.609).

The practical implications of the 1 mm pupil size and a measurable decrease in log CCS have several practical implications for clinicians. When measuring elderly patients or those with pharmacologically constricted pupils, where smaller pupil sizes may artificially lower scores, this finding emphasizes the importance of considering pupil size when interpreting contrast sensitivity test results. Also, clinicians should consider these implications when administering miotic drugs (e.g., pilocarpine) or testing contrast sensitivity under non-standard lighting conditions, as these can reduce pupil diameter and potentially mask true visual function. Finally, understanding this relationship may help manage the expectations of patients with underlying neural or retinal disorders where contrast sensitivity is already compromised. This reiterates the value of assessing both structural and functional vision, including contrast sensitivity, as part of a holistic visual evaluation [17,18,25].

Although the normal or natural pupil size ranged from 4 mm to 5 mm for all participants, it was interesting to note that, with a few exceptions (M-cone for females and S-cones for males), generally, the mean log CCS produced by the normal pupil for both sexes was still greater than the log CS for the 4 mm and 5 mm artificial pupil sizes for all chromaticities. It is possible that, for artificial pupils created by apertures placed in the spectacle plane, field-of-view restrictions may result from vignetting with the eye pupil. Thus, smaller artificial pupil sizes can act as pinholes, causing the target resolution to become impaired, which can adversely affect CCS [26].

Nevertheless, when comparing results from this study to that by Cisarik and Kampwerth with a 2.5 pupil size for all chromaticities (L-cone: large stimulus: 0.309, small stimulus: 0.260; M-cone: large stimulus: 0.297, small stimulus: 0.273; S-cone: large stimulus: 0.163, small stimulus: 0.197), it was found that, for the L-cone and S-cone, results were similar to the mean difference in log CCS between the normal for the 3 mm pupil size for both sexes (L-cone: male: 0.394, female: 0.294; S-cone: male: 0.292, female: 0.211). Regarding M-cones, the results were similar for the 2 mm pupil size for both sexes (male: 0.280, female: 0.261) [14].

It can be seen that the S-cone, generally, had smaller mean Log contrast sensitivity for all pupil sizes as compared to M- and L-cone sensitivities. One reason for this could be longitudinal chromatic aberration. With larger pupils, peripheral rays are affected, and there is an increase in optical blurring and light scattering. This worsens the chromatic aberrations, thus reducing contrast sensitivity [27].

The smallest artificial pupil size (1 mm) reduced retinal illumination by approximately 75%. This shifted the testing conditions from photopic to mesopic retinal light levels. Nevertheless, the 75% decrease from the original monitor luminance of 65 cd/m² to 16 cd/m² remained within the photopic range (defined as >3.0 cd/m²) [28]. Under these conditions, the rod cells likely play a negligible role in detecting S-wavelength stimuli. This minimal rod involvement holds across all tested stimulus sizes because photopic vision (dominated by cone cells) typically suppresses rod activity in bright environments.

Standardized and documented testing conditions are essential to ensure that visual function tests can effectively track disease progression [29]. Although a patient's natural pupil size under consistent lighting remains relatively stable over time, clinicians must account for variations in retinal illumination caused by pupil dilation. For instance, when monitoring diabetic retinopathy progression via CCS, comparing the results from a dilated pupil visit versus those from an undilated visit could lead to a misinterpretation of retinal health. Differences in illumination may artificially alter the CCS scores, potentially masking or exaggerating disease-related changes. Thus, clinicians should maintain consistent protocols (e.g., controlling the dilation status) to avoid false positive diagnostic errors.

5. Strengths, Limitations, and Recommendations

The findings of this study were limited by the homogeneous age range of the participants. Age-related retinal dysfunction, which can affect color perception, and cataract development, which reduces retinal illuminance, are more common in older populations. It is essential to extend this study to include older adults with healthy retinas and visual pathways [30]. Future research should encompass a broader age range and include populations with retinal or visual pathway disorders. This approach would enhance our understanding of how retinal illuminance and stimulus size influence clinical contrast sensitivity (CCS) measurements. Such studies would improve the reliability of CCS as a diagnostic tool and help distinguish between changes related to aging, disease, or testing artifacts. Despite these limitations, this study provided valuable insights into how pupil size interacts with CCS. This information is particularly important in aging eyes that experience natural lens changes and illumination deficits, as it is critical for adopting CCS as a screening tool for retinal or neural visual pathway disorders in older individuals. Without this understanding, age-related physiological changes could obscure or mimic pathological trends, compromising the diagnostic accuracy of the test in this demographic group.

6. Conclusions

This study evaluated the impact of different retinal illumination sizes on cone contrast sensitivity (CCS) using ColorDx technology. The results contributed to the development of optimal guidelines for clinicians regarding pupil management and ambient lighting conditions during CCS testing. Additionally, emerging technologies that assess individual cone pathway functions show promise for detecting early or progressive pathologies that affect color vision pathways from the retina to the brain. To reduce the risk of data misinterpretation, it is recommended to use standardized testing conditions, including consistent retinal illumination.

Author Contributions: Conceptualization, A.A. (Ali Almustanyir) and M.S.A.; methodology, formal analysis, investigation, and data curation, A.A. (Amal Aldrwish), A.A. (Ali Almustanyir), B.A.A., F.F. and B.A.; writing—original draft, A.A. (Ali Almustanyir), B.A., N.H. and A.A. (Amal Aldrwish); writing—review and editing, A.A. (Ali Almustanyir), B.A., B.A.A., M.A. (Muteb Alanazi), E.A., T.A., F.F., M.A. (Mansour Alghamdi) and M.A. (Mosaad Alhassan); supervision, A.A. (Ali Almustanyir),

B.A. and M.A. (Mosaad Alhassan) All authors have read and agreed to the published version of the manuscript.

Funding: This research was funded by the Ongoing Research Funding Program (ORF-2025-1168), King Saud University, Riyadh, Saudi Arabia.

Institutional Review Board Statement: This study was conducted in accordance with the Declaration of Helsinki and was approved by the Institutional Review Board of the College of Medicine at King Saud University (E-23-8123; date: 23 September 2023).

Informed Consent Statement: All the participants provided written informed consent after the nature and purpose of the study were described.

Data Availability Statement: Data are contained within the article.

Acknowledgments: Ongoing Research Funding Program (ORF-2025-1168), King Saud University, Riyadh, Saudi Arabia.

Conflicts of Interest: The authors declare no conflicts of interest.

References

1. Birch, J. Worldwide prevalence of red-green color deficiency. *J. Opt. Soc. Am. A Opt. Image Sci. Vis.* **2012**, *29*, 313–320. [CrossRef] [PubMed]
2. Birch, J. Identification of red-green colour deficiency: Sensitivity of the Ishihara and American Optical Company (hard, Rand and Rittler) pseudo-isochromatic plates to identify slight anomalous trichromatism. *Ophthalmic Physiol. Opt.* **2010**, *30*, 667–671. [CrossRef]
3. Vemala, R.; Sivaprasad, S.; Barbur, J.L. Detection of early loss of color vision in age-related macular degeneration—With emphasis on drusen and reticular pseudodrusen. *Investig. Ophthalmol. Vis. Sci.* **2017**, *58*, BIO247–BIO254. [CrossRef] [PubMed]
4. Papaconstantinou, D.; Georgalas, I.; Kalantzis, G.; Karmiris, E.; Koutsandrea, C.; Diagourtas, A.; Ladas, I.; Georgopoulos, G. Acquired color vision and visual field defects in patients with ocular hypertension and early glaucoma. *Clin. Ophthalmol.* **2009**, *3*, 251–257.
5. Melamud, A.; Hagstrom, S.; Traboulsi, E. Color vision testing. *Ophthalmic Genet.* **2004**, *25*, 159–187. [CrossRef] [PubMed]
6. Walsh, D.V.; Robinson, J.; Jurek, G.M.; Capó-Aponte, J.E.; Riggs, D.W.; Temme, L.A. A performance comparison of color vision tests for military screening. *Aerosp. Med. Hum. Perform.* **2016**, *87*, 382–387. [CrossRef]
7. Rabin, J. Cone-specific measures of human color vision. *Investig. Ophthalmol. Vis. Sci.* **1996**, *37*, 2771–2774.
8. Rabin, J.; Gooch, J.; Ivan, D. Rapid quantification of color vision: The cone contrast test. *Invest. Ophthalmol. Vis. Sci.* **2011**, *52*, 816–820. [CrossRef]
9. Rabin, J. Quantification of color vision with cone contrast sensitivity. *Vis. Neurosci.* **2004**, *21*, 483–485. [CrossRef]
10. Rabin, J.C.; Kryder, A.C.; Lam, D. Diagnosis of normal and abnormal color vision with cone-specific VEPs. *Transl. Vis. Sci. Technol.* **2016**, *5*, 8. [CrossRef]
11. Rabin, J.; Adams, A.J. Visual acuity and contrast sensitivity of the S cone pathway: Preliminary measures with letter charts. *Optom. Vis. Sci.* **1990**, *67*, 799–802. [CrossRef] [PubMed]
12. Trieschmann, M.; van Kuijk, F.J.; Alexander, R.; Hermans, P.; Luthert, P.; Bird, A.C.; Pauleikhoff, D. Macular pigment in the human retina: Histological evaluation of localization and distribution. *Eye* **2008**, *22*, 132–137. [CrossRef] [PubMed]
13. Gaska, J.; Winterbottom, M.; van Atta, A. *Operational Based Vision Assessment Cone Contrast Test: Description and Operation*; Report No. FRL-SA-WP-SR-2016-0007; USAF School of Aerospace Medicine, Aeromedical Research Department: Wright-Patterson AFB, OH, USA, 2016.
14. Cisarik, P.M.; Kampwerth, J.E. Cone-isolation contrast sensitivity–do pupil and stimulus sizes matter? *Clin. Exp. Optom.* **2024**, *107*, 307–312. [CrossRef] [PubMed]
15. Coletta, N.J.; Sharma, V. Effects of luminance and spatial noise on interferometric contrast sensitivity. *J. Opt. Soc. Am. A Opt. Image Sci. Vis.* **1995**, *12*, 2244–2251. [CrossRef]
16. Hastings, G.D.; Marsack, J.D.; Thibos, L.N.; Applegate, R.A. Combining optical and neural components in physiological visual image quality metrics as functions of luminance and age. *J. Vis.* **2020**, *20*, 20. [CrossRef]
17. Pelli, D.G.; Bex, P. Measuring contrast sensitivity. *Vis. Res.* **2013**, *90*, 10–14. [CrossRef]
18. Owsley, C. Contrast sensitivity. *Ophthalmol. Clin. N. Am.* **2003**, *16*, 171–177. [CrossRef]
19. Nio, Y.K.; Jansonius, N.M.; Fidler, V.; Geraghty, E.; Norrby, S.; Kooijman, A.C. Age-related changes of defocus-specific contrast sensitivity in healthy subjects. *Ophthalmic Physiol. Opt.* **2000**, *20*, 323–334. [CrossRef]

This case report describes a unique instance of bilateral choroidal effusion following the administration of oral acetazolamide for the treatment of pseudophakic cystoid macular edema (PCME), also known as Irvine–Gass Syndrome.

2. Case Report

An 87-year-old Caucasian male was admitted to our clinic with sudden, painless vision loss of his left eye. His medical history was unremarkable except for uneventful cataract surgery in both eyes two months prior. Two months postoperatively, he developed macular edema in the left eye, which was confirmed on optical coherence tomography (OCT, SOCT-Copernicus, Revo NX, Software version 11.5.1, Optopol Technology Ltd., Zawiercie, Poland) (Figure 1). Treatment for PCME was initiated with topical pranoprofen and oral acetazolamide (250 mg twice a day).

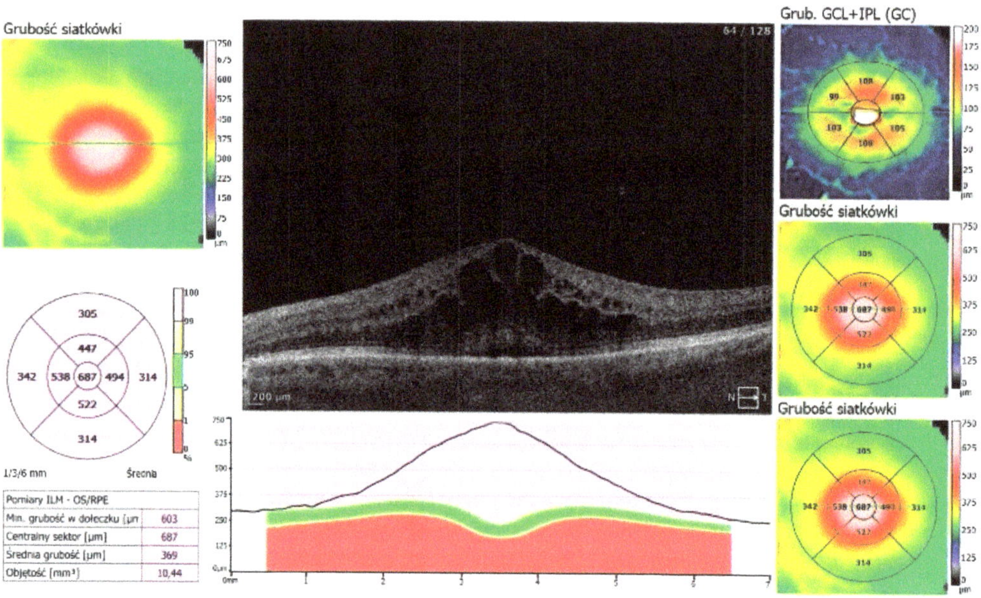

Figure 1. PCME—Irvin–Gass Syndrome in the LE. Best corrected visual acuity (BCVA) = 0.4.

After one week of treatment for PCME, the patient returned with a bilateral vision decline. Fundoscopy revealed bilateral, infero-temporal and infero-nasal choroidal detachment (fundus photo with the use of confocal scanner Eidon, CenterVue, ICare Finland Oy, Vantaa, Finland); Figure 2A. Ultrasound examination confirmed bullous choroidal detachments (Ultrasound B-scan, Pirop, Echo-SonSA, Puławy, Poland) in both eyes (Figure 2B). OCT scans showed subretinal fluid (SRF) and choroidal folds in both eyes but complete resolution of the macular edema in the LE (Figure 2C). The intraocular pressure (IOP) measured with Tono-Pen AVIA (Reichert Technologies, Reichert Inc., Depew, NY, USA) was 16 mmHg (RE) and 14 mmHg (LE).

Ophthalmological examination details are depicted in Table 1.

Anterior segment OCT revealed iris plateau configuration, a possible contributing factor to the choroidal effusion (Figure 3).

Acetazolamide was discontinued immediately. Treatment included topical dexamethasone 0.1% every two hours, atropine 1% twice daily, and bromfenac twice daily. Significant improvement was observed within eigh days. Best corrected visual acuity (BCVA) improved to 0.5 Snellen (RE) and 0.6 Snellen (LE). OCT showed resolution of choroidal effusion and almost complete resorption of subretinal fluid (Figure 2).

At 29 days, the patient was stable, BCVA was 0.7 Snellen (RE) and 0.6 Snellen (LE), and treatment was discontinued.

Following the immediate discontinuation of acetazolamide and the initiation of topical therapy, the patient showed rapid improvement. Within eight days, visual acuity significantly improved. Imaging confirmed the complete resolution of choroidal effusion (Table 2 and Figure 4). At a follow-up visit on Day 29, the patient remained stable, with no recurrence of symptoms (Table 3).

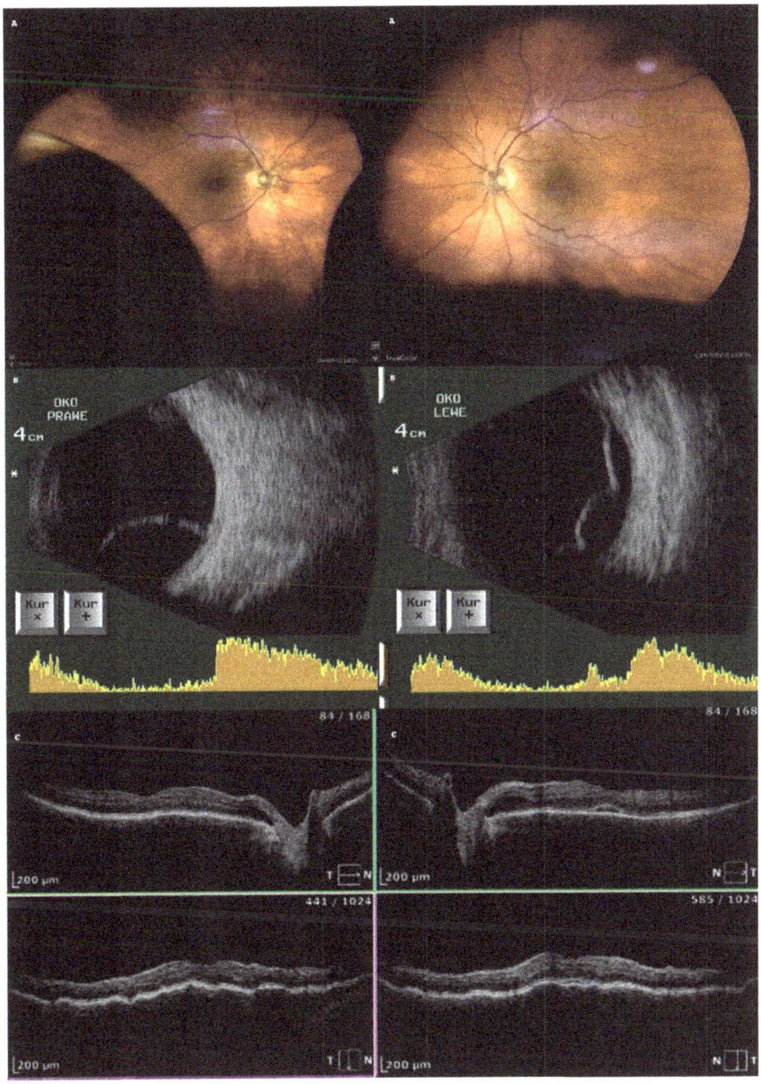

Figure 2. Imaging of choroidal effusion in both eyes: (**A**): Fundus photographs showing bullous choroidal detachment; (**B**): ultrasonography showing more pronounced detachment in the right eye; A scan is depicted on the bottom of the B scan (yellow diagram), top of the ultrasound probe is indicated as (*) (**C**): OCT showing choroidal folds and resolution of PCME in the left eye.

Table 1. Summary of findings on Day 1 (onset of choroidal effusion).

	Day 1
Chief Complaint (CC)	acute, painless bilateral vision deterioration
BCVA	BCVA RE = 0.3 cc − 1.5 sph, −1.25 cyl ax 88 BCVA LE = 0.4 cc + 0.25 sph, −1.0 cyl ax 107
Anterior Segment	Moderately shallow anterior chambers in both eyes (confirmed on anterior segment OCT)
Posterior Segment Figure 2A	Choroidal effusion in the inferior–temporal and inferior–nasal quadrants in both eyes
USG ScanB Figure 2B	Inferior–temporal and inferior–nasal choroidal detachment, more pronounced in RE
OCT Figure 2C	No cystoid macular edema in the left eye; residual subretinal fluid (SRF) and choroidal folds in both eyes; fluid next to the optic disk and macular choroidal folds in both eyes
IOP	RE 16 mmHg LE 14 mmHg
Treatment	1. Immediate discontinuation of acetazolamide; 2. 0.1% dexamethasone eye drops every two hours—both eyes; 3. 1% Atropine eye drops twice a day—both eyes; 4. Bromfenac twice a day—left eye.

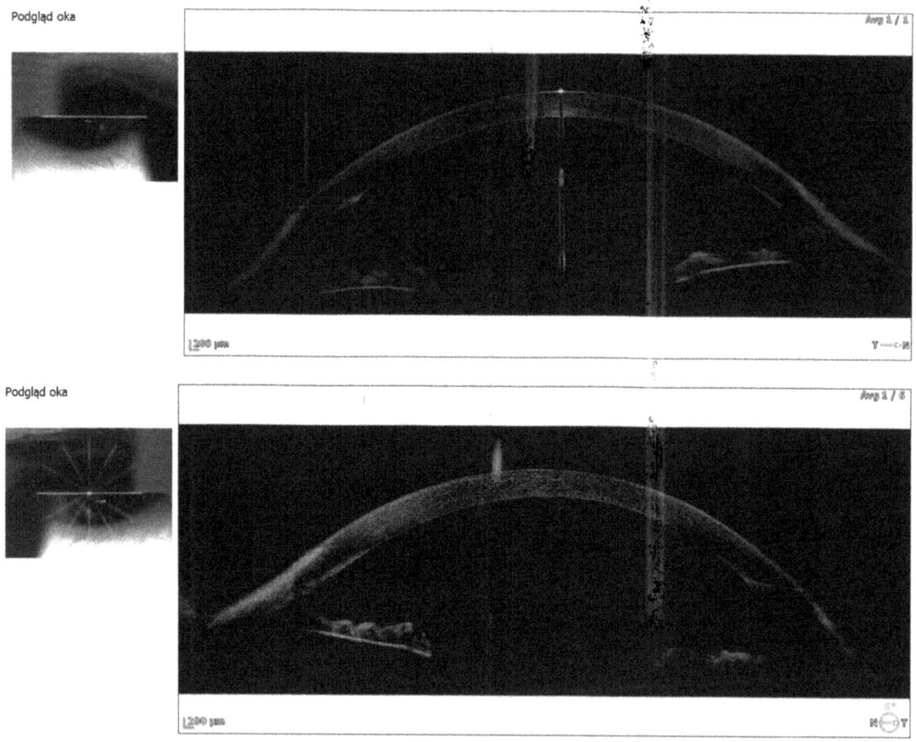

Figure 3. Anterior segment OCT—iris plateau configuration RLE (right eye: upper image, left eye: lower image).

Table 2. Case presentation summary at day 8—following one week of treatment for choroidal effusion.

	Day 8
CC	Visual acuity improvement
BCVA	BCVA RE = 0.5 cc 0 sph, −1.5 cyl ax 88 BCVA LE = 0.6 + 0.5 sph, −1.0 cyl ax 107
Slit lamp exam and fundoscopy	AC deepened; Complete resolution of choroidal effusion
OCT	Residual submacular subretinal fluid persisted in the left eye, fluid next to the optic disk resolved, and choroidal folds disappeared
IOP	RE 16 mmHg, LE 16 mmHg
Treatment	1. 0.1% dexamethasone eye drops 4 times a day to both eyes for 7 days; 2. topical bromfenac 2xdaily—both eyes; 3. 1% atropine eye drops were discontinued.

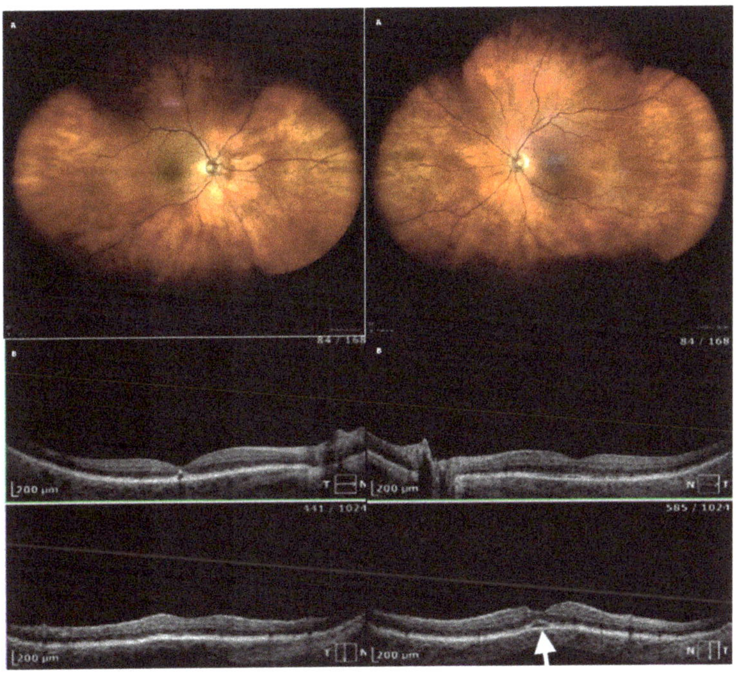

Figure 4. Resolution of choroidal effusion at day 8. (**A**) Fundus photograph—choroid and retina attached, bullous detachment disappeared; (**B**) OCT—no folds, remnants of the subretinal fluid in the LE (arrow).

Table 3. Follow-up visit at Day 29.

	Day 29
CC	No complains
BCVA	BCVA RE = 0.7 cc 0 sph, −1.5 cyl ax 90, cyl ax 88 BCVA LE = 0.6 + 0.5 sph, −1.0 cyl ax 107
Treatment	All medications discontinued

3. Discussion

Choroidal effusion is a complex and multifactorial condition marked by the accumulation of fluid in the suprachoroidal space, often resulting in serous choroidal detachment. If not diagnosed and treated promptly, it may cause significant and potentially irreversible visual impairment. Although rare, choroidal effusion has been associated with systemic conditions (e.g., hypertension and altitude sickness), ocular surgeries (e.g., glaucoma procedures), and pharmacological agents, including carbonic anhydrase inhibitors (CAIs) [2].

Acetazolamide, a widely used carbonic anhydrase inhibitor (CAI), is commonly prescribed for glaucoma, idiopathic intracranial hypertension, and macular edema. It is commonly used for altitude sickness [7]. Acetazolamide is routinely prescribed in addition to non- steroidal anti-inflammatory drugs (NSAIDs) in PCME. Despite its effectiveness in reducing intraocular pressure and retinal fluid, acetazolamide has been linked to rare adverse effects, including choroidal effusion and secondary angle-closure glaucoma [6,8]. This report describes a rare instance of bilateral choroidal effusion in an elderly patient treated with oral acetazolamide for PCME.

3.1. *Proposed Pathophysiological Mechanisms of Acetazolamide-Induced Choroidal Effusion*

Several mechanisms have been proposed to explain the pathogenesis of acetazolamide-induced choroidal effusion. These mechanisms likely act in combination, leading to the accumulation of fluid in the suprachoroidal space.

3.2. *Increased Choroidal Vascular Permeability and Endothelial Dysfunction*

Acetazolamide, a sulfonamide derivative, may compromise the endothelial integrity of choroidal blood vessels, leading to plasma leakage and fluid accumulation in the suprachoroidal space [9].

3.3. *Alteration in Hydrostatic and Osmotic Pressure*

As a diuretic, acetazolamide reduces systemic fluid retention by inhibiting carbonic anhydrase activity. This may decrease systemic venous pressure, disturbing the hydrostatic balance between intraocular and extraocular compartments. The resulting pressure gradient may promote fluid accumulation in the choroidal space. Additionally, acetazolamide's suppression of aqueous humor production may lead to a rapid drop in intraocular pressure (IOP), potentially causing ciliochoroidal detachment [4].

3.4. *Direct Effect on the Ciliary Body and Choroidal Blood Flow*

The inhibition of carbonic anhydrase isoenzymes within the ciliary body leads to decreased aqueous humor secretion, but it may also impact the fluid dynamics within the choroidal circulation. Carbonic anhydrase plays an important role in the regulation of pH and ionic balance in ocular tissues. Its inhibition may disrupt the normal function of the choroidal capillaries, leading to increased extravasation of fluid into the suprachoroidal space [1].

3.5. *Idiosyncratic Drug Reaction and Immune-Mediated Response*

Some patients may experience an idiosyncratic hypersensitivity reaction to carbonic anhydrase inhibitors. This reaction is defined as an abnormal susceptibility to a drug peculiar to the individual [8,10]. This phenomenon has been observed with both systemic (e.g., acetazolamide) and topical (e.g., dorzolamide and brinzolamide) CAIs [11]. These reactions may cause uveal effusion, anterior segment inflammation, and choroidal detachment, particularly in elderly individuals with altered pharmacokinetics and decreased drug clearance [12].

4. Review of Previous Literature and Comparisons

Choroidal effusion associated with carbonic anhydrase inhibitors (CAIs) has been documented in previous case reports and studies, supporting the hypothesis that CAIs can trigger fluid accumulation in the suprachoroidal space. There are examples presented below. There was a case report in which a 76-year-old patient developed bilateral angle-closure glaucoma and extensive choroidal detachment following oral acetazolamide administration after routine cataract surgery. The condition improved rapidly upon discontinuation of acetazolamide and initiation of high-dose intravenous steroid therapy. This case highlights the importance of early steroid intervention in CAI-induced choroidal effusion [13].

An echographic study was conducted evaluating the incidence of uveal effusion after cataract surgery. The findings indicated that the postoperative combination of oral acetazolamide and topical pilocarpine gel significantly increased the risk of choroidal effusion, suggesting that certain pharmacological combinations may exacerbate this condition [14]. A case of a 60-year-old male with plateau iris configuration who developed bilateral cilio-choroidal effusion syndrome after acetazolamide use was described. The patient presented with a myopic shift, elevated intraocular pressure, and shallow anterior chambers. Upon discontinuation of acetazolamide and the initiation of topical therapy, the choroidal effusion resolved. This case demonstrates how predisposing anatomical factors may contribute to the severity of acetazolamide-induced choroidal detachment [15]. Liyanage et al. reported two cases of uveal effusion following acetazolamide administration, one after cataract surgery and another following prophylactic treatment for altitude sickness. In both cases, timely discontinuation of the drug led to complete resolution of symptoms, underscoring the reversibility of CAI-induced effusions with appropriate management [16].

5. Clinical Implications and Recommendations for Management

Awareness of acetazolamide-induced choroidal effusion is vital for ophthalmologists, especially when prescribing this medication in postoperative settings or in elderly and anatomically predisposed patients [8,15,17]. Elderly individuals and those with a history of choroidal detachment, angle-closure glaucoma, or uveal effusion should be carefully monitored when prescribed acetazolamide or other CAIs. Regular follow-up with ultrasonography and optical coherence tomography (OCT) can aid in the early detection of subclinical choroidal effusion before symptomatic vision loss occurs [12,14].

The combination of acetazolamide with miotics like pilocarpine may increase the risk of uveal effusion and secondary angle closure [14]. Alternative treatments for postoperative macular edema should be considered for patients with known risk factors [1].

If choroidal effusion is suspected, acetazolamide should be discontinued immediately to prevent worsening of the condition. Alternative anti-inflammatory therapy, including topical corticosteroids (dexamethasone) and cycloplegics (atropine), should be initiated to reduce inflammation and promote fluid resolution [2].

In cases with significant visual impairment or extensive choroidal detachment, systemic or periocular corticosteroids may be beneficial in hastening resolution [1].

6. Conclusions

This case demonstrates that CAIs can rarely lead to choroidal effusion—a potentially sight-threatening complication, particularly in elderly or anatomically predisposed patients.

To the best of our knowledge, this is the first reported case of bilateral choroidal effusion following oral acetazolamide treatment specifically for PCME. Prompt discontinuation of the CAI and initiation of topical corticosteroids and mydriatics resulted in complete clinical and anatomical resolution.

Further research is warranted to identify risk factors and underlying mechanisms, including idiosyncratic or hypersensitivity reactions, that may predispose certain patients to CAI-induced choroidal effusion. Improved understanding may help prevent such adverse events in the postoperative course of susceptible individuals.

Elderly patients receiving acetazolamide after cataract surgery are potentially at risk for bilateral choroidal effusion. Careful monitoring, immediate cessation of the drug, and prompt anti-inflammatory therapy can ensure complete recovery.

In case of PCME in elderly patients, topical therapy with steroids and NSAIDs could be considered first prior to the initiation of systemic oral acetazolamide therapy.

7. Plain Language Summary

This case report describes an 87-year-old man who suddenly lost his vision in both eyes after taking a medication called acetazolamide for a common eye condition known as pseudophakic cystoid macular edema (PCME), which can occur after cataract surgery. The drug was meant to reduce swelling in the eye, but it caused an unexpected problem—fluid built up behind both of his eyes, a condition called choroidal effusion.

The patient was treated with acetazolamide and anti-inflammatory eye drops due to PCME (Irvin–Gass syndrome) in the left eye. About a week after starting the medication, he began to lose his vision. Eye scans showed that fluid had collected under the choroid in both eyes. The doctors immediately stopped the acetazolamide and started treatment with steroids and atropine eye drops. Within eight days, his vision improved significantly, and the fluid had cleared up.

This report highlights a rare but serious side effect of acetazolamide. While it is commonly used to lower eye pressure or treat swelling, it can sometimes cause fluid under the choroid, leading to its detachment. Older adults may be more at risk for this side effect. Recognizing the problem early and stopping the medication is important to prevent permanent vision loss.

This appears to be the first reported case of both eyes being affected by choroidal effusion after using acetazolamide to treat PCME. It also indicates that in case of PCME, particularly in elderly patients, topical therapy with steroids and NSAIDs could be considered first prior to initiation of systemic oral acetazolamide therapy.

Author Contributions: Conceptualization, A.K.-K. and M.O.; methodology, T.U.; software, T.U.; validation, A.K.-K., M.O., T.U. and S.C.; formal analysis, S.C.; investigation, M.O. and T.U.; resources, A.K.-K.; data curation, M.O.; writing—original draft preparation, A.K.-K.; writing—review and editing, M.O., T.U. and S.C.; visualization, A.K.-K.; supervision, S.C.; project administration, M.O.; funding acquisition, A.K.-K. All authors have read and agreed to the published version of the manuscript.

Funding: This research received no external funding.

Institutional Review Board Statement: This project did not require any institutional review board statement.

Informed Consent Statement: Informed consent was obtained from the Subjects involved in the study. Written informed consent has been obtained from the patient(s) to publish this paper.

Data Availability Statement: The authors declare that all data supporting the report are available upon request to the corresponding author.

Conflicts of Interest: The authors declare no conflicts of interest.

References

1. Ying, S.; Sidoti, P.A.; Panarelli, J.F. Risk factors and management of choroidal effusions. *Curr. Opin. Ophthalmol.* **2023**, *34*, 162–167. [CrossRef] [PubMed]
2. Waheed, N.K.; Mendonça, L.S.M.; Young, L.H. *Albert and Jakobiec's Principles and Practice of Ophthalmology*; Albert, D.M., Miller, J.W., Azar, D.T., Young, L.H., Eds.; Springer: Cham, Switzerland, 2022. [CrossRef]
3. Phylactou, M.; Matarazzo, F.; Jones, E. Indapamide-induced bilateral choroidal effusion in pseudophakic patient. *BMJ Case Rep.* **2018**, *2018*, bcr-2018-225920. [CrossRef] [PubMed]
4. Bakir, B.; Pasquale, L.R. Causes and treatment of choroidal effusion after glaucoma surgery. *Semin. Ophthalmol.* **2014**, *29*, 409–413. [CrossRef] [PubMed]
5. Koenigstein, D.; Neudorfer, M.; Goldenberg, D.; Habot-Wilner, Z. Choroidal Effusion as an Ocular Manifestation of Immunoglobulin G4-Related Disease. *Retin. Cases Brief Rep.* **2016**, *10*, 197–200. [CrossRef] [PubMed]
6. Khanam, Z.; Krishnamoorthy, S.; Baskaran, V.; Mashruwala, A. Acetazolamide—Friend to foe. *Indian J. Ophthalmol. Case Rep.* **2024**, *4*, 98–100. [CrossRef]
7. Rothwell, A.; Anderson, O. Bilateral choroidal effusions after taking acetazolamide for altitude sickness. *BMJ Case Rep.* **2022**, *15*, e246145. [CrossRef] [PubMed]
8. Atisundara, S.M.; Rifada, R.M.; Umbara, S.; Gustianty, E.; Prahasta, A. Acetazolamide-induced secondary angle closure glaucoma: A rare case report. *Ophthalmol. Indones.* **2024**, *49*. [CrossRef]
9. Yang, J.G.; Li, J.J.; Tian, H.; Li, Y.H.; Gong, Y.J.; Su, A.L.; He, N. Uveal effusion following acute primary angle-closure: A retrospective case series. *Int. J. Ophthalmol.* **2017**, *10*, 406–412. [PubMed]
10. Malagola, R.; Arrico, L.; Giannotti, R.; Pattavina, L. Acetazolamide-induced cilio-choroidal effusion after cataract surgery: Unusual posterior involvement. *Drug Des. Devel. Ther.* **2013**, *7*, 33–36. [PubMed]
11. Mehta, A.; Lewis, A. Multimodal etiology of drug-induced angle closure with topical glaucoma therapy. *Am. J. Ophthalmol. Case Rep.* **2021**, *23*, 101152. [CrossRef] [PubMed]
12. Malagola, R.; Giannotti, R.; Pattavina, L.; Arrico, L. Acute cilio-choroidal effusion due to acetazolamide: Unusual posterior involvement (OCT aspects). *Eye* **2013**, *27*, 781–782. [CrossRef] [PubMed]
13. Mancino, R.; Varesi, C.; Cerulli, A.; Aiello, F.; Nucci, C. Acute bilateral angle-closure glaucoma and choroidal effusion associated with acetazolamide administration after cataract surgery. *J. Cataract Refract. Surg.* **2011**, *37*, 415–417. [CrossRef] [PubMed]
14. Sabti, K.; Lindley, S.K.; Mansour, M.; Discepola, M. Uveal effusion after cataract surgery: An echographic study. *Ophthalmology* **2001**, *108*, 100–103. [CrossRef]
15. Man, X.; Costa, R.; Ayres, B.M.; Moroi, S.E. Acetazolamide-induced bilateral ciliochoroidal effusion syndrome in plateau iris configuration. *Am. J. Ophthalmol. Case Rep.* **2016**, *3*, 14–17. [CrossRef] [PubMed]
16. Liyanage, G.; Bertin, S.; Villaret, J.; Paques, M. Acetazolamide and uveal effusion: Report of two cases. *J. Fr. Ophtalmol.* **2023**, *ahead of print*.
17. Ashok, A.; Bhat, M.; Shetty, R. Acetazolamide-induced bilateral uveal effusion after cataract surgery. *TNOA J. Ophthalmic Sci. Res.* **2023**, *61*, 357. [CrossRef]

life

MDPI

Article

Clinical Outcomes and Optical Bench Analysis of a Novel Enhanced Monofocal Intraocular Lens

Giovanni Romualdi [1,*], Matilde Buzzi [1], Pier Giuseppe Ruggeri [1], Federico Tommasi [2], Alessio Giorgetti [2], Stefano Cavalieri [2] and Rita Mencucci [1]

1 Eye Clinic, Department of Neuroscience, Psychology, Pharmacology and Child Health (NEUROFARBA), University of Florence, Largo Brambilla 3, 50134 Florence, Italy; matilde.buzzi@gmail.com (M.B.); piergiuseppe.ruggeri@unifi.it (P.G.R.); rita.mencucci@unifi.it (R.M.)

2 Department of Physics and Astronomy, University of Florence, via Giovanni Sansone 1, 50019 Sesto Fiorentino, Italy; federico.tommasi@unifi.it (F.T.); alessio.giorgetti@unifi.it (A.G.); stefano.cavalieri@unifi.it (S.C.)

* Correspondence: romualdigiovanni@gmail.com

Abstract: Purpose: A novel enhanced monofocal intraocular lens (IOL) has been developed to improve functional intermediate vision, maintaining a distance vision comparable to a standard monofocal lens and avoiding the drawbacks of multifocal IOLs. The aim of this study is to perform optical bench analysis and to evaluate refractive and visual outcomes and patient satisfaction. **Methods**: This prospective comparative single-center study was conducted in Careggi Hospital, University of Florence (Italy). We included 100 eyes from 50 patients who underwent bilateral cataract surgery. One group received the standard monofocal Tecnis GCB00 IOL, while the other group received the novel enhanced monofocal Evolux IOL. We evaluated binocular visual and refractive outcomes at 6 months after surgery. Binocular defocus curves and contrast sensitivity (CS) were also assessed. Optical quality was also analyzed in terms of higher-order aberrations (HOAs), modulation transfer function (MTF), objective scatter index (OSI), Strehl ratio, effective lens position (ELP), and halo analysis. A Patient-Reported Spectacle Independence Questionnaire (PRSIQ) was performed to assess spectacle independence outcomes. Finally, we analyzed the optical bench of both lenses. **Results**: All eyes implanted with Evolux achieved excellent distance vision, comparable to that achieved with GCB00. Evolux showed better intermediate and near vision, without any loss of visual quality, contrast sensitivity, or the presence of halos and photic phenomena. The optical bench analysis confirmed the different optical properties of the two lenses and supported the behavior obtained with the clinical defocus curve. **Conclusions**: These preliminary results show good refractive accuracy and visual outcomes for the enhanced monofocal IOL Evolux after cataract surgery. Further studies are needed to confirm our findings in terms of the number of patients and the period of follow-up.

Keywords: cataract surgery; IOL; enhanced IOL; EDOF IOL; Evolux; halos; optical quality

1. Introduction

Monofocal lenses are the most frequently implanted intraocular lenses (IOLs) in cataract surgery, because of their relatively low cost, excellent outcomes for distance visual performance, and low values of photic phenomena (glare, halos) compared to multifocal IOLs [1]. Nevertheless, monofocal IOLs have a very limited depth of field and thus do not provide the functional intermediate and near vision required for most daily activities, which nowadays involve tablets, smartphones, and computers [2,3]. Patients' expectations of a highly successful cataract surgery outcome with additional presbyopia correction are constantly increasing in terms of visual quality and postoperative functional vision, aiming to achieve a total, or nearly total, spectacle independence [4].

For these reasons, the number of IOLs with an augmented range of vision has significantly increased in recent years. There is an increasing focus on emerging technologies aimed at enhancing the intermediate visual outcomes of IOLs, while mitigating the undesired side effects associated with multifocal IOLs [5–8]. As a result, Extended Depth of Focus (EDOF) IOLs were introduced to improve intermediate visual acuity while minimizing photic phenomena [4,9]. Lately, a new class of monofocal IOLs, named "enhanced monofocal IOLs", has been developed, providing the same excellent distance vision of a monofocal with improved intermediate vision [10–14].

In this increasingly diverse context, classifying IOLs has become progressively more challenging. Recently, a new evidence-based functional classification has been developed [15,16]. Two principal categories can be distinguished based on the defocus curve's range of focus (RoF) and its configuration: PARTIAL-RoF and FULL-RoF. Within the PARTIAL-RoF group, three subtypes are defined according to the extent of the RoF achieved: narrow, enhanced, and extended. Conversely, subcategories of FULL-RoF IOLs are classified based on the steepness of the visual acuity (VA) improvement from intermediate to near distances: continuous, smooth transition, and steep transition.

In this new context, the aim of the current study is to compare visual outcomes, optical quality (including optical bench analysis), and patient satisfaction between eyes implanted with a new enhanced monofocal IOL, Evolux (SIFI S.p.A., Catania, Italy), and the standard monofocal IOL, Tecnis GCB00 (Johnson & Johnson Vision Care, Santa Ana, CA, USA). These IOLs are classified as PARTIAL-RoF: PARTIAL-RoF narrow for Tecnis GCB00 and PARTIAL-RoF enhance for Evolux.

2. Materials and Methods

2.1. Study Design and Patients

A single-center, prospective, non-randomized, comparative clinical trial was conducted at the Eye Clinic, Department of NEUROFARBA, University of Florence, Italy. From June 2023 to July 2024, 100 eyes of 50 study participants were included. Each patient was bilaterally implanted with the same type of intraocular lens. Prior to the study, local ethics committee approval (protocol number Ethics Committee FA000459, ID study 24175) was obtained. In accordance with the tenets of the Declaration of Helsinki, each study participant received a careful explanation of the intended procedure and signed an informed consent form prior to inclusion.

The inclusion criteria for our analysis were: patients with lens opacification and cataract grade greater than II, according to the Lens Opacities Classification System III (LOCS III); and patients aged 60 years or older. The exclusion criteria comprised an axial length greater than 26.0 mm or less than 21.00 mm, corneal astigmatism higher than $\pm$0.75 D, angle Kappa > 0.5 mm, post-surgical refractive outcome exceeding $\pm$0.50 D, prior ocular surgeries (including corneal or refractive procedures), and ocular comorbidities such as uveitis, external or internal infections, diabetes mellitus with retinal complications, pathological miosis, amblyopia, use of alpha-blockers that could cause floppy-iris syndrome, choroidal hemorrhage, keratoconus, corneal endothelial dystrophy, diabetic retinopathy, uncontrolled glaucoma and/or IOP > 24 mmHg, traumatic cataract, pseudoexfoliation syndrome, pupillary abnormalities including aniridia and/or pupillary diameter in photopic conditions $\leq$ 2.5 mm and in mesopic conditions $\geq$ 6 mm, microphthalmia, strabismus, nystagmus, pregnancy or lactation period for female patients, degenerative visual disorders (e.g., macular degeneration, optic nerve atrophy, or other retinal disorders).

2.2. Patient Evaluation

Prior to surgery, all participants underwent a thorough preoperative ophthalmic evaluation, which encompassed the assessment of monocular and binocular Uncorrected Distance Visual Acuity (UDVA) and best-corrected distance visual acuity (CDVA) analyzed in photopic conditions using 85 cd/m^2 illumination with 100% contrast with the Early Treatment Diabetic Retinopathy Study (ETDRS) charts at a distance of 4 mt, optical biometry (IOL Master 500, Carl Zeiss Meditec AG, Jena, Germany), subjective and objective refraction, biomicroscopy (Accuref K-900, Shin-Nippon, Tokyo, Japan), Goldmann applanation tonometry, corneal topography and anterior segment optical coherence tomography (AS-OCT) (MS-39, CSO, Florence, Italy), macular OCT (DRI OCT Triton 3D, Topcon Medical Systems, Inc., Oakland, NJ, USA), and dilated fundoscopy. The IOL power and predicted postoperative refraction were based on biometric data (IOL Master 500, Carl Zeiss Meditec, Jena, Germany), calculated using the Barret Formula with an A-constant of 118.35. The IOL power was selected to achieve the predicted postoperative refraction closest to emmetropia. Postoperatively, patients were evaluated at 1 day, 1 month, 3 months, and 6 months. Visual acuity was recorded under photopic conditions and included monocular and binocular UDVA, best-corrected distance visual acuity (BCDVA) at 4 mt, uncorrected intermediate visual acuity (UIVA) and distance-corrected intermediate visual acuity (DCIVA) at 66 cm, and uncorrected near visual acuity (UNVA) and distance-corrected near visual acuity (DCNVA) at 40 cm. Distance visual acuities (UDVA and CDVA) were assessed at 4 m using high-contrast (100%) ETDRS charts illuminated by a calibrated 85 cd/m^2 light source (Precision Vision, Woodstock, IL, USA). Intermediate and near acuity tests were performed using printed high-contrast ETDRS charts (Precision Vision) at 66 cm and 40 cm, respectively. Photopic lighting conditions were standardized using a halogen lamp with a controlled potentiometer, aligned with ambient brightness values measured by a digital light meter (ST-1300, STANDARD Instruments Co., Ltd., Hong Kong). Defocus curves were acquired binocularly using the subject's best distance correction. Defocus was simulated by incrementally introducing trial lenses in 0.50 diopter steps, ranging from +2.00 D to −4.00 D, and assessing visual acuity after each step. Binocular contrast sensitivity was tested under photopic conditions using the Optec 6500 Vision Tester (Stereo Optical Co., Inc., Chicago, IL, USA). Objective evaluation of ocular optical quality was carried out using the AcuTarget HD Analyzer (Visiometrics USA, Costa Mesa, CA, USA), a device based on double-pass imaging technology. Measurements were obtained with a 4.0 mm pupil and included the objective scatter index (OSI), modulation transfer function (MTF) cutoff, and the Strehl ratio derived from the point spread function (PSF) [17,18]. Moreover, we measured HOAs at 4.0 mm pupil size using an Osiris-T aberrometer (CSO, Florence, Italy).

At the end of the last follow-up visit, halometry was also performed to assess the presence of lens-induced halos, using the Aston App Halometer [19]. The examination is conducted in a dark room with the patient positioned 2 m away from an LED device located at the center of an iPad. The operator controls the iPad using an iPhone connected via Bluetooth and projects 0.3 LogMAR letters, proceeding from the periphery towards the center of the iPad, where the light source is located, until the patient can recognize the letter. This evaluation is repeated in each of the 8 or 6 directions (at the operator's discretion) to determine the objective area of obscuration caused by the patient's halo. For each patient, a halometer glare map was created to represent the halo area.

Effective lens position (ELP) was evaluated at 1, 3, and 6 months using AS-OCT imaging in a single-line scan mode. Patients were seated and instructed to fixate on the internal target. Two images were captured at 0 degrees and 90 degrees, and the image with the highest quality from each pair was selected for analysis. No topical cycloplegic agent was administered during the exams, and all scans were conducted by the same examiner, who was blinded to the IOL model [20]. Finally, the Patient-Reported Spectacle Independence Questionnaire (PRSIQ) was conducted to evaluate spectacle independence during daily life [21].

2.3. Intraocular Lenses

The Evolux (SIFI Spa, Catania, Italy) lens is a novel enhanced monofocal IOL, based on a non-diffractive profile, designed to provide better intermediate vision and equivalent distance vision when compared to a standard monofocal IOL. It is a preloaded hydrophobic acrylic IOL with a 6 mm optic diameter and an overall diameter of 13 mm. It is characterized by a biconvex optical design based on positive/negative spherical aberration (SA) distributed in the central 4.5 mm zone of the anterior surface of the IOL, with an aspheric monofocal periphery. It is available in powers ranging from +5.0 D to 30.0 D, with 0.50 D steps. Evolux was developed on a patented technology platform, creating a single elongated focal point to enhance the depth of the field in order to improve intermediate vision.

The Tecnis one-piece GCB00 (Johnson & Johnson Vision Care, Santa Ana, CA, USA) is a standard monofocal IOL. It is an aspherical acrylic hydrophobic IOL with a 6 mm optic and an overall diameter of 13 mm.

2.4. Surgery

The surgical interventions were performed by the same highly experienced surgeon (R.M.), all using topical anesthesia. After the creation of a temporal self-sealing corneal incision and a capsulorrhexis of about 5.5 mm, phacoemulsification of the nucleus and irrigation/aspiration were performed (Centurion, Alcon Laboratories Inc., Geneva, Switzerland). The IOL was implanted and, at the end of the surgery, intracameral cefuroxime was injected into the anterior chamber. Routine postoperative treatment included topical nonsteroidal anti-inflammatory, steroidal, and antibiotic eye drops for 2–4 weeks. No intraoperative or postoperative complications occurred.

2.5. Statistical Analysis

The data analysis for this study was performed using Stata 18.0 (StataCorp, College Station, TX, USA). To summarize the numerical data, descriptive statistics were applied, including the calculation of mean values and standard deviations. Both groups exhibited normally distributed data, with the assumption of normality assessed using the Shapiro–Wilk test. A two-tailed Student's t-test with 95% confidence intervals was used to compare the clinical characteristics of the two treatment groups. A p-value of <0.05 was set as the threshold for statistical significance.

2.6. Optical Bench Analysis

The optical characterization of the IOLs was performed with the optical benches PMTF (LambdaX) and NIMO (Lambda X), and then analyzed with our software written in the Matlab programming language. We measured the modulation transfer function (MTF) of the IOLs and the images of the USAF (United States Air Force) resolution target as a function of the defocus using the PMTF in through-focus mode. We also measured the power map using the NIMO optical bench, based on phase-shifting and Schlieren techniques. The MTF measures the degradation of contrast in an image compared to the contrast of the original object, quantifying the image quality of an optical system. USAF is a standard image system used as an evaluation tool to test the resolution. Moreover, the power map represents the spatially resolved power of the IOL.

3. Results

The final study sample included 100 eyes from 50 patients who underwent bilateral cataract surgery. Twenty-five patients were bilaterally implanted with Evolux IOL, while the other twenty-five patients received the GCB00 IOL. Cataract surgery in the second eye of the same patient was performed at least 1 month apart. The rate of posterior capsular opacification (PCO) observed at 6 months was 2% (one eye) in both groups. Table 1 shows the patient's characteristics at inclusion. Both groups of patients exhibited homogeneous preoperative characteristics, with no statistically significant differences. No patients were lost during the follow-up period.

Table 1. Preoperative demographic and clinical characteristics of study participants in the 2 groups.

Characteristics	Evolux IOL	GCB00 IOL	*p*-Value *
Patients (n)	25	25	
Eyes (n)	50	50	
Age (years)	66.3 ± 2.5	65.6 ± 2.1	0.145
AL (mm)	23.32 ± 0.56	24.17 ± 0.63	0.089
CYL (D)	0.48 ± 0.21	0.40 ± 0.33	0.064
SE (D)	1.54 ± 0.73	1.34 ± 0.68	0.076
UDVA (logMAR)	0.48 ± 0.15	0.45 ± 0.09	0.110
BCDVA (logMAR)	0.41 ± 0.12	0.42 ± 0.10	0.097
Anterior chamber depth (mm)	3.02 ± 0.25	3.11 ± 0.18	0.104
IOL power (D)	22.2 ± 2.0	22.0 ± 1.8	0.143

Results are expressed as mean ± standard deviation. AL = axial length; CYL = Cylinder; SE = Spherical Equivalent; UDVA = binocular Uncorrected Distance Visual Acuity; BCDVA = binocular Best Corrected Distance Visual Acuity. * Statistical analysis: Student's *t*-test. No statistically significant differences were observed between groups ($p > 0.05$).

3.1. Refractive and Visual Outcomes

Six months postoperatively, all patients reached good levels of UDVA and BCDVA, but the UIVA and DCIVA were significantly better in the Evolux compared to the GCB00 group (*p*-value, respectively, <0.001 and 0.004). Table 2 summarizes visual outcomes for the 2 groups.

Table 2. Visual performance and subjective refraction 6 months following implantation of Evolux and GCB00 IOLs.

Outcome	Evolux IOL	GCB00 IOL	*p*-Value *	CI
SE (D)	−0.14 ± 0.31	−0.22 ± 0.20	0.098	[0.01; −0.17]
UDVA (LogMAR)	0.03 ± 0.03	0.03 ± 0.02	0.953	[−0.01; 0.01]
BCDVA (LogMAR)	0.01 ± 0.02	0.01 ± 0.02	0.811	[−0.01; 0.01]
UIVA (LogMAR)	0.10 ± 0.06	0.26 ± 0.09	<0.001 *	[−0.21; −0.11]
CIVA (LogMAR)	0.02 ± 0.02	0.03 ± 0.03	0.106	[−0.03; 0.01]

Table 2. *Cont.*

Outcome	Evolux IOL	GCB00 IOL	p-Value *	CI
DCIVA (LogMAR)	0.14 ± 0.06	0.20 ± 0.06	0.004 *	[−0.09; −0.02]
UNVA (LogMAR)	0.36 ± 0.12	0.44 ± 0.17	0.071	[−0.16; 0.01]
CNVA (LogMAR)	0.02 ± 0.03	0.05 ± 0.06	0.067	[−0.05; 0.01]
ADD NEAR (D)	1.35 ± 0.43	2.57 ± 0.23	0.143	[0.41; 2.85]

Results are expressed as mean ± standard deviation. CI = Confidence Interval; UIVA = binocular Uncorrected Intermediate Visual Acuity; CIVA = binocular Corrected Intermediate Visual Acuity; DCIVA = binocular Distance-Corrected Intermediate Visual Acuity; UNVA = binocular Uncorrected Near Visual Acuity; CNVA = binocular Corrected Near Visual Acuity. * Statistical analysis: Student's t-test.

3.2. ELP

Effective lens position was evaluated at 1 month, 3 months, and 6 months postoperatively with AS-OCT in a single-line scan mode. The ELP, defined as the distance from the central corneal endothelium to the anterior surface of the IOL, was measured using AS-OCT MS-39 (CSO, Florence, Italy) with the aid of caliper function. Table 3 shows that there are no statistically significant differences between the Evolux and GCB00 groups.

Table 3. ELP for Evolux and GCB00 IOLs at 1, 3, and 6 months postoperatively.

Postoperative Time	Evolux ELP (mm)	GCB00 ELP (mm)	p-Value *
1 month	4.10 ± 0.23	4.03 ± 0.18	0.298
3 months	4.12 ± 0.24	4.08 ± 0.17	0.123
6 months	4.15 ± 0.21	4.10 ± 0.22	0.145

Results are expressed as mean ± standard deviation. * Statistical analysis: Student's t-test. ELP = effective lens position.

3.3. Aberrometric Parameters and Optical Quality

Table 4 shows the results of higher-order aberrations (HOAs) evaluated at 4.0 mm pupil size, 6 months postoperatively. All parameters were lower than 0.300 microns, with no significant differences in the two groups. Internal spherical aberration (SA) and internal HOAs showed no statistically significant differences in the two groups (p-value 0.098 and 0.124, respectively). Table 4 also shows optical quality parameters measured with the OQAS system at 4.0 mm pupil size. The comparison between the two groups revealed no statistically significant differences in the objective scatter index (OSI), modulation transfer function (MTF) cutoff, or Strehl ratio (p-value = 0.179, 0.129, and 0.096, respectively).

Table 4. Aberrometric parameters and optical quality results 6 months after implantation of Evolux and GCB00 IOLs.

Characteristics	Evolux IOL	GCB00 IOL	p-Value *
Internal HOA (RMS)	0.16 ± 0.03	0.15 ± 0.02	0.098
Internal SA (RMS)	0.08 ± 0.03	0.05 ± 0.04	0.124
OSI	1.39 ± 0.63	1.41 ± 0.51	0.179
MTF cutoff (c/deg)	30.4 ± 7.5	31.0 ± 4.1	0.129
Strehl ratio	0.16 ± 0.03	0.16 ± 0.05	0.096

Results are expressed as mean ± standard deviation. HOA = higher-order aberration, SA = spherical aberration, OSI = objective scatter index, MTF = modulation transfer function. * Statistical analysis: Student's t-test.

3.4. Binocular Defocus Curve

The binocular defocus curve, illustrated in Figure 1, showed the highest visual acuity at 0.00 D (4 m) in both groups, with a gradual decline in visual acuity as defocus shifted to both negative and positive values. While the GCB00 IOL exhibited a notable drop in the curve with increasing negative defocus, the Evolux IOL displayed a smoother trend, particularly within the intermediate defocus range (−1 to −2 D), demonstrating superior performance at intermediate distances compared to the GCB00 IOL. *p*-values reached statistical significance at −1.00 D, −1.50 D, and −2.00 D.

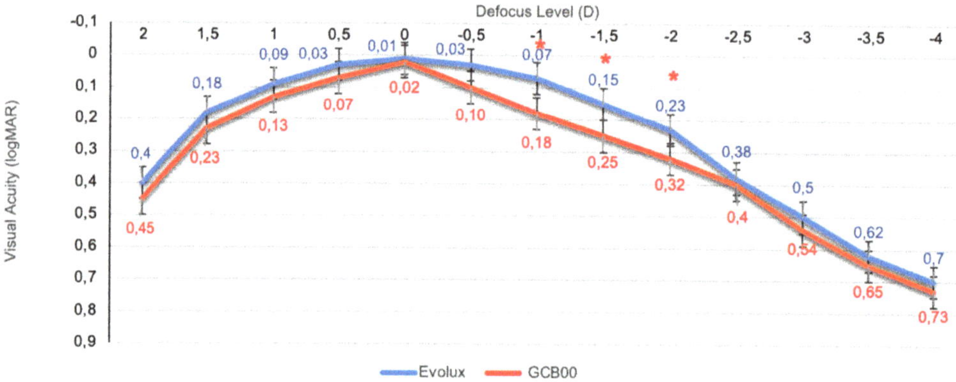

Figure 1. Comparison between mean defocus curves in the IOL groups (logMAR). * *p*-values for −1.00 D, −1.50 D, and −2.0 D are statistically significant (0.038, 0.023, and 0,035, respectively).

3.5. Binocular Contrast Sensitivity

Figure 2 shows contrast sensitivity (CS) under photopic conditions. No statistically significant differences were found between the GCB00 IOL group and the Evolux IOL group across all spatial frequencies.

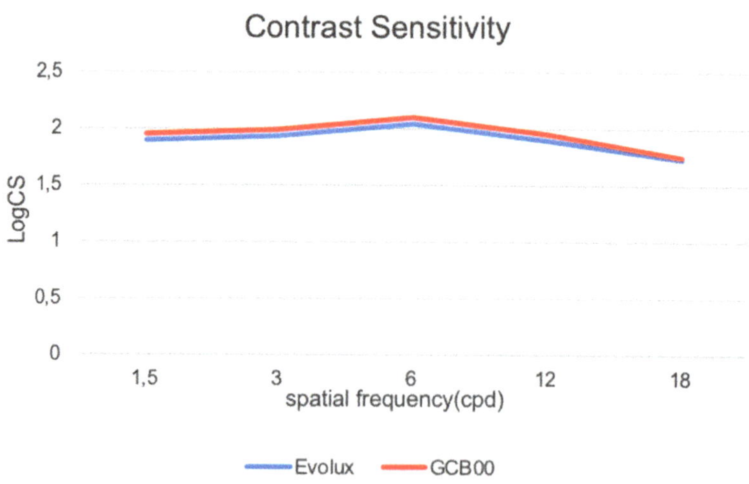

Figure 2. Binocular contrast sensitivity measured with the Optec 6500 Vision Tester under photopic conditions at different spatial frequencies (cycles per degree) (LogCS = Log Contrast Sensitivity).

3.6. Halometry

In terms of halo assessment, the Evolux IOL group achieved an average halo size of 0.44 ± 0.03 degs^2, while the GCB00 IOL group achieved 0.42 ± 0.04, with a p-value of 0.098, which was not statistically significant. Figure 3 shows, on the left side, the result of a single examination with a halometer glare map and a numerical result indicating the corresponding area. On the right side, there is an explanatory image of the instrument.

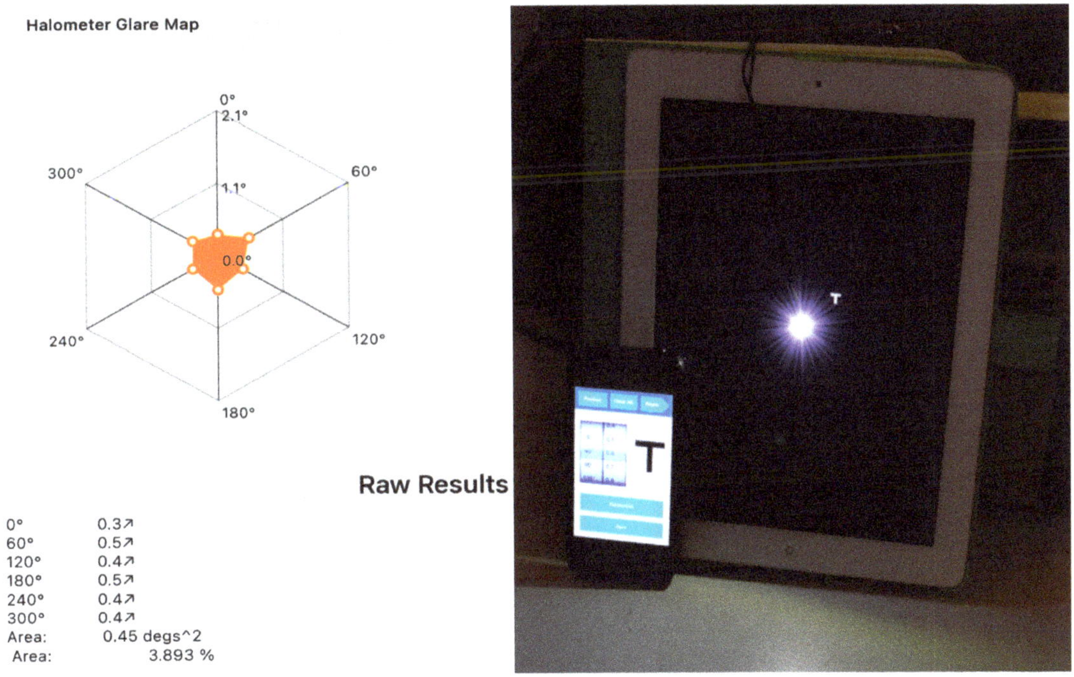

Figure 3. On the left side is the halometer glare map with area expressed in degrees^2. On the right side is an explanatory image of the halometer.

3.7. Optical Bench Analysis Results

In Figure 4, we report the MTF as a function of defocus for three spatial frequencies: 20 cycles/mm (blue line), 50 cycles/mm (red line), and 100 cycles/mm (yellow line). As an upper limit, we also report the pure diffraction case (labelled as MTF0), with blue, red, and yellow markers in the focus. The three dashed vertical lines represent the values of the defocus that correspond to the far (infinite distance), intermediate (60 cm), and near (40 cm) vision. For these same vision distances, the images of the USAF are shown for the two IOLs, providing visual information about the contrast degradation of the image. In both cases, the power of the IOL is 21 D and the pupil size is 3.0 mm. The results show a larger depth of field with Evolux IOL, providing better performance for the near-intermediate vision compared to the GCB00 IOL. The GCB00 IOL instead presents a better contrast preservation in distance vision.

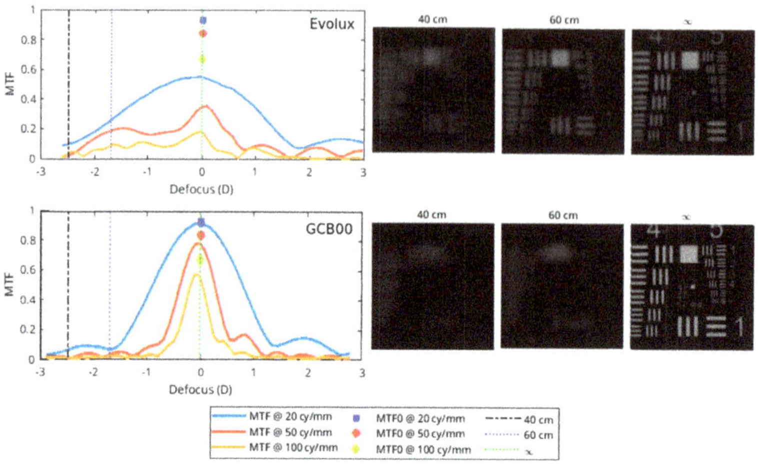

Figure 4. MTF (**left side**) and USAF chart (**right side**) for Evolux IOL (**upper image**) and GCB00 IOL (**lower image**).

Figure 5 shows the power map of the IOLs with the same power (21 D). The scale is relative to the central value. The characteristics both in shape and in the range of the power show the differences in the two IOLs, in agreement with the optical performances shown in Figure 4. In fact, the large range of power values in the Evolux IOL results in a larger depth of field compared to the GCB00. Furthermore, the power map reflects the optical/geometric design of the two IOLs described in Section 2.3. The GCB00 has a nearly constant power in the central part with a periphery aspheric region with a negative value that can compensate for the natural spherical aberration to obtain a true monofocal lens. The Evolux presents an alternate variation of power in the central part to give an enhanced depth of field that characterizes this IOL. In the lower part of Figure 5, the power is reported as a function of the radial coordinate obtained by averaging two perpendicular meridians.

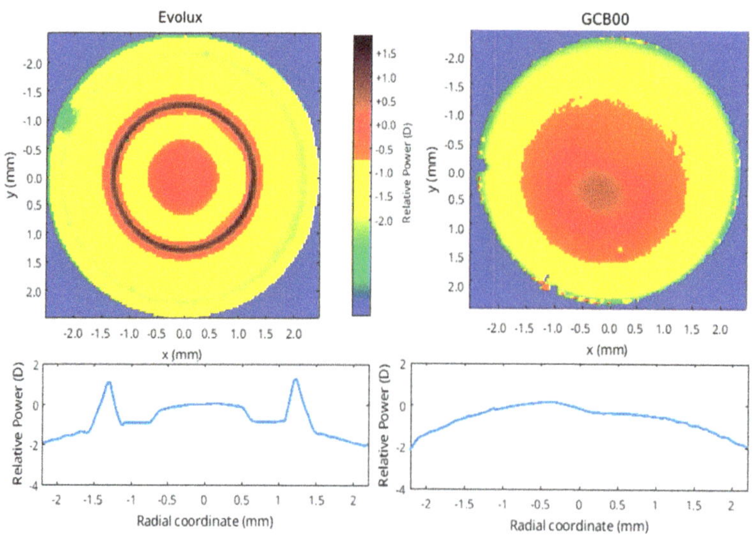

Figure 5. Power Map comparison of Evolux IOL (**left side**) and GCB00 IOL (**right side**). In the lower part of the image, the IOL power is reported as a function of the radial coordinate.

3.8. Questionnaire

The PRSIQ (Patient-Reported Spectacle Independence) assesses the level of spectacle independence in daily activities. None of the patients reported needing spectacles for distance vision. The Evolux IOL group demonstrated greater spectacle independence, particularly for intermediate distances, with only 23% of patients requiring intermediate correction during daily tasks, compared to 87% in the GCB00 IOL group. Notably, question 3 ("How often did you wear glasses for intermediate vision?") revealed that 70% of patients in the Evolux IOL group reported being able to comfortably perform intermediate tasks without spectacles, whereas no patients in the GCB00 IOL group expressed such satisfaction.

4. Discussion

In modern cataract surgery, patients increasingly seek not only improved visual acuity but also greater functional vision and spectacle independence, aiming for a significant enhancement in quality of life. This evolution in patient expectations has fueled advances in IOL technologies, leading to the development of a broad array of options, including bifocal, trifocal, EDOF, and enhanced monofocal IOLs. Multifocal IOLs can provide uncorrected vision across all distances; however, numerous studies have highlighted their drawbacks—particularly reduced contrast sensitivity and increased visual disturbances such as glare and halos [22]. These side effects, which may be exacerbated under certain lighting conditions, remain among the most frequently reported patient complaints in both the early and late postoperative phases [23–25]. These limitations, along with the high cost of multifocal lenses, underscore the importance of careful patient selection and have restricted the widespread adoption of these technologies.

In response, enhanced monofocal and extended depth of field IOLs—categorized under partial RoF lenses [16]—have emerged as viable alternatives. The Evolux IOL is a recent entrant in this category, designed to expand the depth of field by employing a 4.5 mm central zone with modulated positive and negative spherical aberrations, thereby supporting both distance and intermediate visual tasks. Though published evidence on the Evolux IOL remains limited [26,27], early reports—including our own—indicate favorable visual outcomes, both corrected and uncorrected, without a significant increase in photic phenomena or decline in contrast sensitivity. Our retrospective, comparative study contributes to this growing body of evidence, demonstrating statistically significant advantages of Evolux over the standard monofocal GCB00, particularly in UIVA and DCIVA. While the UNVA results were unexpectedly strong and better in the Evolux group without being statistically significant, we acknowledge these findings must be interpreted with caution and validated in larger, prospective trials [28]. The defocus curve further supports these results, showing visual acuity better than 0.2 logMAR across a defocus range of +1.00 D to −2.00 D, with a notably smoother performance between −1.00 and −2.00 D in the Evolux group. These findings align with greater functional range at intermediate distances. Moreover, PRSIQ results showed that 70% of patients implanted with Evolux reported independence from spectacles for intermediate tasks. Additionally, the Evolux IOL exhibited favorable aberrometric and contrast sensitivity profiles, comparable to those of GCB00. Our incorporation of halometry offers further value, demonstrating no significant increase in halos among Evolux patients—an objective assessment not previously reported in the literature. Optical bench analysis corroborated the clinical findings, showing greater depth of field for Evolux. Power mapping revealed spatial modulation in the lens center, consistent with its engineered spherical aberration profile. This optical structure directly supports the observed clinical performance in near and intermediate vision. Refractive predictability was high in both groups, with all patients achieving a postoperative SE within ±0.50 D. Evolux eyes showed a mean SE of −0.14 ± 0.31, similar to the GCB00 group. The ELP remained stable throughout follow-up, reflecting the mechanical and material stability of the Evolux IOL.

We acknowledge several limitations of our study. The non-randomized, unmasked design may introduce bias, particularly in subjective outcomes. Additionally, the relatively small and selective sample size may limit generalizability. Pupillary characteristics may also play a role in lens performance—especially for designs like Evolux that rely on central zone modulation—yet this was not directly analyzed in our study. These factors underscore the need for randomized, masked studies with broader inclusion criteria.

In conclusion, the Evolux IOL demonstrated favorable outcomes in intermediate vision. However, these improvements should be interpreted with caution, as the observed benefit at intermediate distances was modest and may be partially attributable to a slight myopic shift. The lens maintained excellent distance vision and demonstrated good overall optical quality, with no significant increase in photic phenomena. Its smooth, non-diffractive design may make it a suitable choice for patients seeking improved visual function across daily tasks without the drawbacks commonly associated with multifocal technologies. Further studies, ideally randomized and with larger populations, are necessary to validate these findings and directly compare Evolux with other PARTIAL-RoF enhanced IOLs.

Author Contributions: Conceptualization, G.R., M.B., A.G. and R.M.; Methodology, G.R., M.B., F.T., A.G., S.C. and R.M.; Software, G.R., A.G., S.C. and R.M.; Investigation, G.R., S.C. and R.M.; Resources, G.R., M.B. and S.C.; Writing—original draft, G.R., M.B., F.T., A.G. and S.C.; Writing—review & editing, G.R., M.B., P.G.R., F.T., S.C. and R.M.; Supervision, R.M.; Funding acquisition, R.M. All authors have read and agreed to the published version of the manuscript.

Funding: This research received no external funding.

Institutional Review Board Statement: The study was approved by Comitato Etico Regione Toscana-Area Vasta Centro (CEAVC) (protocol number Ethics Committee FA000459, ID study 24175, approved on 06.02.2024).

Informed Consent Statement: Each study participant received a careful explanation of the intended procedure and signed an informed consent form prior to inclusion.

Data Availability Statement: The data presented in this study are available on request from the corresponding author. The data is not publicly available due to ethical reason.

Conflicts of Interest: The authors declare no conflicts of interest.

References

1. Rosen, E.; Alió, J.L.; Dick, H.B.; Dell, S.; Slade, S. Efficacy and safety of multifocal intraocular lenses following cataract and refractive lens exchange: Metaanalysis of peer-reviewed publications. *J. Cataract Refract. Surg.* **2016**, *42*, 310–328. [CrossRef] [PubMed]
2. Li, J.; Sun, B.; Zhang, Y.; Hao, Y.; Wang, Z.; Liu, C.; Jiang, S. Comparative efficacy and safety of all kinds of intraocular lenses in presbyopia-correcting cataract surgery: A systematic review and meta-analysis. *BMC Ophthalmol.* **2024**, *24*, 172. [CrossRef] [PubMed]
3. Dell, S.J.; Hannan, S.J.; Venter, J.A.; Teenan, D.; Hannan, N.C.; Raju, D.; Berry, C.W.; Kiss, H.J.; Schallhorn, J.M. Comparative analysis of clinical and patient-reported outcomes of a new enhanced monofocal IOL and a conventional monofocal IOL. *Clin. Ophthalmol.* **2024**, *18*, 1157–1169. [CrossRef]
4. Breyer, D.R.H.; Kaymak, H.; Ax, T.; Kretz, F.T.A.; Auffarth, G.U.; Hagen, P.R. Multifocal intraocular lenses and extended depth of focus intraocular lenses. *Asia-Pac. J. Ophthalmol.* **2017**, *6*, 339–349.
5. Alio, J.L.; Plaza-Puche, A.B.; Piero, D.P.; Amparo, F.; Rodríguez-Prats, J.L.; Ayala, M.J. Quality of life evaluation after implantation of 2 multifocal intraocular lens models and a mon-ofocal model. *J. Cataract Refract. Surg.* **2011**, *37*, 638–648. [CrossRef]

6. Wan, K.H.; Au, A.C.K.; Kua, W.N.; Ng, A.L.K.; Cheng, G.P.M.; Lam, N.M.; Chow, V.W.S. Enhanced Monofocal Versus Conventional Monofocal Intraocular Lens in Cataract Surgery: A Meta-analysis. *J. Refract. Surg.* **2022**, *38*, 538–546. [CrossRef]
7. Sachdev, G.S.; Sachdev, M. Optimizing outcomes with multifocal intraocular lenses. *Indian J. Ophthalmol.* **2017**, *65*, 1294–1300. [CrossRef]
8. De Silva, S.R.; Evans, J.R.; Kirthi, V.; Ziaei, M.; Leyland, M. Multifocal versus monofocal intraocular lenses after cataract extraction. *Cochrane Database Syst. Rev.* **2016**, *12*, CD003169. [CrossRef]
9. Coassin, M.; Di Zazzo, A.; Antonini, M.; Gaudenzi, D.; Gallo Afflitto, G.; Kohnen, T. Extended depth-of-focus intraocular lenses: Power calculation and outcomes. *J. Cataract Refract. Surg.* **2020**, *46*, 1554–1560. [CrossRef]
10. Mencucci, R.; Cennamo, M.; Venturi, D.; Vignapiano, R.; Favuzza, E. Visual outcome, optical quality, and patient satisfaction with a new monofocal IOL, enhanced for intermediate vision: Preliminary results. *J. Cataract Refract. Surg.* **2020**, *46*, 378–387. [CrossRef] [PubMed]
11. Mencucci, R.; Morelli, A.; Cennamo, M.; Roszkowska, A.M.; Favuzza, E. Enhanced monofocal intraocular lenses: A retrospective, comparative study between three different models. *J. Clin. Med.* **2023**, *12*, 3588. [CrossRef] [PubMed]
12. Fernández, J.; Rocha-de-Lossada, C.; Zamorano-Martín, F.; Rodríguez-Calvo-de-Mora, M.; Rodríguez-Vallejo, M. Positioning of enhanced monofocal intraocular lenses between conventional monofocal and extended depth of focus lenses: A scoping review. *BMC Ophthalmol.* **2023**, *23*, 101. [CrossRef] [PubMed]
13. Beltraminelli, T.; Rizzato, A.; Toniolo, K.; Galli, A.; Menghini, M. Comparison of visual performances of enhanced mon-ofocal versus standard monofocal IOLs in a mini-monovision approach. *BMC Ophthalmol.* **2023**, *23*, 170. [CrossRef] [PubMed]
14. Mencucci, R.; Romualdi, G.; De Vitto, C.; Cennamo, M. Enhanced Monofocal Intraocular Lenses in Fuchs' Endothelial Dystrophy Patients: Results from Triple Descemet Mem-brane Endothelial Keratoplasty Procedure. *Life* **2024**, *14*, 243. [CrossRef] [PubMed] [PubMed Central]
15. Ribeiro, F.; Dick, H.B.; Kohnen, T.; Findl, O.; Nuijts, R.; Cochener, B.; Fernández, J. Evidence-based functional classification of simultaneous vision intraocular lenses: Seeking a global consensus by the ESCRS Functional Vision Working Group. *J. Cataract Refract. Surg.* **2024**, *50*, 794–798. [CrossRef] [PubMed]
16. Fernández, J.; Ribeiro, F.; Rocha-de-Lossada, C.; Rodríguez-Vallejo, M. Functional Classification of Intraocular Lenses Based on Defocus Curves: A Scoping Review and Cluster Analysis. *J. Refract. Surg.* **2024**, *40*, e108–e116. [CrossRef] [PubMed]
17. Güell, J.L.; Pujol, J.; Arjona, M.; Diaz-Douton, F.; Artal, P. Optical Quality Analysis System; Instrument for objective clinical evaluation of ocular optical quality. *J. Cataract Refract. Surg.* **2004**, *30*, 1598–1599. [CrossRef]
18. Castro, J.J.; Jiménez, J.R.; Ortiz, C.; Alarcón, A.; Anera, R.G. New testing software for quantifying discrimination capacity in subjects with ocular pathologies. *J. Biomed. Opt.* **2011**, *16*, 015001. [CrossRef]
19. Buckhurst, P.J.; Naroo, S.A.; Davies, L.N.; Shah, S.; Buckhurst, H.; Kingsnorth, A.; Drew, T.; Wolffsohn, J.S. Tablet App halometer for the assessment of dysphotopsia. *J. Cataract Refract. Surg.* **2015**, *41*, 2424–2429. [CrossRef] [PubMed]
20. Eom, Y.; Kang, S.Y.; Song, J.S.; Kim, H.M. Comparison of the actual amount of axial movement of 3 aspheric intraocular lenses using anterior segment optical coherence tomography. *J. Cataract Refract. Surg.* **2013**, *39*, 1528–1533. [CrossRef] [PubMed]
21. Morlock, R.; Wirth, R.J.; Tally, S.R.; Garufis, C.; Heichel, C.W.D. Patient-Reported Spectacle Independence Questionnaire (PRSIQ): Development and Validation. *Am. J. Ophthalmol.* **2017**, *178*, 101–114. [CrossRef] [PubMed]
22. Mojzis, P.; Majerova, K.; Hrckova, L.; Piñero, D.P. Implantation of a diffractive trifocal intraocular lens: One-year follow-up. *J. Cataract Refract. Surg.* **2015**, *41*, 1623–1630. [CrossRef] [PubMed]
23. Gil, M.A.; Varón, C.; Cardona, G.; Vega, F.; Buil, J.A. Comparison of far and near contrast sensitivity in patients symmetrically implanted with multifocal and monofocal IOLs. *Eur. J. Ophthalmol.* **2014**, *24*, 44–52. [CrossRef] [PubMed]
24. Wang, S.Y.; Stem, M.S.; Oren, G.; Shtein, R.; Lichter, P.R. Patient-Centered and visual quality outcomes of premium cataract surgery: A Systematic Review. *Eur. J. Ophthalmol.* **2017**, *27*, 387–401. [CrossRef]
25. Mencucci, R.; Favuzza, E.; Caporossi, O.; Savastano, A.; Rizzo, S. Comparative analysis of visual outcomes, reading skills, contrast sensitivity, and patient satisfaction with two models of trifocal diffractive intraocular lenses and an extended range of vision intraocular lens. *Graefes Arch. Clin. Exp. Ophthalmol.* **2018**, *256*, 1913–1922. [CrossRef]
26. Cano-Ortiz, A.; Sánchez-Ventosa, Á.; González-Cruces, T.; Villalba González, M.; López Pérez, M.D.; Díaz-Ramos, J.C.; Prados Carmona, J.J.; Tejerina Fernández, V.; Elies Amat, D.; Villarrubia, A. Evaluation of Evolux™ Intraocular Lenses in Cataract Surgery: Clinical Outcomes and Patient Satisfaction. *J. Clin. Med.* **2024**, *13*, 7404. [CrossRef] [PubMed] [PubMed Central]

27. Spagnuolo, V.; Vicini, G.; Marincolo, G.; Franchini, A.; Giansanti, F.; Mazzini, C. Comparison of 3-month clinical outcomes between two enhanced monofocal intraocular lenses: A single-center prospective study. *Eur. J. Ophthalmol.* **2024**, *15*, 11206721241298031. [CrossRef] [PubMed]
28. Fernández, J.; Ribeiro, F.; Burguera, N.; Rodríguez-Calvo-de-Mora, M.; Rodríguez-Vallejo, M. Visual and patient-reported outcomes of an enhanced versus monofocal intraocular lenses in cataract surgery: A systematic review and meta-analysis. *Eye* **2025**, *39*, 883–898. [CrossRef] [PubMed] [PubMed Central]

life

MDPI

Case Report

An Unusual Manifestation of HSV-1 Uveitis Transforming into an Acute Iris Transillumination-like Syndrome with Pigmentary Glaucoma: A Reminder of Treatment Pitfalls in Herpetic Uveitis

Marin Radmilović, Goran Marić, Ante Vukojević, Mia Zorić Geber * and Zoran Vatavuk

Department of Ophthalmology, Sestre milosrdnice University Hospital Center, Vinogradska cesta 29, 10000 Zagreb, Croatia; radmilovic.marin@gmail.com (M.R.); goran.maric10@gmail.com (G.M.); ante.vukojevic1@gmail.com (A.V.); zo.vatavuk@gmail.com (Z.V.)

* Correspondence: miazoricgeber@gmail.com

Abstract

We report a case of herpes simplex virus type 1 (HSV-1) anterior uveitis evolving into an acute iris transillumination-like syndrome with secondary pigmentary glaucoma, highlighting diagnostic challenges and treatment considerations. A 61-year-old immunocompetent woman presented with unilateral anterior uveitis characterized by keratic precipitates and mild anterior chamber inflammation. The condition was initially treated with topical and subconjunctival corticosteroids without antiviral therapy. After an initial resolution of symptoms, upon the cessation of treatment, the patient developed features resembling unilateral acute iris transillumination (UAIT) syndrome with elevated intraocular pressure, diffuse pigment dispersion, and progressive iris transillumination defects. Aqueous polymerase chain reaction (PCR) testing confirmed the presence of HSV-1. Despite the initiation of antiviral therapy, the condition progressed to severe pigmentary glaucoma, with unreliable intraocular pressure measurements due to prior LASIK surgery. Cataract extraction, pars plana vitrectomy, and Ahmed valve implantation were performed, with only partial recovery of visual acuity. This case illustrates that HSV-1 uveitis can mimic or transition into a UAIT-like syndrome, possibly due to steroid use without concurrent antiviral treatment, which may exacerbate viral replication and damage to the iris pigment epithelium. Aqueous PCR testing aids in differential diagnosis, but indicative medical history and clinical findings should remain instrumental. Clinicians should maintain a high index of suspicion for herpetic etiology in anterior uveitis cases and initiate prompt antiviral treatment to prevent potentially sight-threatening complications.

Keywords: Herpes simplex virus (HSV-1); anterior uveitis; acute iris transillumination; pigmentary glaucoma; antiviral therapy

1. Introduction

Herpes simplex virus (HSV) has been established as a cause of acute anterior uveitis, usually with unilateral presentation, with possible sectoral iris atrophy, pigment dispersion, and secondary ocular hypertension [1–3]. The main differential diagnoses in such cases include pigment dispersion syndrome, Fuchs heterochromic iridocyclitis, and acute bilateral or unilateral iris transillumination syndrome (BAIT/UAIT). These entities can usually be distinguished with a careful evaluation of medical history, laterality, iris atrophy patterns, as well as the presence or lack of inflammatory findings, which are especially stressed when discerning herpetic uveitis from BAIT/UAIT [4]. The latter presents similarly to

 https://doi.org/10.3390/life15081164

herpetic uveitis, albeit almost always bilaterally, with acute onset of ocular pain, redness, and photophobia. However, it is characterized by diffuse pigment dispersion from the iris pigment epithelium (IPE), its deposition in anterior chamber structures, and the absence of keratic precipitates, anterior chamber inflammatory cells, or vitritis [4–6]. While the etiopathogenesis of BAIT/UAIT is still not fully understood, it has been attributed to the toxic effect of systemic or local antibiotic therapy, most commonly fluoroquinolones, on IPE [7–11]. Given the existence of antecedent viral infections in two-thirds of these patients, viral etiology has also been suggested to play a role [4,12].

We report a case of acute anterior uveitis due to herpes simplex virus type 1 (HSV-1), developing clinically from a typical herpetic uveitis into an acute iris transillumination-like syndrome with pigmentary glaucoma, necessitating cataract surgery, vitrectomy, and glaucoma filtration surgery.

2. Case Report

A 61-year-old woman presented to the emergency department with redness, pain, and blurred vision in her left eye. Her ocular history included amblyopia in the right eye, and LASIK performed for high myopia 12 years prior on the left eye. Her systemic history included Hashimoto thyroiditis, an episode of pericarditis 4 years prior, and an episode of viral pneumonia 2 years prior. She was otherwise healthy, took no antibiotics or other medications, had no recent vaccinations, and experienced no viral prodrome or other symptoms. At the time of the initial evaluation, her best corrected visual acuity (BCVA) was hand motion (HM) in the right, amblyopic eye, and 20/40 in the left eye. Her intraocular pressure (IOP) measured 12 mmHg in the right eye and 14 mmHg in the left eye on Goldmann applanation tonometry (GAT). Her left eye was documented (only textually, with no available photodocumentation) to show ciliary injection, fine keratic precipitates, and anterior chamber cells, with normal pupils and no other pathological findings except for a mild nuclear cataract. No signs of vitritis were noted, and a dilated fundus examination showed a slightly tilted optic disc with myopic fundus tessellation and an inferior type of posterior staphyloma (Curtin type V) but was otherwise unremarkable. The right eye showed no signs of inflammation or any other pathological finding aside from a dense nuclear cataract, a slightly tilted optic disc, fundus tessellation, and a posterior pole staphyloma (Curtin type I).

The general ophthalmologist who saw the patient applied a subconjunctival dexamethasone injection and prescribed treatment with dexamethasone drops and ointment, tropicamide drops, and oral ibuprofen. Over the course of one month, the patient reported an almost complete resolution of symptoms; her left eye BCVA improved to 20/25, and signs of inflammation regressed, with only a few keratic precipitates and no cells observed in the anterior chamber. The treatment was tapered and subsequently discontinued. However, within a couple of days after treatment cessation, the patient returned complaining of blurred vision once again. Her left eye BCVA was now 20/50, and slit lamp examination revealed diffuse pigmented precipitates on the corneal endothelium and the anterior iris surface, an abundant convection current of dispersed pigment in the anterior chamber, and dense pigment deposition on the anterior hyaloid membrane and posterior lens capsule in the visual axis and temporally (Figures 1 and 2). Additionally, the IOP of the left eye was now elevated and measured 31 mmHg. No corneal infiltration or non-pigmented keratic precipitates, anterior chamber cells, vitritis, or posterior synechiae were noted. The patient was administered another subconjunctival dexamethasone injection, restarted on topical dexamethasone and tropicamide, with added dorzolamide/timolol drops, and referred to a uveitis specialist.

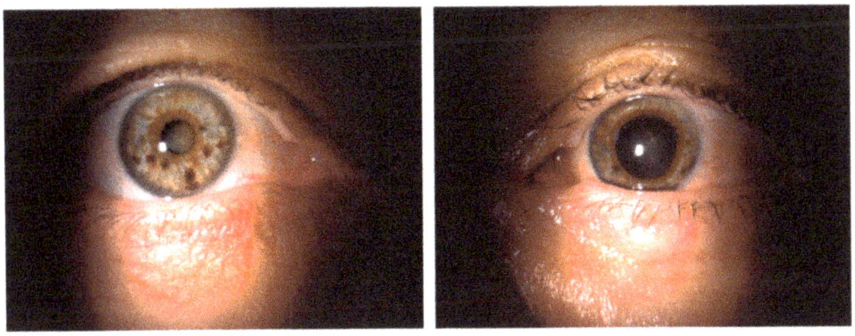

(**a**) (**b**)

Figure 1. Clinical appearance upon referral to the uveitis service. (**a**) Unaffected (right) eye. (**b**) Affected (left) eye with irregular, mid-dilated, unresponsive pupil, mild bulbar hyperemia, pigmented corneal precipitates, and pigment deposits posterior to the crystalline lens.

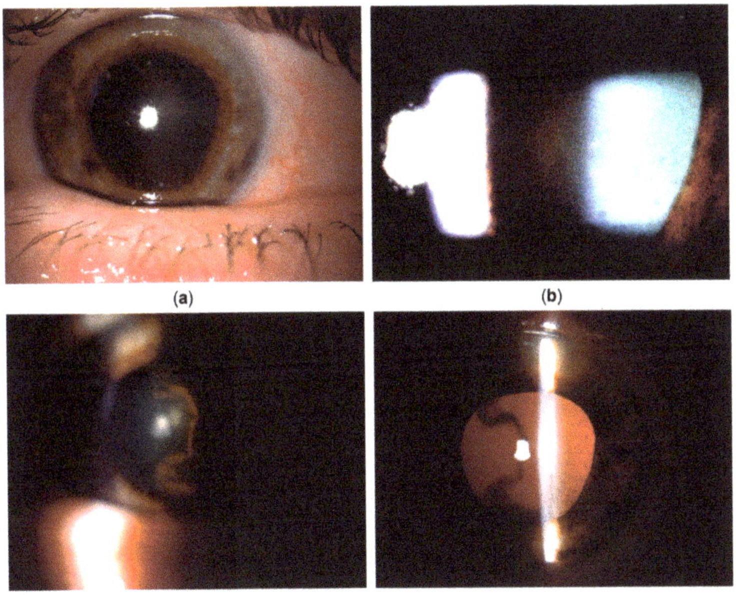

(**a**) (**b**) (**c**) (**d**)

Figure 2. Clinical appearance upon referral to the uveitis service (details, left eye). (**a**) Pigmented corneal precipitates with fine and stellate morphology. (**b**) Marked pigment dispersion in the anterior chamber. (**c**) Pigment deposits on the anterior hyaloid surface and posterior lens capsule, indicating the temporal origin of pigment dispersion. (**d**) Iris transillumination defects showing sectoral, patchy morphology in the temporal portion of the iris.

Upon referral, a mid-dilated, irregular pupil with poor light reaction was additionally noted, with the iris showing pronounced sectoral transillumination defects in the temporal quadrant (Figures 1 and 2). A working diagnosis of UAIT syndrome seemed possible for the abundance of pigment dispersion and a current lack of inflammatory cells in the anterior chamber or vitritis. However, given the likely differential diagnosis of herpetic uveitis, especially due to previously described findings and a good response to dexamethasone treatment, as well as a typical finding of sectoral iris transillumination and the stellate morphology of pigmented corneal precipitates, the patient was started on oral acyclovir (800 mg five times daily, which was planned to be maintained long-term) with continued topical therapy and dexamethasone injections. An anterior chamber tap for polymerase chain reaction (PCR) was performed to test for Herpes simplex virus type 1 and 2, the Varicella-Zoster virus (VZV), Cytomegalovirus (CMV), and Epstein–Barr virus (EBV), returning positive for HSV-1.

Despite the ongoing treatment, and despite the continuous lack of inflammatory cells in the anterior chamber or vitreous, BCVA further deteriorated to 20/400 with increasing retrolental pigment deposition. The transillumination defects progressed to encompass the entire iris, and gonioscopy showed an open angle with circumferential dense pigmentation obscuring all structures (Figure 3). Intraocular pressure mounted, prompting the addition of brimonidine and bimatoprost drops with oral acetazolamide, which maintained IOP variably between 14 and 28 mmHg, as measured by GAT. However, discrete retinal arterial pulsations were occasionally observed at the optic disc in the left eye, suggesting that the true IOP may have been higher than the measured values, especially considering the known challenges of accurate IOP measurement in post-LASIK eyes [13,14].

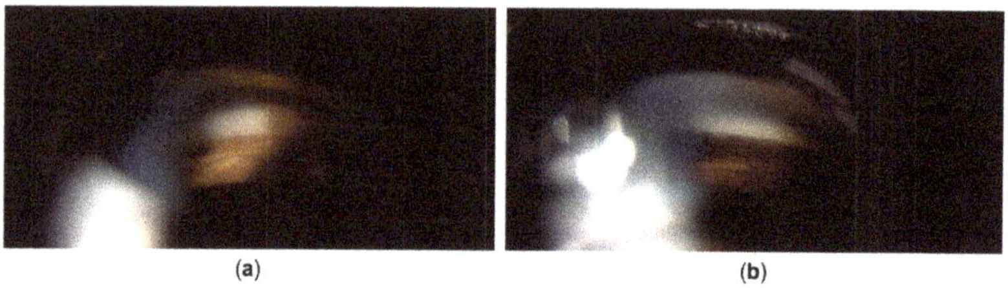

Figure 3. Gonioscopy. (**a**) Right eye showing open angle with mild pigmentation. (**b**) Left eye with heavy pigmentation obscuring all angle structures.

After three months of the documented absence of anterior chamber cells and complete resolution of keratic precipitates, with ongoing antiviral, corticosteroid, and IOP-lowering therapy, the patient underwent combined phacoemulsification cataract surgery with pars plana vitrectomy to remove the pigment obstructing the visual axis. Despite an unremarkable surgical course, the eye was hypotonic on postoperative day one, with multiple choroidal detachments and several intraretinal hemorrhages. While the hemorrhages persisted longer, the choroidal detachments and hypotony resolved within days (Figure 4), with BCVA improving only to 20/125. Optical coherence tomography (OCT) revealed no macular edema or overt foveal pathology (Figure 5). The thin extrafoveal hemorrhages (not visible in the central OCT scans), primarily localized to the outer plexiform layer with occasional extension into the subretinal space, may have indicated ischemia of the deep retinal capillary plexus. Nevertheless, as far as could be determined from the available scans, no definitive hyperreflective bands or thinning within the inner nuclear, outer plexiform, or outer nuclear layers were identified, and these layers appeared uniformly thick. A few pinpoint hyperreflective foci within the outer nuclear layer and outer photoreceptor segments, also extrafoveal, may have indicated focal ischemia at the level of the choriocapillaris. However, the outer nuclear layer, external limiting membrane, ellipsoid zone, and RPE/Bruch's membrane complex appeared normal and continuous within the fovea. The most striking finding was the diffuse thinning of the ganglion cell complex, including the papillomacular region (Figure 5). The optic nerve head OCT demonstrated a glaucomatous pattern of retinal nerve fiber layer thinning, with inferotemporal involvement extending into the papillomacular bundle, likely related to a more oblique angle between the optic disc and the fovea (Figure 5). These findings supported glaucomatous optic neuropathy with a papillomacular bundle defect as the primary cause of the reduced BCVA, with possible additional functional impairment from the generalized hypoperfusion of the retinal and choroidal vascular beds. The IOP measurements continued fluctuating between 16 and

30 mmHg, despite ongoing IOP-lowering therapy, and as reliable IOP assessment was compromised due to the post-LASIK status of the eye, further clinical decisions were aided by digital tonometry and monitoring the status of the optic nerve head via fundoscopy and OCT. Within several weeks, however, signs of corneal decompensation with epithelial edema developed (Figure 6), reducing BCVA to counting figers (CF) at 1 meter. As no signs of inflammation were present, with antiviral and anti-inflammatory therapy still ongoing, and as recent specular microscopy had shown normal corneal endothelial morphology, this decompensation was considered likely secondary to elevated IOP. The patient subsequently underwent an Ahmed glaucoma valve implant. Postoperatively, IOP values were reduced to measurements between 6 and 13 mmHg, with only a partial resolution of corneal edema, and BCVA improved to 20/400. The patient was maintained on antiviral therapy (acyclovir 800 mg five times daily for two postoperative months, followed by a reduced dose of 400 mg twice daily for long-term prophylaxis), along with additional IOP-lowering treatment, with close monitoring for further changes in corneal edema and IOP.

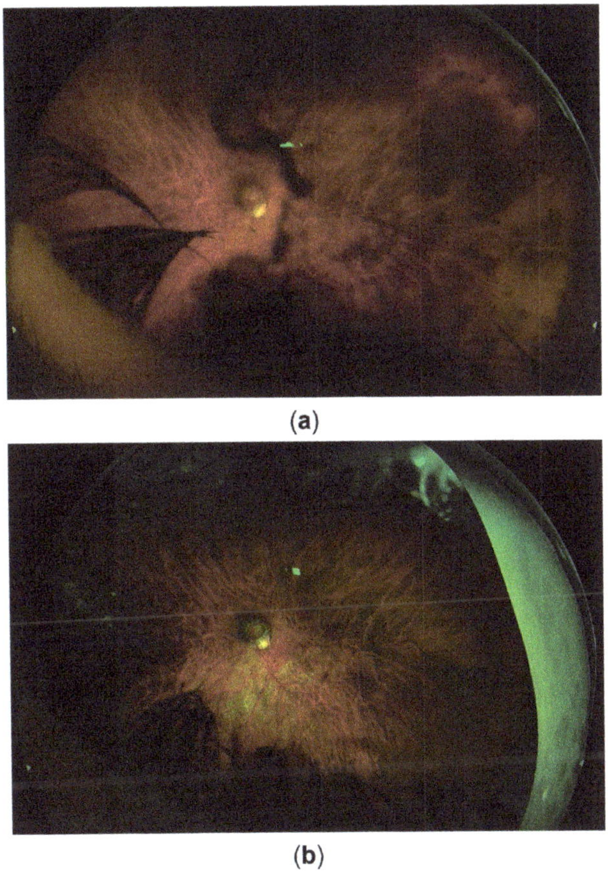

Figure 4. Fundus image. (**a**) Appearance upon referral to the uveitis service. (**b**) Appearance 3 months later after recovery from combined cataract surgery and vitrectomy. Signs of glaucomatous optic atrophy are visible. Postoperative intraretinal hemorrhages can also be seen.

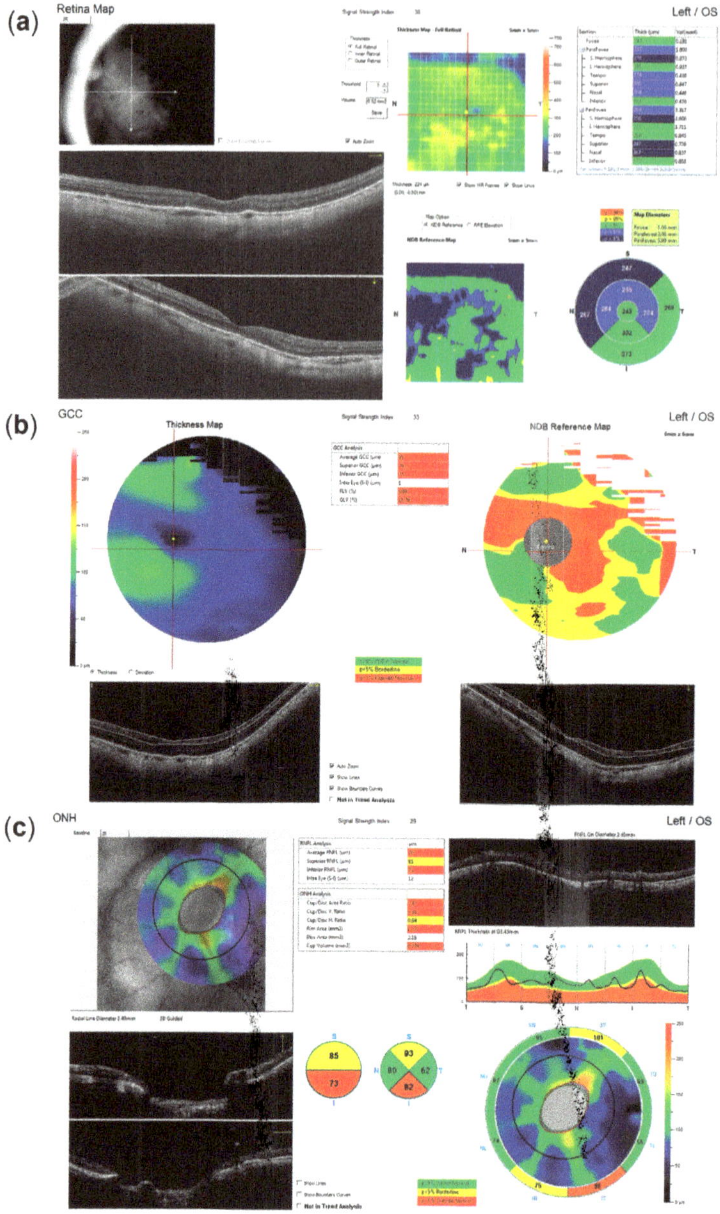

Figure 5. Optical coherence tomography (OCT) imaging following recovery from combined cataract surgery and vitrectomy, indicating glaucomatous optic neuropathy as the most likely primary cause of reduced visual acuity. (**a**) Macular OCT reveals no evidence of edema or other foveal pathology. (**b**) Ganglion cell complex (GCC) analysis demonstrates diffuse thinning, including the entire papillomacular bundle (note: segmentation artifacts that may underestimate GCC loss in the inferior portion of the papillomacular bundle may be observed in the horizontal B-scan). (**c**) The optic nerve head (ONH) OCT shows inferotemporal retinal nerve fiber layer (RNFL) thinning (note: reduced RNFL reflectivity and internal limiting membrane (ILM) thickening may be observed in the circular B-scan, contributing to segmentation artifacts that may underestimate the extent of overall RNFL loss).

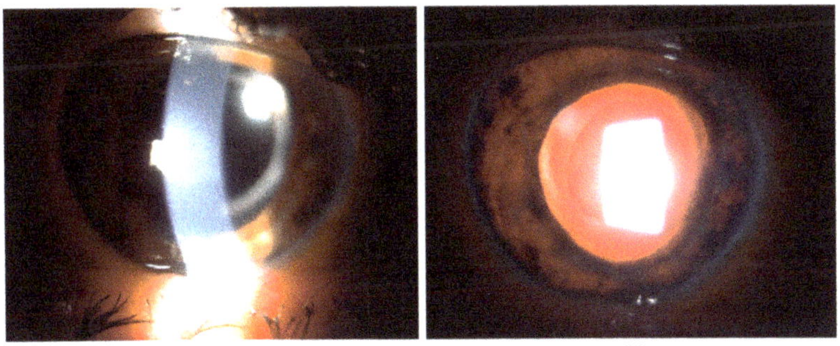

(a) (b)

Figure 6. Clinical appearance several weeks after cataract surgery and pars plana vitrectomy. (**a**) Corneal edema developed. Pigmented corneal precipitates are no longer present. (**b**) Iris transillumination defects are now present circularly.

3. Discussion

Herpetic uveitis can lead to significant pigment dispersion and iris transillumination defects, especially in cases with systemic immunosuppression, where bilateral presentation may also occur [3]. In such cases, the distinction between herpetic uveitis and acute iris transillumination syndrome can become problematic by means of clinical signs alone, and indicative medical history is instrumental. So far, as we know it, only a few acute iris transillumination-like cases have been described with confirmed HSV association [15,16]. This contrasts with the vast majority of BAIT/UAIT cases, which seem to have a distinct etiopathogenesis, primarily implicating the toxic effect of fluoroquinolones or other drugs on iris pigment epithelium [7]. And although viral etiology, including the herpesvirus infections, has also been suggested to play a role in BAIT/UAIT, conclusive evidence is lacking, with anterior chamber PCR for the herpesvirus family being negative in almost all published cases [4–6,12,17]. A conclusion could be drawn that cases with confirmed HSV association may be misinterpreted as falling within the scope of iris transillumination syndrome due to not being seen in the inflammatory phase, such as in the case described by Gonzalez Martinez et al. [15], or due to significant discrepancy between the amount of iris epithelial pigment dispersion and signs of inflammation, as in the case reported by Dastrup et al. [16]. This is reinforced by the reported history, although non-descriptive, of preceding acute iritis in the former case, and by the finding of keratic precipitates in the latter case. Both studies acknowledge herpetic etiology as uncommon for this syndrome. However, given the suggested role of viral infections in BAIT/UAIT, these studies imply the possible existence of a common pathway for virally mediated iris pigment loss. Our case also illustrates such a possibility through a well-documented shift from a clinical picture typical of herpetic uveitis to one suggestive of UAIT. However, while the apparent absence of inflammatory cells in the anterior chamber and vitreous during the latter phase could have suggested this alternative diagnosis, it is more likely that corticosteroid treatment masked these clinical findings, thereby blurring the distinction between the two entities.

In our case, a suggestive clinical presentation and a supportive medical history led to the diagnosis of herpetic anterior uveitis, which was further reinforced by PCR testing. However, while aqueous PCR testing is a highly specific and valuable diagnostic tool for identifying viral etiologies in anterior uveitis, its sensitivity can vary depending on factors such as the timing of sampling relative to symptom onset, viral load, and prior antiviral treatment [2], with reported detection rates ranging from 81% with real-time PCR to as low as 50–55% using conventional PCR, highlighting the need for clinical correlation when interpreting the results [18–20].

Regardless, the unabated progression of IPE atrophy and pigment dispersion during the phase with no visible inflammation suggests a distinct pathophysiological process either unrelated to general inflammatory activity, such as the direct viral cytopathic effect, or related to its inappropriate modulation. This opens up the possibility of the iatrogenic exacerbation of such processes. As previously mentioned, herpetic uveitis under systemic immunosuppression can manifest bilaterally and with more severe sequelae, as corticosteroid treatment without adequate antiviral coverage may reduce the host's ability to control viral replication, potentially exacerbating cytopathic damage [3]. The delayed initiation of antiviral therapy in herpetic anterior uveitis can result from diagnostic challenges, errors, and under-recognition in both typical and atypical cases, leading to inappropriate corticosteroid monotherapy and increasing the risk of recurrences and long-term complications [3,21–24]. The lack of standardized guidelines further contributes to variability in treatment initiation, agent selection, administration route, dosage, and duration [23]. Although systematic studies quantifying undertreatment in real-world settings are lacking, the authors' clinical impression is that these challenges remain relevant, particularly at the primary care and general ophthalmology levels. This underscores the need for heightened clinical suspicion and structured antiviral stewardship, especially given the potential for antiviral resistance in immunocompromised patients, which can range from 2.5% to over 30% depending on immunosuppression severity and underlying conditions [24].

It is noteworthy that manifestations of ocular herpetic disease such as retinal necrosis or iris atrophy are believed to result from a combination of direct viral effects on multiple cell types, including endothelial cells, and immune-mediated inflammation, leading to occlusive vasculitis [25,26]. Although our patient was treated only with topical and subconjunctival steroids, and was otherwise immunocompetent, these were at first used without appropriate antiviral treatment. This may have led to uncontrolled viral replication and delayed exacerbation mimicking UAIT due to cytopathic or ischemic damage and the necrosis of the IPE. While we did not obtain intraoperative iris samples for histological analysis in our study, in the study of Gonzalez Martinez et al., the histological examination of an enucleated eye demonstrated a pronounced absence of the IPE and iris dilator muscle, with extensive necrosis and focal vascular occlusion of the iris sphincter muscle, but no evidence of active vasculitis or nuclear viral cytopathic changes typical of herpesvirus infection [15]. Additionally, the inflammatory infiltrate in the uveal tract was extremely mild and predominantly lymphocytic. The authors noted possible limitations due to sampling, and the possible modification of histological findings due to topical steroids administered to the patient. It should be emphasized that their patient presented in the late, quiet phase, several months after the initial iritis episode (n.b. also treated with topical corticosteroids and without antiviral therapy), which likely influenced the histological findings.

HSV-1 infection can also cause mitochondrial DNA depletion and dysfunction through the action of the UL12.5 isoform, leading to increased oxidative stress and impaired mitochondrial energy production [27]. Fluoroquinolones, in turn, can form a chelate with essential cations such as magnesium and calcium, disrupt the electron transport chain, reduce mitochondrial membrane potential, and increase reactive oxygen species production within the mitochondria [28]. These mechanisms result in disrupted ATP synthesis, oxidative damage, and disturbances in cellular homeostasis, which may trigger apoptotic pathways and contribute to the pigment epithelium damage and acute pigment dispersion observed in both HSV-1 and fluoroquinolone-induced cases. Given this overlap, targeted antioxidant therapies may be considered as supportive strategies. Agents such as alpha-lipoic acid, coenzyme Q10, N-acetylcysteine, and vitamins C and E have been described to help stabilize mitochondrial function, lower oxidative stress, and support tissue recovery. However, caution is warranted, as the clinical benefit, timing, and dosing of antioxidants in these indications remain unproven, and excessive antioxidant use during viral illnesses could disrupt the physiological redox signaling or immune responses necessary for viral control [28]. Further research is needed to elucidate the role of these mitochondrial and oxidative stress mechanisms in the pathogenesis of both these clinical entities, and to clarify whether and how antioxidant support might be integrated into the comprehensive management of these complex cases.

4. Conclusions

Both our case and the previously mentioned cases highlight the unusual presentation of HSV-1 uveitis with acute iris transillumination-like findings. However, this observation only suggests a potential pathway for HSV-1-mediated IPE loss, which could be shared with other viruses, though this remains theoretical. Also, current clinical evidence for acute iris transillumination syndrome favors an alternative, toxic mechanism as the likely cause of IPE damage, distinguishing it from the mechanism postulated for HSV-1-related IPE loss. Therefore, it would be appropriate to use the descriptor "acute iris transillumination-like" in such cases, clearly differentiating between these entities. When clinical signs alone are insufficiently distinctive, aqueous tap and PCR testing for herpesviruses can provide additional diagnostic support. However, given the possibility of false-negative results, PCR testing should be viewed as confirmatory rather than exclusionary, and an indicative medical history should remain instrumental. More importantly, the potential for complications, such as those described here, arising from the use of corticosteroid treatment alone or from the delayed initiation of antiviral therapy, should be carefully considered. It may be prudent to apply a low threshold for the immediate introduction of antiviral therapy in any case of uveitis unattributed to other clear causes, particularly if clinical signs are consistent with possible herpetic etiology. Additionally, testing for antiviral resistance should be made readily available to allow for the timely adjustment of therapy in complicated or unresponsive cases.

Author Contributions: Conceptualization and writing—original draft preparation, M.R.; writing—review and editing, G.M., A.V., M.Z.G. and Z.V.; visualization, M.R.; supervision, M.Z.G. and Z.V. All authors have read and agreed to the published version of the manuscript.

Funding: This research received no external funding.

Institutional Review Board Statement: No institutional review board statement was required.

Informed Consent Statement: Written consent to publish the case report was obtained. This report does not contain any personal information that could lead to the identification of the patient.

Data Availability Statement: The authors declare that all data supporting the report are available upon request to the corresponding author.

Conflicts of Interest: The authors declare that they have no known competing financial interests or personal relationships that could have appeared to influence the work reported in this paper.

References

1. Liesegang, T.J. Herpes Simplex Virus Epidemiology and Ocular Importance. *Cornea* **2001**, *20*, 1–13. [CrossRef] [PubMed]
2. Chan, N.S.; Chee, S. Demystifying Viral Anterior Uveitis: A Review. *Clin. Experiment. Ophthalmol.* **2019**, *47*, 320–333. [CrossRef] [PubMed]
3. de-la-Torre, A.; Valdes-Camacho, J.; Foster, C.S. Bilateral Herpes Simplex Uveitis: Review of the Literature and Own Reports. *Ocul. Immunol. Inflamm.* **2017**, *25*, 497–502. [CrossRef] [PubMed]
4. Tuğal-Tutkun, İ.; Altan, Ç. Bilateral Acute Depigmentation of Iris (BADI) and Bilateral Acute Iris Transillumination (BAIT)-An Update. *Turk. J. Ophthalmol.* **2022**, *52*, 342–347. [CrossRef] [PubMed]

5. Tugal-Tutkun, I.; Onal, S.; Garip, A.; Taskapili, M.; Kazokoglu, H.; Kadayifcilar, S.; Kestelyn, P. Bilateral Acute Iris Transillumination. *Arch. Ophthalmol.* **2011**, *129*, 1312–1319. [CrossRef] [PubMed]
6. Perone, J.M.; Chaussard, D.; Hayek, G. Bilateral Acute Iris Transillumination (BAIT) Syndrome: Literature Review. *Clin. Ophthalmol.* **2019**, *13*, 935–943. [CrossRef] [PubMed]
7. Tranos, P.; Lokovitis, E.; Masselos, S.; Kozeis, N.; Triantafylla, M.; Markomichelakis, N. Bilateral Acute Iris Transillumination Following Systemic Administration of Antibiotics. *Eye* **2018**, *32*, 1190–1196. [CrossRef] [PubMed]
8. Gonul, S.; Eker, S. Unilateral Acute Iris Transillumination Syndrome Following Uneventful Phacoemulsification Surgery with Intracameral Moxifloxacin. *Ocul. Immunol. Inflamm.* **2022**, *30*, 1984–1987. [CrossRef] [PubMed]
9. Sánchez-Sánchez, C.; Puerto, B.; López-Caballero, C.; Contreras, I. Unilateral Acute Iris Depigmentation and Transillumination after Glaucoma Surgery with Mitomycin Application and Intracameral Moxifloxacin. *Am. J. Ophthalmol. Case Rep.* **2020**, *18*, 100639. [CrossRef] [PubMed]
10. Zubicoa, A.; Echeverria-Palacios, M.; Mozo Cuadrado, M.; Compains Silva, E. Unilateral Acute Iris Transillumination like Syndrome Following Intracameral Moxifloxacin Injection. *Ocul. Immunol. Inflamm.* **2022**, *30*, 318–319. [CrossRef] [PubMed]
11. Mahanty, S.; Kawali, A.A.; Dakappa, S.S.; Mahendradas, P.; Kurian, M.; Kharbanda, V.; Shetty, R.; Gangi Setty, S.R. Aqueous Humor Tyrosinase Activity Is Indicative of Iris Melanocyte Toxicity. *Exp. Eye Res.* **2017**, *162*, 79–85. [CrossRef] [PubMed]
12. Kawali, A.; Mahendradas, P.; Shetty, R. Acute Depigmentation of the Iris: A Retrospective Analysis of 22 Cases. *Can. J. Ophthalmol.* **2019**, *54*, 33–39. [CrossRef] [PubMed]
13. Berrett, G.B.; Hogg, J.; Innes, W. Retinal Arterial Pulsation as an Indicator of Raised Intraocular Pressure. *SAGE Open Med. Case Rep.* **2021**, *9*, 2050313X211054633. [CrossRef] [PubMed]
14. Helmy, H.; Hashem, O. Intraocular Pressure Calculation in Myopic Patients After Laser-Assisted In Situ Keratomileusis. *Clin. Ophthalmol.* **2020**, *14*, 509–516. [CrossRef] [PubMed]
15. Gonzalez Martinez, O.G.; Shields, C.L.; Shields, J.A.; Chévez-Barrios, P.; Walley, D.R.; Eagle, R.C.; Milman, T. Unilateral Acute Iris Transillumination Syndrome with Glaucoma and Iris Pigment Epithelium Dispersion Simulating Iris Melanoma. *Am. J. Ophthalmol. Case Rep.* **2023**, *32*, 101912. [CrossRef] [PubMed]
16. Dastrup, B.T. An Unusual Manifestation of Herpes Simplex Virus–Associated Acute Iris Depigmentation and Pigmentary Glaucoma. *Arch. Ophthalmol.* **2011**, *129*, 253–254. [CrossRef] [PubMed]
17. Altan, C.; Basarir, B.; Bayraktar, S.; Tugal-Tutkun, I. Bilateral Acute Depigmentation of Iris (BADI) and Bilateral Acute Iris Transillumination (BAIT)Following Acute COVID-19 Infection. *Ocul. Immunol. Inflamm.* **2023**, *31*, 1163–1168. [CrossRef] [PubMed]
18. De Groot-Mijnes, J.D.F.; Rothova, A.; Van Loon, A.M.; Schuller, M.; Ten Dam-Van Loon, N.H.; De Boer, J.H.; Schuurman, R.; Weersink, A.J.L. Polymerase Chain Reaction and Goldmann-Witmer Coefficient Analysis Are Complimentary for the Diagnosis of Infectious Uveitis. *Am. J. Ophthalmol.* **2006**, *141*, 313–318. [CrossRef] [PubMed]
19. Van der Lelij, A.; Ooijman, F.M.; Kijlstra, A.; Rothova, A. Anterior Uveitis with Sectoral Iris Atrophy in the Absence of Keratitis. *Ophthalmology* **2000**, *107*, 1164–1170. [CrossRef] [PubMed]
20. Sugita, S.; Shimizu, N.; Watanabe, K.; Mizukami, M.; Morio, T.; Sugamoto, Y.; Mochizuki, M. Use of Multiplex PCR and Real-Time PCR to Detect Human Herpes Virus Genome in Ocular Fluids of Patients with Uveitis. *Br. J. Ophthalmol.* **2008**, *92*, 928–932. [CrossRef] [PubMed]
21. Al-Ani, H.H.; Niederer, R.L. Zoster Sine Herpete: A disease that ophthalmologists should be aware of. *Korean J. Pain* **2020**, *33*, 403–404. [CrossRef] [PubMed]
22. Seki, K.; Yoneda, K.; Yoneda, Y.; Takenaka, Y.; Kaburaki, T.; Takeuchi, M. Clinical Features of Varicella-Zoster Virus-Associated Anterior Uveitis with or without Ophthalmic Herpes Zoster. *Ocul. Immunol. Inflamm.* **2025**, *33*, 662–669. [CrossRef] [PubMed]
23. Testi, I.; Aggarwal, K.; Jaiswal, N.; Dahiya, N.; Thng, Z.X.; Agarwal, A.; Ahuja, A.; Duggal, M.; Kankaria, A.; Ling Ho, S.; et al. Antiviral Therapy for Varicella Zoster Virus (VZV) and Herpes Simplex Virus (HSV)-Induced Anterior Uveitis: A Systematic Review and Meta-Analysis. *Front. Med.* **2021**, *8*, 686427. [CrossRef] [PubMed]
24. Majewska, A.; Mlynarczyk-Bonikowska, B. 40 Years after the Registration of Acyclovir: Do We Need New Anti-Herpetic Drugs? *Int. J. Mol. Sci.* **2022**, *23*, 3431. [CrossRef] [PubMed]
25. Zhu, S.; Viejo-Borbolla, A. Pathogenesis and Virulence of Herpes Simplex Virus. *Virulence* **2021**, *12*, 2670–2702. [CrossRef] [PubMed]
26. Kawaguchi, T.; Spencer, D.B.; Mochizuki, M. Therapy for Acute Retinal Necrosis. *Semin. Ophthalmol.* **2008**, *23*, 285–290. [CrossRef] [PubMed]

27. Saffran, H.A.; Pare, J.M.; Corcoran, J.A.; Weller, S.K.; Smiley, J.R. Herpes Simplex Virus Eliminates Host Mitochondrial DNA. *EMBO Rep.* **2007**, *8*, 188–193. [CrossRef] [PubMed]
28. Michalak, K.; Sobolewska-Włodarczyk, A.; Włodarczyk, M.; Sobolewska, J.; Woźniak, P.; Sobolewski, B. Treatment of the Fluoroquinolone-Associated Disability: The Pathobiochemical Implications. *Oxid. Med. Cell. Longev.* **2017**, *2017*, 8023935. [CrossRef] [PubMed]

MDPI AG
Grosspeteranlage 5
4052 Basel
Switzerland
Tel.: +41 61 683 77 34

Life Editorial Office
E-mail: life@mdpi.com
www.mdpi.com/journal/life

www.ingramcontent.com/pod-product-compliance
Lightning Source LLC
Chambersburg PA
CBHW061502210926
51850CB00008B/1797
* 9 7 8 3 7 2 5 8 7 3 2 2 7 *